THE RE-CENTER METHOD
NATURAL DIET
COOKBOOK

Hareldau Argyle King

Also Available from
Refinement Publishing & Media

Quotes to Habits
Remember
Hareldau Argyle King

The Re-center Method
Natural Diet
Hareldau Argyle King

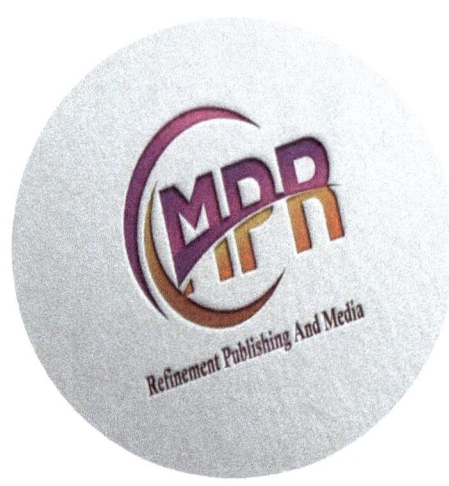

© Copyright August 2022 by Refinement Publishing & Media
Published by Refinement Publishing &Media - All rights reserved.

Web site:www.beingelevatedlifestyle.com
Email: support@beingelevatedlifestyle.com

As with all exercises and dietary programs, you should get your doctor's approval before beginning. The information here is to help you make an informed decision about your health.

This book is not intended as a substitute for any treatment that may have been prescribed by your doctor. The reader should regularly consult a doctor in matters about his/her health and particularly concerning any symptoms that may require diagnosis or medical attention.

This book is intended as a reference manual and not a medical manual. The exercises and dietary programs in the book are not intended as a substitute for any exercise routine or dietary regimen that may have been prescribed by your doctor.

**Copyright © 2022 by Refinement Publishing & Media
All rights reserved.**

All rights reserved. No part of the publication may be reproduced or transmitted in any form or by any means. Without the express written permission of the publisher except for the use of brief quotations in a book review.

The scanning, uploading, and distribution of this book via the internet or any other means without the permission of the publisher are illegal and punishable by law. Please by law Please purchase only authorized electronic editions and do not participate in or encourage electronic piracy of copyrighted materials. Your support of the author's rights is appreciated.

www.beingelevatedlifestyle.com
ISBN 978-1-950838-18-9 Ebook
ISBN- 978-1-9508 38-19-6 Hardcover
ISBN 978-1-950838-20-2 Paperback

Dedication

In honor of

DAVID "Dave" MODESTE

In honor of my dear friend, Talented Musician, & Food Connoisseur!

Mr. David Modeste lives a life of Dedication, Adventure, and Focusness

You are a constant source of humanity, progress & enlightenment

A trusted voice to many: whether as an entertainer, adviser, or an encourager

A man of conviction, compassion & character

I love the way you find solutions, care about international justice, and befriend people from all nations

When I think about someone who lives out the essence of this book, uses international food & flavors as connectors of people of all nations, honors diverse people groups from all cultures, and lives a healthy lifestyle. I think of you.

Your Desire to make this world a better, place is inspirational!

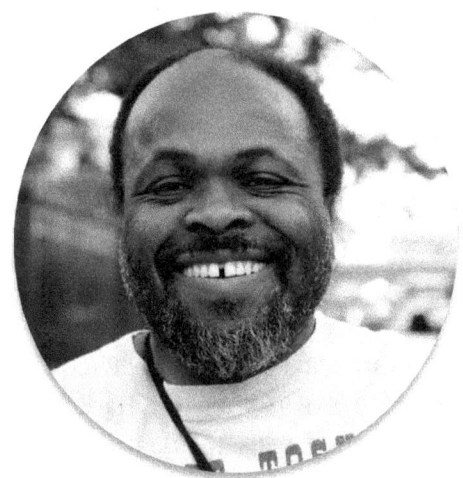

David Modeste

Foreword

Hang on for a wonderful and tastHareldau and I both hail from Guyana, which is a multicultural nation with Asians, Africans, Native Americans, and European influences that are hard to miss.

As a Chemical Engineer working and living in Baton Rouge Louisiana, it was a huge benefit of living close to the Louisiana State University the state flagship university where I could meet and interact with people from all around the world. In this environment, I met Hareldau, and since then we have been friends.

The weekend is a time for socializing as much as it is for academic pursuits when it comes to a university campus, but for many international students, socializing offers the opportunity not only to enjoy the company of others but also, share music and most of all food.

Many International students who have attended Louisiana State University (LSU) know of the International Cultural Center, and the famous parties and potluck socials involving students from all around the world. It is here that Hareldau as a top-class athlete at one of the high-ranking NCAA rack & Field teams in the country, and myself as a local resident of Baton Rouge and connoisseur of good foods met, socialized created friendships, and enjoyed some of the most exotic foods we had ever tasted.

It is a real joy and an honor to be asked to write this foreword because I know that the stories, the food and recipes will paint a picture of how Hareldau has interacted with people of many cultures. At the time I am sure we weren't thinking of how important the setting and the food created the the atmosphere for building such great relationships; however, as I look back cuisine played a big part in connecting people of different backgrounds and cultures.

I am sure the readers of this book will be just as excited as I am to learn how a young athlete from Guyana far away from home and under the pressures of academic and athletic performance was able to benefit from the wonderful food and social gatherings. Hareldau will take you around the world with stories recipes and food.

Hang on for a wonderful and tasty trip!

David Modeste, Chemical

Engineer, Chicago.

How to use this Book
Take Obedient Action

This book is a guide to a higher quality of life, through building relationships and varying your food choices. Whether you never had an international meal or friend or whether this is your way of life, there are words of encouragement, new ideas & solutions to enhance your quality of life.

The book is divided into weekly challenges, with a to-do list at the beginning of the week and a follow-up checklist at the end of the week.

In addition to encouragement to try new recipes whether there are for lunch, Dinner, or Breakfast, personal devotions for prayer, meditation, and gratitude journaling along with physical activities.

You are tasked with completing each week's challenge by taking obedient action, before starting week one.

This is not a diet book, a weight loss book, or a meal plan. On your first attempt to prepare these dishes, your meal may or may not look like the photo of the meal in this book..

This book is designed to enhance your tastebud, exposing you to different textures and tastes of food from all the continents of the world. After you would complete this 4-part of series international recipe books you experience cuisines from 195 countries in 7 continents.

It also challenges you to increase your physical activity, and your spiritual growth and make connections with old & new relationships.

I invite you to get started today. Don't Procrastinate!!

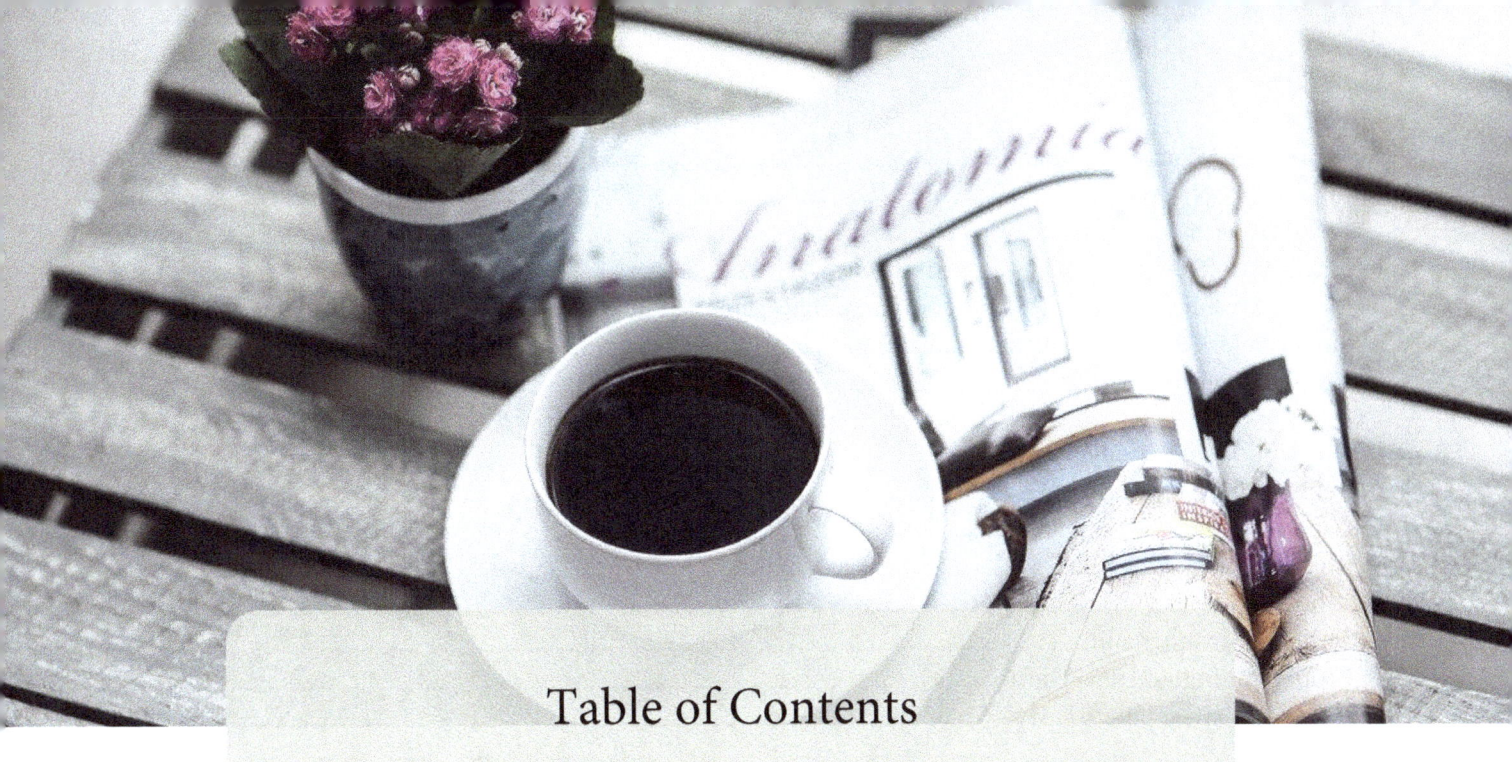

Table of Contents

Introduction 1

Week 1: Setting Real Goals
Beignets - Louisiana, USA 8
Piri-Piri Chicken - Mozambique 9
Japanese Sushi - Japan 10
Coconut Kau Kau – Papua New Guinea 11
Spanakopita Bites: Spinach and Feta Cheese Appetizers - Greece 12
Trini Pelau – Trinidad & Tobago 13
Brazilian Cheese Bread (Pão De Queijo) – Brazil 14

Week 2: Commit to Change
Oregon Salmon Patties - Oregon 21
Malawian Chicken Curry with Nsima - Malawi 22
Tofu Pudding - China 23
Barfi Recipe - Palau 24
Spanish Fabada: Chorizo Stew & White Bean - Spain 25
Tortilla recipe - Panama 26
Lomo saltado - Peru 27

Week 3: Rise Early and Go
Baked Paper Salmon – Washington DC 34
Chicken Muamba - Angola 35
Al Harees - UAE 36
Aussie Fried Rice - Australia 37
Brioches - Italy 38
Colombo - Martinique 39
Vegetarian Locro - Argentina 40

Week 4: Create Mile Markers

Moon over Miami egg - Miami 47
Jollof Rice - Nigeria 48
Lentil Spinach and Lemon Stew - Lebanon 49
Fijian Roro (Stew of Greens) + Boiled Cassava - Fiji 50
Basque-Style Fish with Green Peppers and Manila Clams - France 51
Jamaican Jerk Sauce Ingredients - Jamaica 52
Arepa - Venezuela 53

Week 5: When you fall, rise again
Texas Chili - Texas 60
Cape Malay curry – South Africa 61
Khao tom - Thailand 62
Whitebait Fritters – New Zealand 63
Stamppot - Netherland 64
Pepper Pot Ingredients - Guyana 65
Vegetarian sweet potato curry - Colombia 66

Week 6: Seek out Accountability
Chicago Style Barbecue Sauce - Illinois 73
Banana Akaras: Sierra Leone Banana Fritters – Sierra Leone 74
Biryani rice (Kuska rice) - India 75
Samoan Raw Fish Salad - Samoa 76
Full English breakfast – The United Kingdom 77
Cou Cou Dish - Barbados 78
Pom - Suriname 79

Week 7: Examine your Progress
Montréal Reuben Breakfast Bagel - Montreal 86
Fufu and goat light soup - Ghana 87
Hainanese chicken rice - Singapore 88
Solomon poi - Solomon 89
Green Pea Soup - Germany 90
Quesito – Pureto Rico 91
Chilean Lentil Soup - Chile 92

Week 8: Re-set your Goals
Tortilla Soup – Mexico City 99
Stewed Kapenta (Matemba) with Sadza - Zimbabwe 100
Al Kabsa – Saudi Arabia 101
Micronesian Salad - Micronesia 102
Menemen - Turky 103
Haitian Pumpkin Soup - Haiti 104
Sopa de Mani - Bolivia 105

Week 9: Identify your Strongholds
Avocado Kale Caesar Salad - Toronto 112
Kwacoco Bible - Cameroon 113
Tahu Gejrot Cirebon - Indonesia 114
Bougna – New Caledonia 115

Vegan Yellow Split Pea Soup - Sweden ... 116
Cayman Fried Crab – Cayman Islands ... 117
Tigrillo - Ecuador ... 118

Week 10: Reframing your Obstacles
Bagel – New York City ... 125
Peanut Soup Rice - Togo ... 126
Crab Curry – Sri Lanka ... 127
Kiribati Palusami - Kiribati ... 128
Gobovajuha (Slovenian Mushroom soup) - Slovenia ... 129
Bahamas conch fritters - Bahamas ... 130
Paraguayan Chipa - Paraguay ... 131

Week 11: Measuring your Gains
Barberton chicken – Ohio, USA ... 138
Injera - Ethiopia ... 139
Shakshuka - Israel ... 140
Chicken Kelaguen – Northern Mariana Islands ... 141
Falklanders lettuce soup – Falkand Islands(Islas Malvinas) ... 142
St Lucia Banana Bread Recipe – St. Lucia ... 143
Uruguayan Asado - Uruguay ... 144

Week 12: Celebrating your Success
Tasty Chicken Mole Enchiladas - Seattle ... 151
Kuli-kuli - Benin ... 152
Pyongyang on an – North Korea ... 153
Wallisian Sweet Potatoes – Wallis and Futuna ... 154
Full Cypriot breakfast bagel - Cyprus ... 155
Ducanna - Antigua ... 156
Fish Fritters – French Guiana ... 157

Bonus Week 13: Go the Extra Mile
Spicy sweet potatoes pancakes - Mississppi ... 164
Zambian fish curry with Nsima - Zambia ... 165
Shakshouka - Palestine ... 166
Traditional Hawaiian kalua pork - Tokelau ... 167
Cauliflower soup - Morocco ... 168
Dominican Location – Dominica Republic ... 169
Plato Tipico – Honduras ... 170

Next Step ... 173

Introduction

Dear Friend,

Celebrating the joy of healthy eating of global cuisine is essential for a sustainable lifestyle.

When was the last time you had a new food experience? Cooked a new healthy meal, dined at different exotic international restaurants, or shopped at a specialty supermarket?

Embracing different textures, types, and touches of food adds to living a full, fit, and fun lifestyle.

It is often said that books you read or don't read reflect your mindset, your bank, and your credit card statement since reflecting your priorities and what you value. Glancing into your shopping basket at the grocery store or farmer's market reflects your waistline, your taste bud, and your food tendencies.

As a fitness professional, nutrition specialist, and food & culture enthusiast, I am constantly observing other people's food habits in grocery stores and restaurants while managing my own. I find myself curiously observing other people's shopping habits in the checkout aisle, much the way friends and family come over to examine what's on my plate and in glass at a cocktail or dinner party. A wiser statement a friend said to me about food choices is "every time I do grocery shopping, I purchase at least one item I have never tried before" This statement inspires me every day.

A glance into your shopping cart will tell me where you spend most of your time shopping and the quality of the food you are buying, whether it is in between the aisle getting lots of cans, frozen meals, and bagged snacks or on the perimeter of the store getting fresh fruits & vegetables, lean cuts of meats or you explored the international aisle add some variety to your healthy meals.

In college is where my love language of international cuisines & curiosities started. I went to school with students from many nations while sticking to a healthy southern meal plan of cafeteria food for track athletes and surviving the tortuous bayou heat. I was starting to desire geera, masala, curry, jerk, and other tantalizing flavors.

I intentionally started seeking out international students making new friends and embracing new cultures. It was my low-budget way of gathering recipes, tasting new cuisines, and sharing stories about the uniqueness of culture from people from around the world. I quickly discovered almost every culture has a unique way of preparing two things: bread and rice & peas.

I was intentional about making new friends, I think I met and had a friend from almost every nation that was represented on the LSU campus. I can still remember the taste, the stories shared, and many friends as we connected over meals. We didn't have many resources, we didn't have much time, yet we found a way to tear down walls of isolation and build bridges with each other through food and stories about family and traditions.

This book is a continuation of the food experiences that have profoundly changed and shaped my lifestyle. This collection of recipes gathered is in a 4-part series. Part 1 – Cookbook, part 2- A Soup book, part 3- Salad book, and Part 4 Smoothie book a total of 195 countries that will be released over 12 months period. It is a gift I have been given in college I now give to you.

Have you ever wondered how unpleasant life would be without good food? Food is an essential requirement for growth and tissue repair. It's equally important that you make nutritious food choices.

It has been proposed that breakfast is the most important food for the day. A healthy choice is another factor. Better breakfast options include a mix of protein, healthy fat, and fiber with little or no added sugar. The food eaten upon waking is used to refuel the body after a prolonged night of fasting and sets the pace for the rest of the day.

Each meal in the day is important to attain and sustain a healthy lifestyle. Research shows that people who eat breakfast have lesser consumption of calories throughout the day, are more likely to gain healthier muscle weight, and are less likely to experience morning fatigue and emotional instabilities.

Lunch is another important part of a day's meal. This is because eating in the afternoon replenishes the depleted energy reserves to enable you to regain focus through the activities of the day. It also supplies glucose to the blood for healthy brain function.

Dinner completes the daily food intake that may be inadequate during the day. Dinner must be also nutritious and lean; to help prepare the body that is going resting stage for a good night's sleep and recovery.

A lifestyle of healthy living is a celebration of healthy eating. Food is good its purpose is to fuel the body with energy to do work, work in the gym or the field, work in the office or at home. Food is also used as a connector, whether among friends at school in the cafeteria or colleagues at lunch in the office, or among families at dinner.

This cookbook consists of 90 recipes for breakfast, lunch, and dinner.

I invite you to explore each continent and all the nations. That exploration journey starts in this cookbook, leads to the international aisle in the supermarket, on towards your table and table bud. The ultimate hope is that this new healthy food experience would lead to purchasing a ticket to visit a nation, build connections and make new friends along the way. If for some reason you are unable to travel to another country because of time, money, safety, or the borders are chosen because of a health crisis. You still have an opportunity to experience a new food experience, a new way of eating, and a new way of living through the pages of this book. The Re-center Method Natural Diet Cookbook

Celebrating the joy of healthy eating of global cuisine is essential for a sustainable lifestyle.

Joyfully

Hareldau Argyle King

Founder of Being Elevated Lifestyle

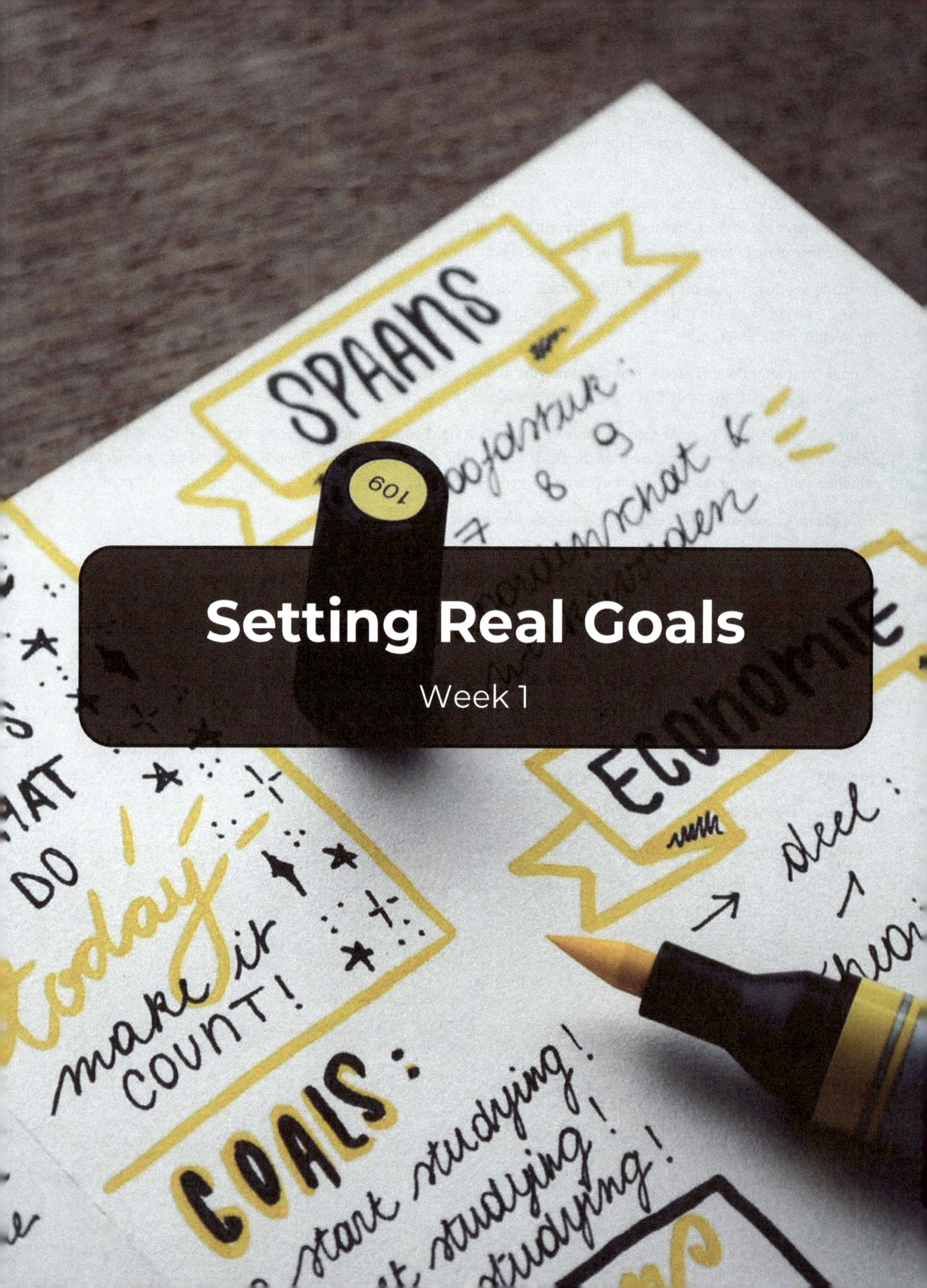

Week - 1
Take Obedient Action

- List 5 things you are grateful for in Life.

_____

_____

_____

_____

_____

_____

_____

- List 5 things you are grateful for in Life.

    Blood Pressure_____

    Heart Rate_____

    Total Weight _____

    Body fat _____

    Girth measurement- waist, hip, chest _____

- List 5 things you are grateful for in Life: _____
- List 5 things you are grateful for in Life.

_____

_____

_____

_____

_____

_____

_____

Louisiana, USA-Breakfast

The ambiance of modern-day Louisiana is a fine mix of cultures including African, French, Native American, Canadian, Haitian and European.

Louisiana (LA) boasts of a population of over 4,657,757 people, with Baton Rouge as the state capital.

The five major cities in LA are New Orleans, Baton Rouge, Shreveport, Metairie, and Lafayette. The largest city in Louisiana is New Orleans, with a population of 388,424.

The Pelican state is famous for its unique Creole and Cajun culture, food, jazz music, and Mari Gras festival.

Louisiana has one of the largest alligator populations in the United States. There are about two million alligators in the wild and another 300,000 on alligator farms.

The vast swamplands and accompanying bird populations, as well as the many outdoor destinations to the north, Creole, or Pelican state.

Take a tour around (LA). You'll tell an exciting story If you go during Mardi Gras, try the official donut of Louisiana, the beignet. Beignets are soft, square-shaped, and vanilla-scented French donuts fried until golden brown.

These are served with chocolate milk or café au lait, at the cafe du Monde.

Beignet contains 188 calories per 45 g serving

Beignets and cafe du lait for breakfast.

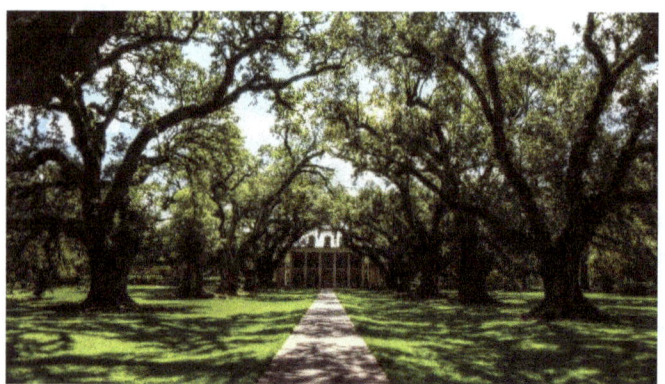

Mozambique-Lunch

An abundance of natural resources, steady water streams from the Zambezi River, rich agriculture (affording staple delicacies, replete with fresh sea foods), and much more are typical of Mozambique.

The East African country has a variety of healthy palettes that will make your stay a memorable one.

The Mozambican lifestyle was largely influenced by the Portuguese and Arab communities, as shown in their cuisine.

The Mozambicans have a knack for binging on staple, and it is a country, of about 30 million people.

These include fresh seafood, stews, corn porridge, rice, millet, and cassava.

If you ever need to explore the richness of capital Maputo, you are in for an unusual treat in terms of commerce, technology, and culture.

You might just want to dash into the cafes to have a first-hand feel of Maputo's beverages.

Feel the attractive aquatic scenery of Maputo Bay and tell the story yourself.

A country in Africa that boasts untamed beaches and beautiful islands.

Mozambique is a destination for all travelers.

It is one of the best places for underwater activities and natural escapades.

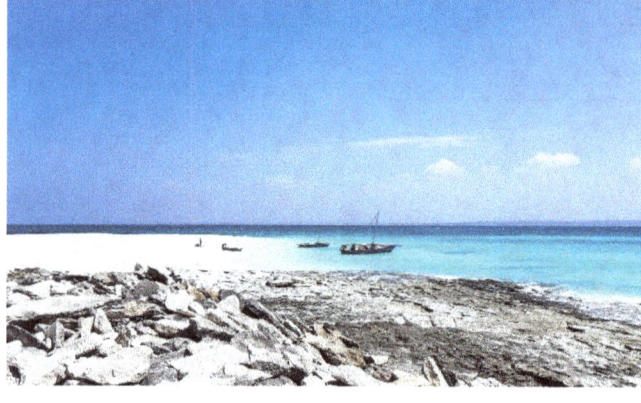

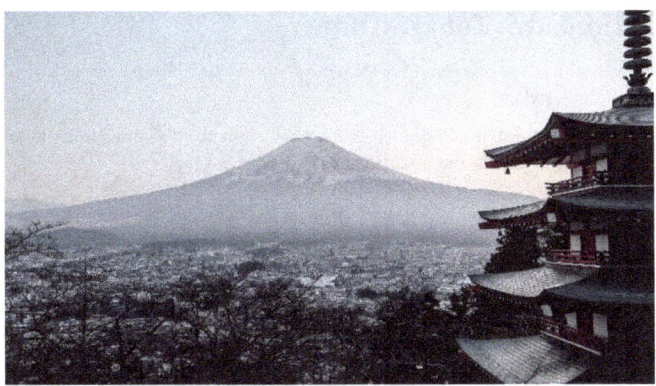

Japan-Dinner

The Land of the Rising Sun is a land of beautiful wonders.

Japan is a top destination for all seasons.

Known for its amazing technology that makes day-to-day tasks easier, natural wonders preserved for centuries, and vibrant, mouth-watering cuisine.

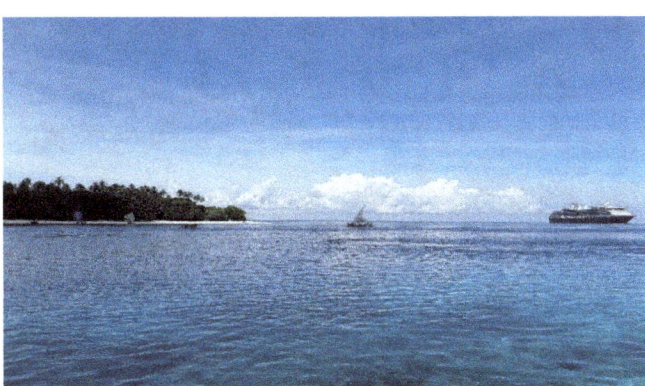

Papua New Guinea-Breakfast

Starchy root crops as a part and parcel of the Papuan's local palette.

Although, impacted on their culture are direct touches from other nations.

Sweet potato has topped the charts concerning the Papuan's preferences for staple meals.

Nonetheless, most of the multilingual/multicultural nation are vegetarians.

Your dreams of sampling the sheer awesomeness of a luxuriant rainforest is valid in Papua New Guinea.

Take a tour to the capital city of Moresby will be worthwhile as it is considered the largest city in the south pacific.

The inhabitants seem quite conservative in their culinary choices as they eat dinner as their main meal for the day, with little or nothing as lunch.

Papuans make do with remnants for breakfast.

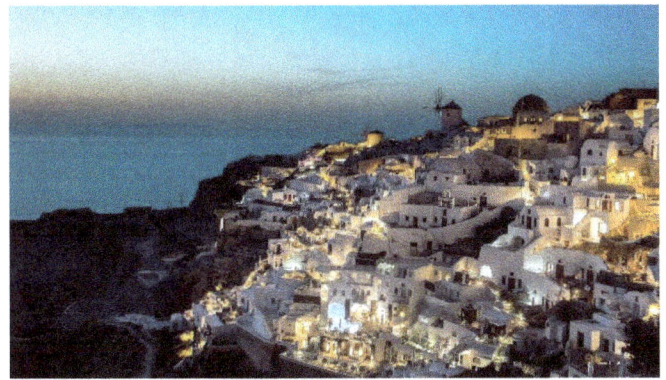

Greece-Lunch

Greece is in the far south of the Balkan Peninsula.

Places to visit in this predominantly mountainous country are cities like Athens (state capital), Piraeus, Elefsina, and many more.

Bread, olives, and wine are ideal constituents of an ideal meal in Greece cuisine.

With an average of 80 percent sunshine per year, Lovers of the sun are sure to have a field day gulping down aromatic drinks like Ouzo, and raki while discovering the aesthetics of Grecian beaches and island.

It has been reported that Winemaking in Greece has been a tradition for 4,000 years, and there are over 600 wineries in Greece.

The estimated population of residents in Greece was estimated as 10.72 million (2020).

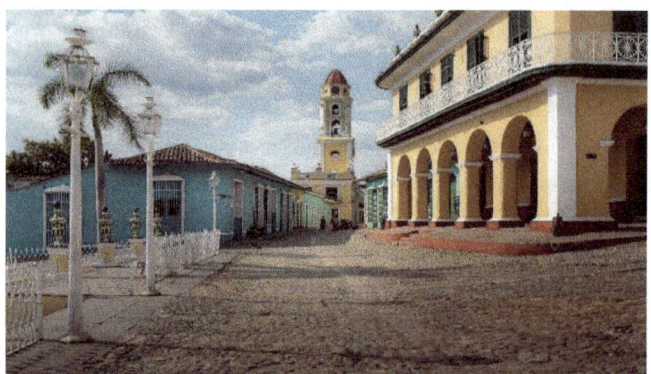

Trinidad & Tobago-Dinner

The wealth of the oil reserves of this country in the Caribbean bears so much to their lifestyle.

The twin island state of Trinidad and Tobago habit boast a population nation of 1.3 million people and uniquely diverse Caribbean recipes.

For such a small island, this country packs a multicultural identity reflected by its adventure toward food.

Trinidad has all the things you can expect from an island paradise – great beaches, virgin forests, and historical sites untouched by time – but it also boasts a fusion of cuisine of Indian, African, Syrian, Lebanese, Italian, Chinese, and Arabian and Creole roots.

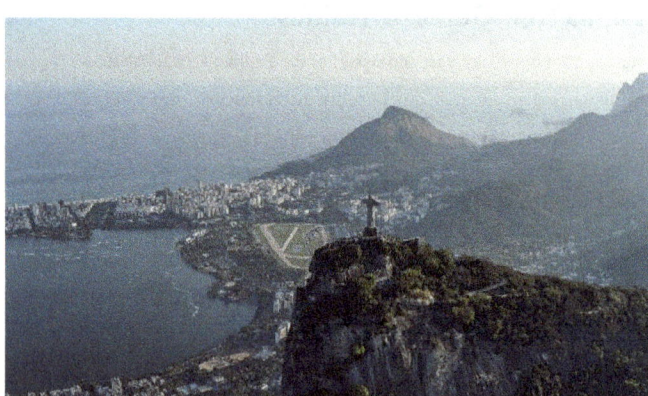

Brazil-Breakfast

With a teeming population of 214,664,519 residents, and major cities like Brasilia (state capital, Sao Paulo (most populated), Rio de Janeiro, etc.

The dense rainforests, exotic beaches, graceful waterfalls, aesthetic carnival fete, and the popular samba dance all feature the main draw to this south American country.

The tropical rainforest vegetations largely support a steady supply of succulent fruits that are featured in most Brazilian dishes. A characteristic Brazilian eats breakfast on the go, on the go-to- easy-to-prepare.

However, coffee is the most essential beverage in Brazilian breakfasts; this is not to exclude juices and smoothies made from whole fruits.

A dense but healthy staple like steamed cornmeal and other starchy lights like, cheese and puffed bread and pound cakes are ideal options for an average Brazilian.

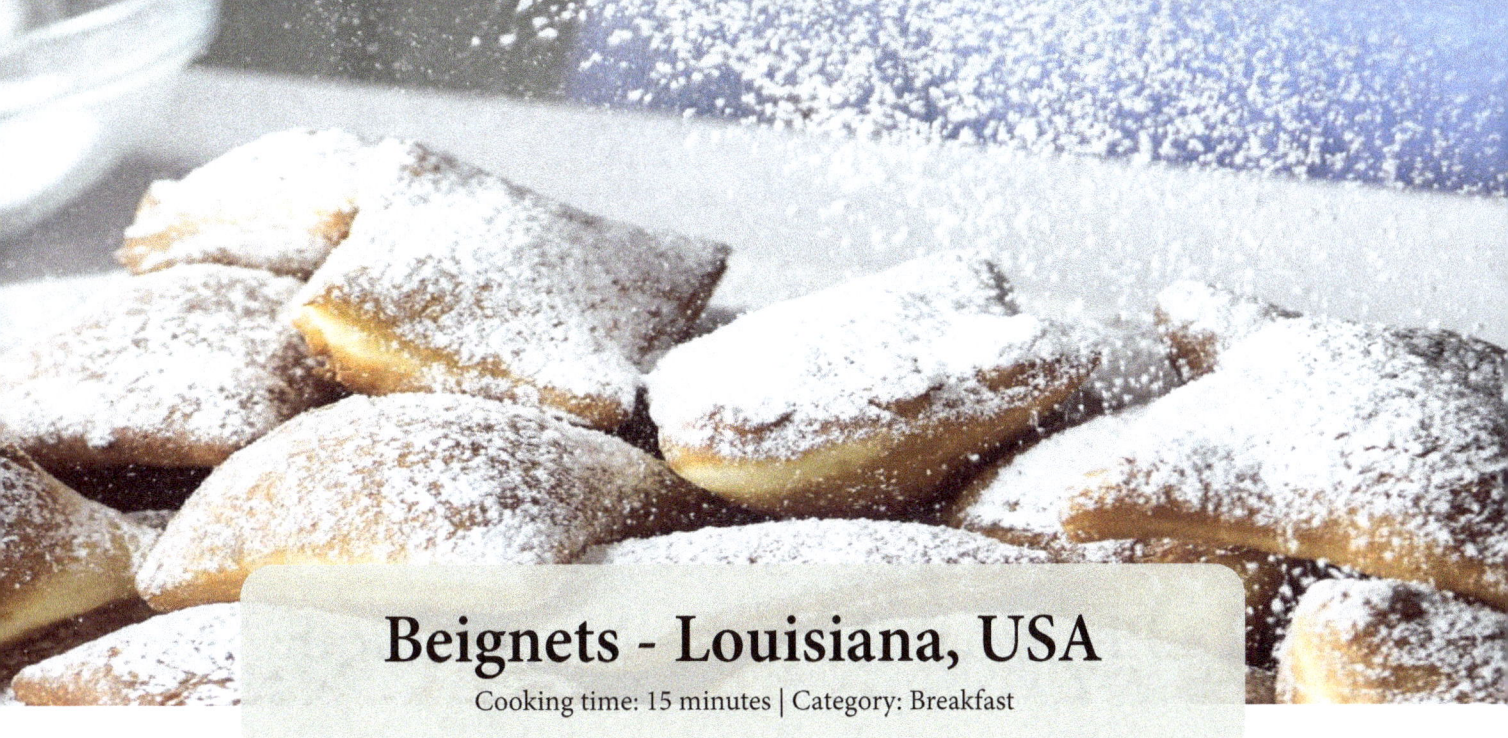

Beignets - Louisiana, USA

Cooking time: 15 minutes | Category: Breakfast

Home-made beignets are very tasty. The incomparable ecstasy of crunching on freshly fried, warm donuts served with a cup of hot coffee. It's simply indescribable!

Ingredients

- Warm water
- Yeast
- All-purpose flour
- Butter
- Whole milk
- Sugar
- Vanilla
- Powdered sugar
- Vegetable oil

Steps to Cook

1. Add the warm water, yeast, and a little sugar to the bowl of a stand mixer and let it activate.
2. Next, add the milk, vanilla, and egg and mix.
3. Add half of the flour and mix until smooth
4. Connect the dough hook and add the remaining flour while mixing on a medium speed. Once the dough comes together add the butter and continues to mix or knead the dough until it comes away from the bowl.
5. Transfer the dough to a lightly oiled bowl and place it in a warm place to rise.
6. Roll the dough into a 1/2-inch-thick rectangle then cut out squares around 2 inches wide
7. Fry the beignets in hot oil making sure to use a candy thermometer to keep an eye on the temperature and drain on kitchen paper.
8. Transfer the donuts to a cooling rack and dust in plenty of powdered sugar, serve immediately

Note:

The Southern Bayou State is well-known as the birthplace of jazz, the home of Mardi Gras, and a melting pot of culinary delights. Louisiana's history is as rich as its people who hailed from France, Spain, Haiti, French Canada, the Caribbean, Africa, and Vietnam. Their love for artistic expression is matched only by their love for food, uniquely Creole/Cajun.

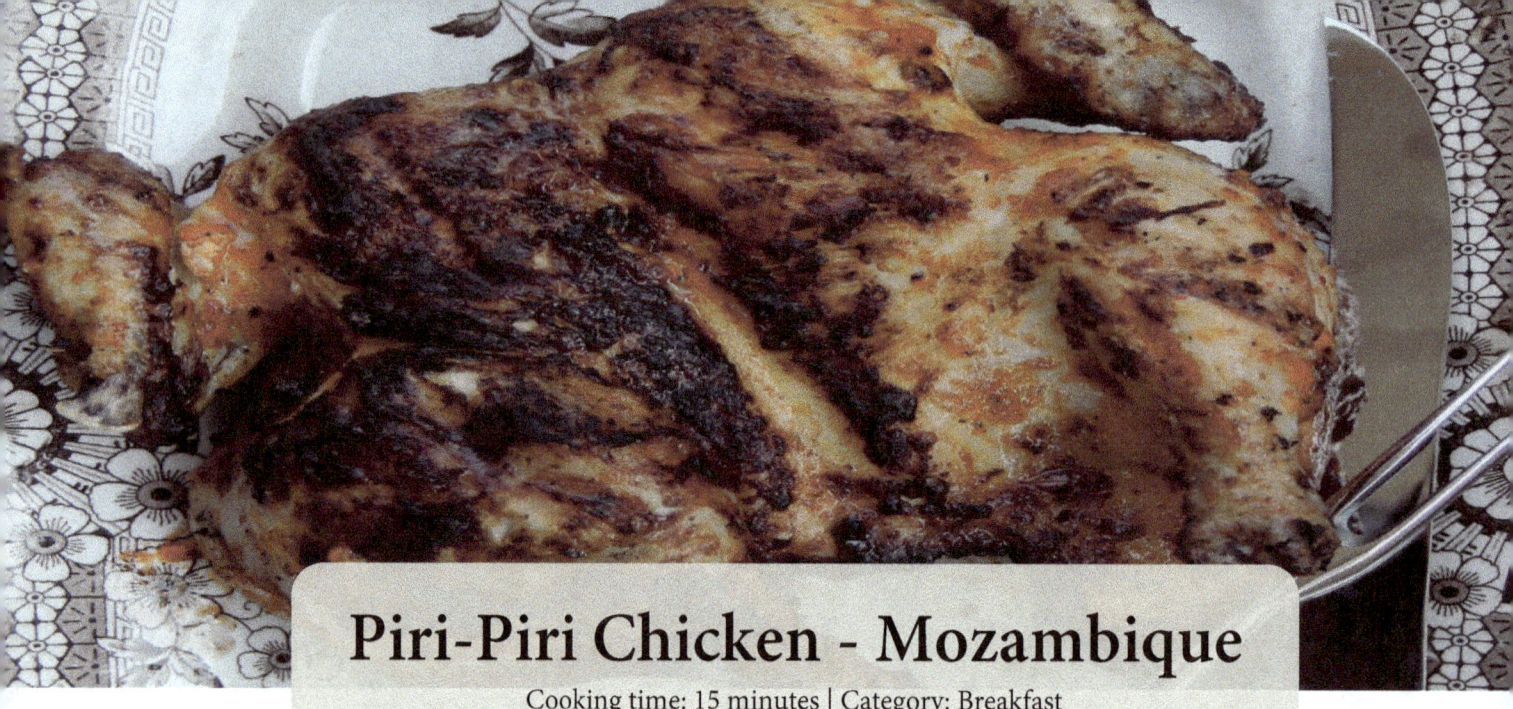

Piri-Piri Chicken - Mozambique

Cooking time: 15 minutes | Category: Breakfast

Piri-Piri is a famous Mozambican spicy sauce. The chicken is mostly grilled and marinated in piripiri gravy (a co-mix of hot pepper, garlic, and parsley) GalinhaAssada (roasted chicken) has strong descent from Africa and Portugal. The multiple varieties of this unique dish make it extremely popular on many eating tables.

Ingredients

- 1 large fresh chicken, about 2kg
- fresh watercress, to garnish
- lemon wedges, to serve

Piri Piri marinade

- 4 plump red chilies, deseeded and roughly chopped
- 2 red bird's-eye chilies, stalks removed, sliced
- 4 garlic cloves, peeled and halved
- 20g bunch of flat leaf parsley (with stalks)
- juice of 2 lemons, about 65ml
- 2 tbsp white wine vinegar
- 1 tsp smoked paprika, sweet or hot
- 1 tsp oregano
- 1 tsp caster sugar
- 2 tsp flaked sea salt

Steps to Cook

1. A To make the marinade, put all the ingredients in a food processor and blitz until everything is well mixed and chopped up small. Remove the bones chicken Discard bones. Cut off the foot joints and wing tips.
2. Strip off all the skin from the bird apart from the ends of the wings.
3. Open the chicken out and place it on the board so the breast side is facing upwards. Press down heavily with the palms of your hands to break the breastbone and flatten the chicken as evenly as possible.
4. Spoon over all the marinade and massage it into both sides of the chicken, marinate in the fridge for at least 4 hours or ideally overnight.
5. Preheat the oven to 210°C/Fan 190°C/Gas 6½. Take the chicken out of the dish and place it on a rack inside a large baking tray, breast-side up. Roast for 50–60 minutes until lightly browned and cooked through.

Note:

Mozambique's Lago Niassa Lake is the third largest and second deepest lake in Africa, with most diverse fish. The impala is a beer locally sourced from staple maize.

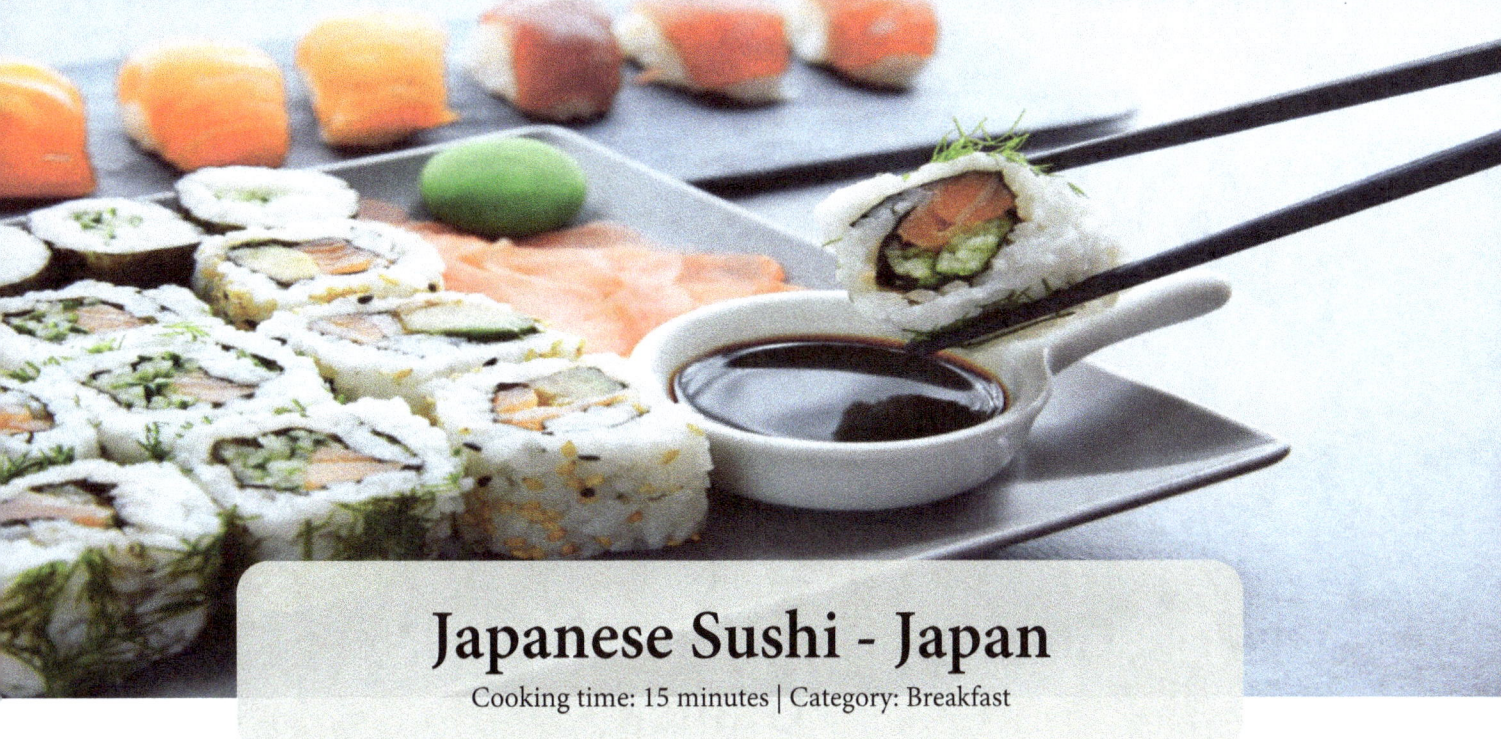

Japanese Sushi - Japan

Cooking time: 15 minutes | Category: Breakfast

Sushi is a combination of vinegar-laden rice, fish, seaweed, or vegetables.

The meal pairs very well with mugicha a non-alcoholic, nutty-flavored beverage made from an infusion of water and water infused with roasted barley grains.

Ingredients

- ⅔ cup uncooked short-grain white rice
- 3 tablespoons rice vinegar
- 3 tablespoons white sugar
- 1 ½ teaspoons salt
- 4 sheets nori seaweed sheets
- ½ cucumber, peeled, cut into small strips
- 2 tablespoons pickled ginger
- 1 avocado
- ½ pound imitation crabmeat, flaked

Steps to Cook

1. In a medium saucepan, bring 1.5 cups of water to a boil. Add rice and stir. Lower the heat, cover, and let it simmer for 20 minutes. In a small bowl, mix the rice vinegar, sugar, and salt. Blend the mixture into the rice.
2. Pre-set the heat in the oven to 300 degrees F (150 degrees C). On a medium baking sheet, heat nori in the preheated oven for 1 to 2 minutes, until warm.
3. Place one sheet of nori on a bamboo sushi mat. Wet your hands. Using your hands spread a thin layer of rice on the sheet of nori and press it into a thin layer.
4. Arrange 1/4 of the cucumber, ginger, avocado, and imitation crabmeat in a line down the center of the rice. Raise the mat ends, and gently roll it over the ingredients, pressing gently.
5. Roll it forward to make a complete roll. Repeat with remaining ingredients.
6. Using a wet knife, Slice the rolls into 4 to 6 slices.

Note:

Japan's financial capital is Tokyo with over 8 million people, while the other 13 cities have over 1 million people.

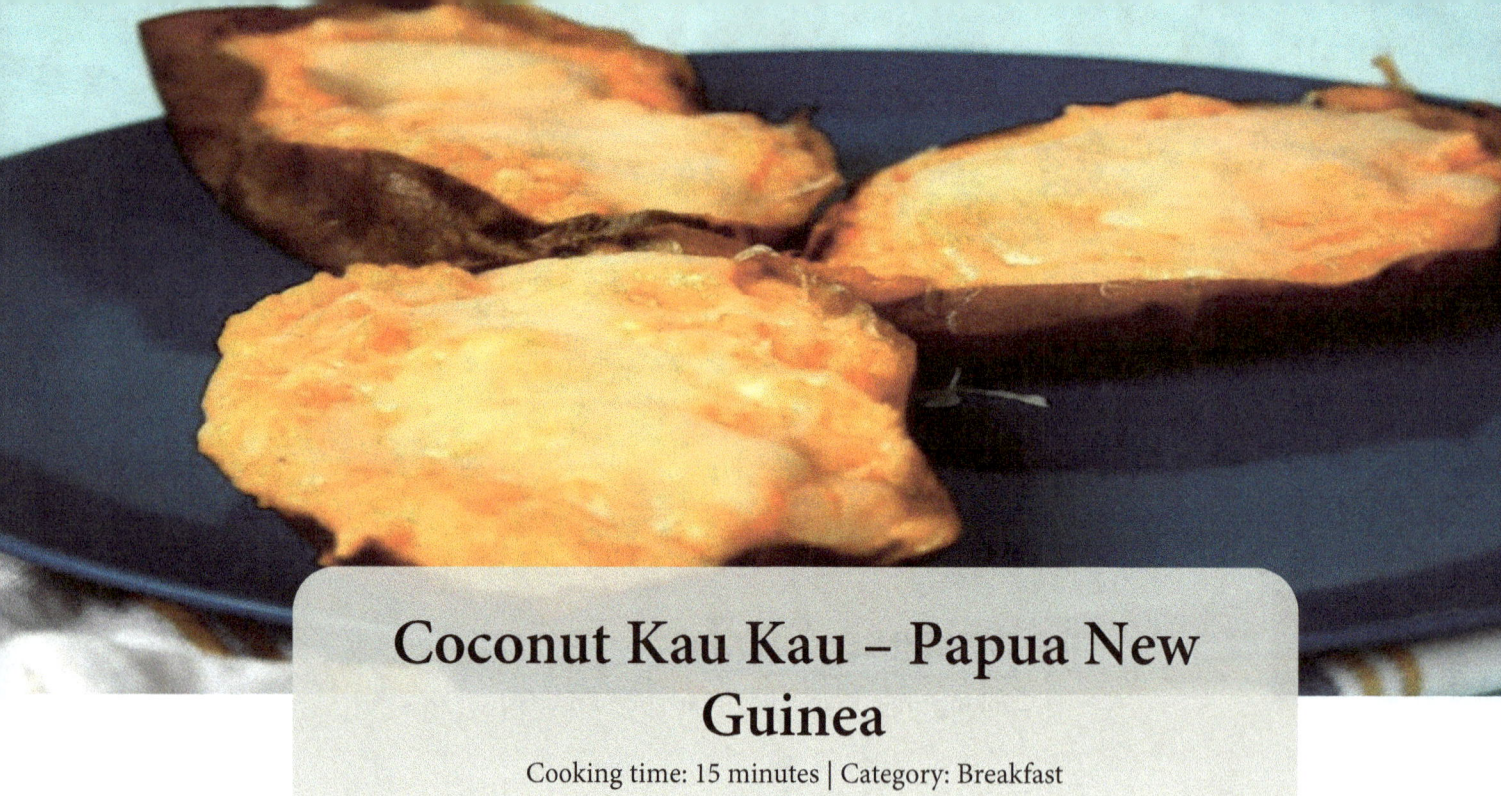

Coconut Kau Kau – Papua New Guinea

Cooking time: 15 minutes | Category: Breakfast

The coconut Kau Kau recipe is a perfect mix of sweet potato, garlic, onions, and coconut cream. Although, variations can be made with mashed potatoes. This recipe is a preferred, healthy breakfast choice for locals for reasons of affordability.

Ingredients

- 2 sweet potatoes (kaukau)
- 4 tablespoons butter, diced
- 3 tablespoons grated fresh coconut (or unsweetened shredded coconut)
- ½ cup coconut cream
- ½ onion, finely chopped
- 2 cloves garlic, crushed
- 1 (1-inch) piece of fresh ginger grated
- 2 tablespoons orange juice
- Salt to taste
- Pepper to taste

Steps to Cook

1. Rinse the sweet potatoes, then wrap each of them in aluminum foil and place them in a plate.
2. Bake in preheated 400F/200C oven for 1 hour or until cooked through.
3. Cut sweet potatoes in two lengthwise.
4. Scoop out about ¾ of the sweet potatoes with a spoon into a bowl.
5. Immediately add the butter. Add salt and pepper, and mash with a fork to get a smooth purée.
6. Set the skins of the half hollowed sweet potatoes on a baking sheet lined with parchment paper.
7. Add the coconut cream, onion, garlic, ginger, and orange juice to the mashed sweet potatoes. Mix well.
8. Fill the hollowed half-sweet potatoes with the mashed mixture.
9. Bake in the oven for another 5 minutes before serving.
10. In this predominantly rural community, cooking is done on an open fire. The food is either wrapped in leaves or placed directly in the fire. Cooking is also done in pits filled with stones called mumu.

Note:

A mixture of the root of kava and water forms a non-alcoholic beverage called the popular kava drink.Coffee is another cash crop and beverage for Papuans.

Currently, the capital of Papua New Guinea is Port Moresby. Papua New Guinea currently boasts of about eight million residents, 800 languages, and over 1,000 distinct ethnic groups. Most of the country's population lives in rural communities.

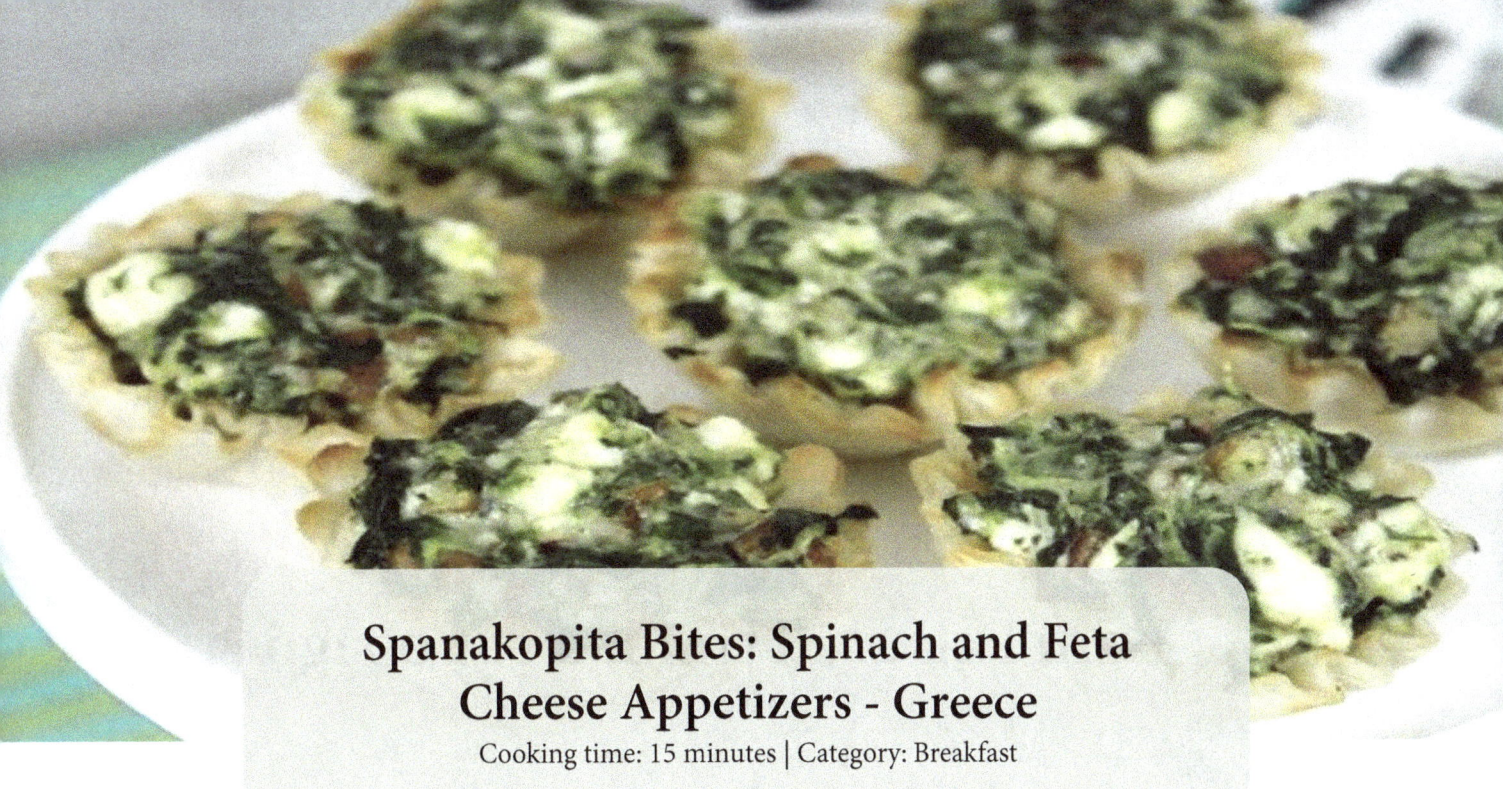

Spanakopita Bites: Spinach and Feta Cheese Appetizers - Greece

Cooking time: 15 minutes | Category: Breakfast

These mini spinach and feta cheese bites will enable you to have a feel of Grecian lunch delights.

Ingredients

- 1-pound fresh spinach, chopped (you can substitute frozen, thawed well)
- 1/4 cup olive oil
- 1 large onion (finely minced)
- 1 bunch of green onion (diced, including 4 inches of the green part)
- 1/4 cup chopped fresh parsley
- 1/4 cup chopped fresh dill
- Pinch of ground nutmeg
- Salt and freshly ground black pepper to taste
- 1/4-pound feta cheese (crumbled)
- 2 eggs, lightly beaten
- 1/2 cup ricotta cheese (or cottage cheese)
- 45 phyllo pastry shells (frozen)

Steps to Cook

1. Gather the ingredients.
2. Wash and drain the chopped spinach very well. If using frozen spinach, thaw completely and squeeze out excess water very well. Spinach should be quite dry.
3. Heat the olive oil in a deep sauté pan or Dutch oven. Sauté the onions and green onions until tender. Add the spinach, parsley, and dill and cook for 5 to 10 minutes until the spinach is wilted and heated through. Add the nutmeg and season with salt and pepper.
4. Cook the spinach mixture until the excess moisture evaporates. You want it to be on the dry side. Remove from heat and set the spinach aside to cool.
5. Once the spinach has cooled, add the crumbled feta, eggs, and ricotta cheese, and mix until combined
6. Preheat the oven to 350 F. Lightly brush the insides of the frozen phyllo shells with olive oil and fill with spinach mixture until approximately 3/4 full.
7. Bake the filled shells on a baking sheet for 15 to 20 minutes, or until the filling is cooked through. Serve immediately.

Note:

You are sure to debunk your prior beliefs about Greek cuisine. Fish and meat addicts as well as vegan lovers are sure to sample a lot of flavorful varieties, apart from moussaka, souvlaki, and the popular Greek Salad choriatiki. Greece has consistently been recognized as a top world destination, attracting as many as 31 million visitors in 2019! Over a hundred archaeological and historical sites bore witness to its glorious past, including the iconic Parthenon. Tourists also flock here for its clean, picturesque beaches and whitewashed towns ensconced on cliffs with amazing views of the Mediterranean Sea.

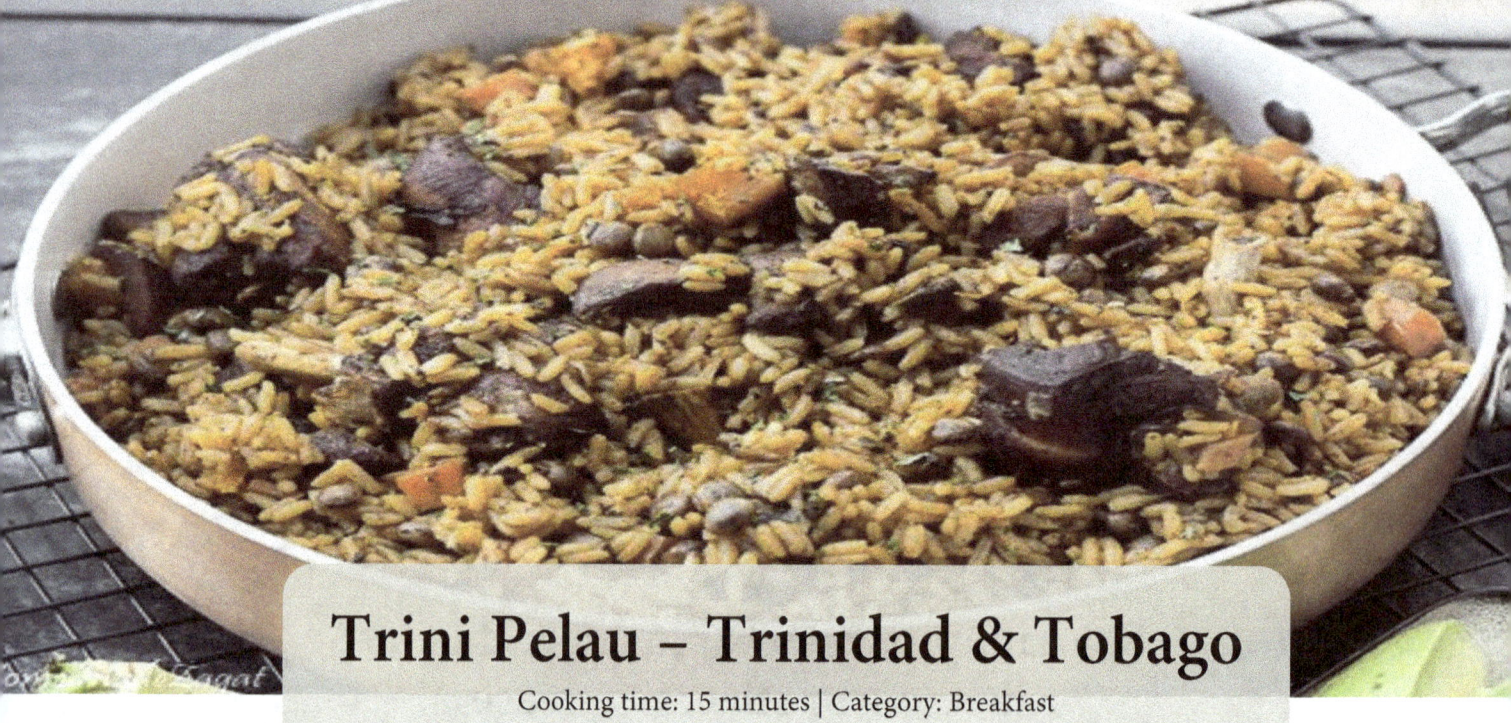

Trini Pelau – Trinidad & Tobago

Cooking time: 15 minutes | Category: Breakfast

Trini Pelau is an iconic recipe from the island of Trinidad & Tabago that is often made on weekends and when family and friends get together for a lime (Caribbean slang word for get-together). This one-dish meal originating in the French West Indies combines pigeon peas, meat or chicken, and rice along with fresh herbs and coconut milk. The entire dish is then flavored and colored with burnt sugar.

Ingredients

- 500g chicken
- 1 tbsp chicken seasoning
- 2 tbsp medium curry powder
- 2 tbsp soy sauce
- 1 onion, sliced
- 2 garlic cloves minced
- 2 sprigs of fresh thyme
- 3 tbsp sunflower oil
- 2 tbsp golden granulated sugar
- 300ml American easy-cook rice
- 410g can black-eyed beans, drained

Steps to Cook

1. Put the chicken into a large, shallow plastic container, ideally with a lid. Carefully stab a knife into each piece of chicken about 3 times. Use a measuring spoon to sprinkle the chicken seasoning and curry powder over the chicken, and then use a fork to turn the chicken and cover in seasoning.

2. Sprinkle with the soy sauce, chopped onion, and crushed garlic. Run your thumb and forefinger down each thyme stem to remove the leaves, then add these to the chicken. Stir with a fork, cover tightly with a lid (if you have one,) and gently shake it all together. You can put this into the fridge for a couple of hours if you want the chicken to be full of flavor it's fine to use it right away.

3. Pour the oil into a 30cm frying pan, add the sugar and put over medium heat for about 5-7 minutes. Keep looking at the mixture, but don't stir it. When it turns a mid-golden brown, it means the sugar has caramelized Stand well back and ask an adult to quickly tip the chicken into the pan. Cover it with a lid, and don't touch it for 5 minutes.

4. Lift the lid, turn the chicken pieces over, cover and cook for another 5 minutes until a lovely, rich golden-brown color.

5. Pour the rice into a measuring jug until it comes up to the 300ml mark, then tip into the pan. Pour 700ml cold water into the plastic container you used to season the chicken, then pour this into the pan, too. Cover and cook for 20 minutes over gentle heat without lifting the lid.

6. Tip the black-eyed beans into a sieve to drain, then add to the pan. Stir it all together, then cover and cook for 3 minutes to warm the beans through. It's now ready to eat.

Note:

The calorie content is 479 calories. Do well to sample the exotic drinks such as sorrels and mauby on the serene islands. It will be worth your time.

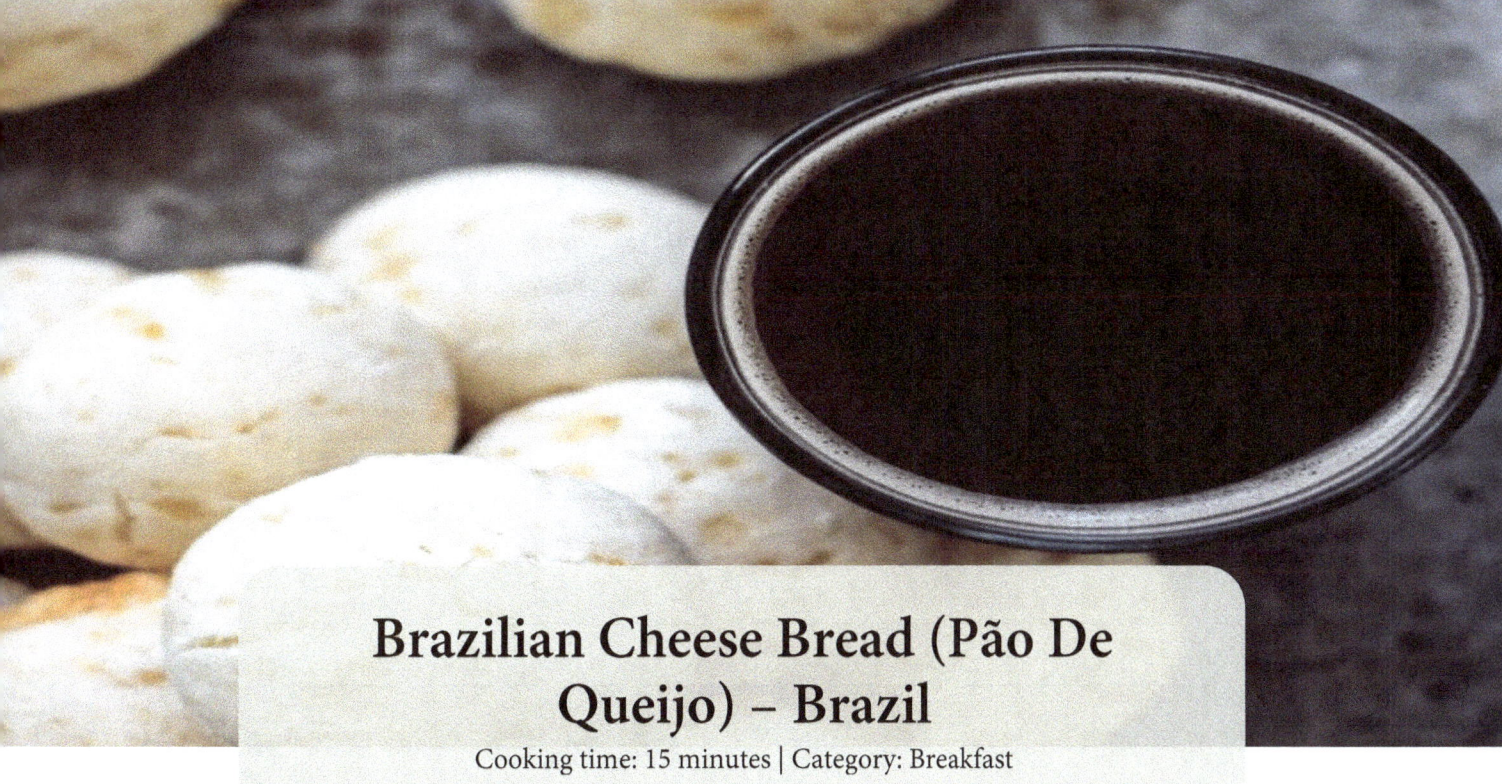

Brazilian Cheese Bread (Pão De Queijo) – Brazil

Cooking time: 15 minutes | Category: Breakfast

The goodness of the Brazilian cheese bread resounds to the gluten-conscious Brazilian.

Ingredients

- 1 ¾ cup tapioca starch
- 1 cup packed grated parmesan
- 1 cup packed grated cheddar
- 1 large egg
- ⅓ cup water
- ⅓ cup vegetable oil
- pinch of salt

Steps to Cook

1. Start by boiling the water with oil and a pinch of salt.
2. In a large bowl, add the tapioca starch and pour the hot water mixture. With a spoon, or using your stand mixer on medium-low, mix it until there's no more dry tapioca starch left. The dough should be grainy and gelatinous. Let it cool for 10 minutes or until you can hold your finger against it.
3. Preheat the oven to 350° F, and rack in the middle.
4. Add the egg and mix with your mixer on medium-low or with a spoon until it is incorporated into the dough. It will look like it won't combine, but it will. If you don't have a mixer and find it too hard to do it with a spoon, you can as well use your hands.
5. After the egg is incorporated, add the cheese and knead the dough until the cheese is fully mixed. The final dough will be similar to cookie dough in consistency, not too sticky, and easy to shape with your hands.
6. To shape the dough into balls, use a spoon or a scoop and shape them a bit smaller than a golf ball. If you find the dough is too sticky to shape, wet your hands with cold water or pour some oil in your hands to help. Don't add more tapioca flour!
7. Place the cheese balls on a baking sheet prepared with parchment paper or a silicone mat, leaving about ½ to 1 inch of space between each one.
8. Bake for 25 minutes on 350°F until they're puffed and golden on top.
9. Serve them warm.

Note:

As a tourist on a visit to Brazil, be sure to indulge yourself in the Carnival festival. You are sure to tell an exciting story. The largest country in South America is also larger than life with its stunning stretches of beaches, exciting carnivals, and breathtaking views. Brazilians simply love to celebrate life and it's hard to resist their charm. Before you know it, you'll keep on coming back.

Week - 1

Reflections

- What 5 things are you grateful for?

_____

_____

_____

_____

_____

_____

- Describe your current health & fitness level?

_____

_____

_____

_____

_____

_____

- What did you like about recipe and is learning about the country?

_____

_____

_____

_____

_____

_____

Commit to Change

Week 2

Week - 2

Take Obedient Action

- Spend 5 -10 minutes writing in your gratitude journal about giving thanks

_____
_____
_____
_____
_____
_____
_____

- Select 1 Lunch recipe and 1 Dinner from this week & prepare them

_____
_____
_____
_____
_____
_____
_____
_____

- Connect with people from the countries you preparing the meals

_____
_____
_____
_____
_____
_____
_____
_____

Select one new fruit_____

Maintain your 1 mile walk or run_____

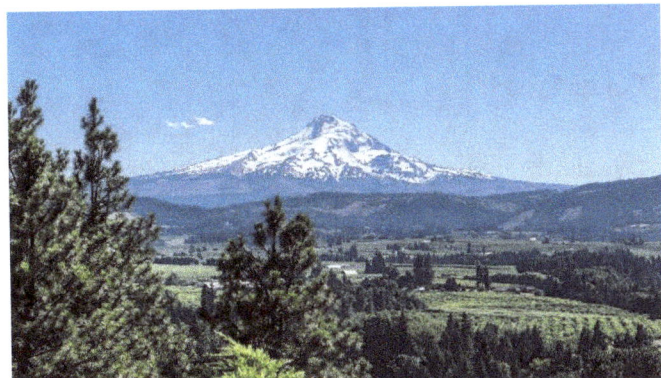

Oregon-Lunch

Oregon has been regarded as a foodie paradise.

This 33rd state of the United States of America boasts several breweries, craft beer is a household name amongst the locals.

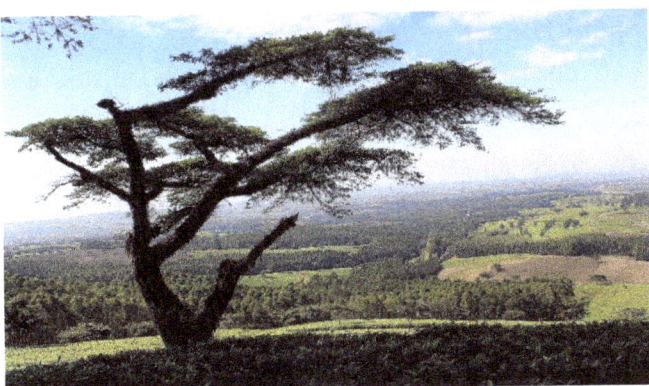

Malawi-Dinner

Little can be said about this East African country without mentioning Lake Malawi. This freshwater lake features interesting fishes that make great cuisine, Malawians are noted for friendliness. Malawi has been considered the county with the big hat, with an estimated population of 17.2 million. Starchy foods like corn, potatoes, sorghum, etc have done wonders in many Malawian staples.

Tourists have not failed to explore the deliciousness of the Nsima dish, which graces the dining table of the locals.

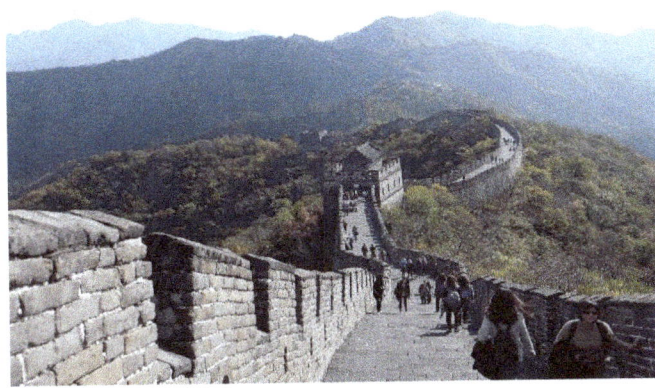

China-Breakfast

China is the world's most populous country with about a 1.4billion residents.

This East Asian nation has been nominated as the second most popular national cuisine worldwide.

China has an expansive repertoire of amazing dishes, having its styles and traditions of cooking.

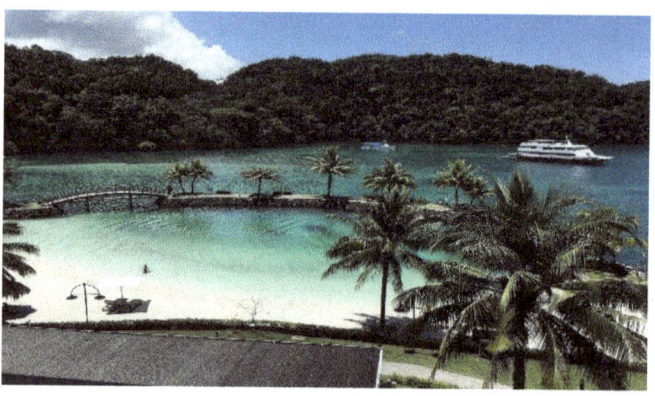

Palau-Lunch

This Island country in the west pacific with a current population of 18,214.

The capital city of Palau is Melekeok taro, pandan, yams, and pumpkin are staples that are commonly eaten by the locals.

There are many Islands and lush waterbodies. This abundance is reflected in Paluan delicacies.

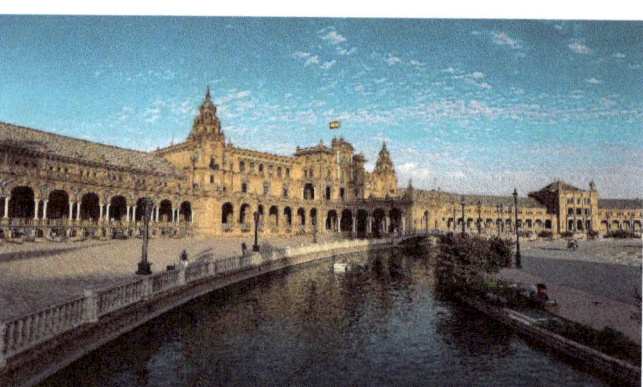

Spain-Dinner

Spain's capital and largest city are Madrid; other major urban areas include Barcelona, Valencia, Seville, and Zaragoza. Spain has a current population of 46,780,022.

There are several beaches, resort centers, and beautiful sceneries to behold on your next visit to Spain. Their dishes also have that touch of Spanish luxury.

Sometimes, you need not say anything about Spain. Just by saying its name evokes a colorful tapestry of history, culture, architecture, festivals, and culinary delights.

Having ranked as one of the top destinations of all time, not visiting Spain when you're in Europe should be considered a crime.

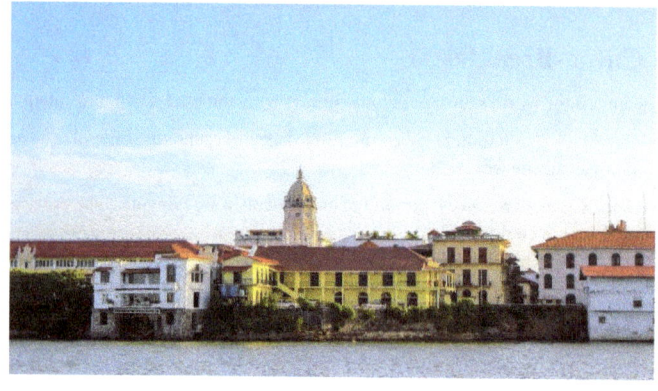

Panama-Breakfast

Cutting-edge skyscrapers, eye-popping taverns, lush rainforest of Natural Metropolitan Park, and many more characters in the beautifully bio-diverse country.

The revered Panama Canal, a man-made, but state-of-the-art masterpiece is another side attraction.

The current estimated population of this Central American country is 4,410,053.

The heartbeat of Panama is in its capital, Panama City.

Breakfasts are usually graced with corn, which is used in a variety of nutritious Panamanian staples.

Roasted or smoked foods are common with the locals.

However, the story is not the same for the capital city, where the inhabitants do more fried foods.

Panamanian Breakfasts are usually accompanied with coffee, chichas (natural juices), or black tea.

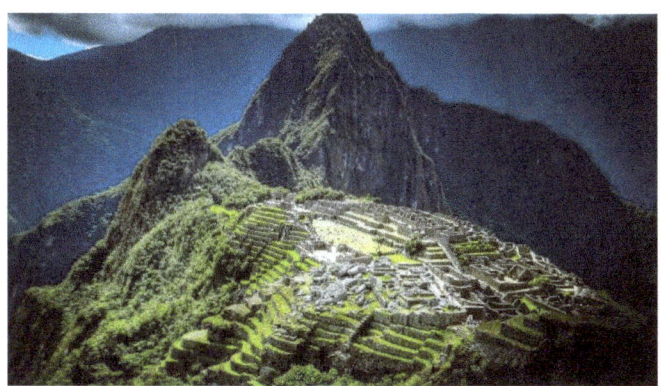

Peru-Lunch

The green rainforest, eye-popping mountainous regions, ancient cities and iconic islands are all characteristic of this South American. The state capital of Peru as well as its commercial and industrial center is Lima.

Beyond exquisite is a perfect description of Peruvian foods. A visit to Peru is not complete without trying the traditional seafood dish called Lomosaltado.

Now, this is a destination that you'd always find on almost everyone's bucket list.

Why? Because it is home to 12 UNESCO World Heritage sites, including the world-famous Machu Pichu, 5000 archaeological sites and 200 protected natural areas.

Travelers of all preferences would always find something in Peru, whether you're a fan of the Great Outdoors, a history geek, an adventurous foodie, or an Instagram star. Peru's got it all.

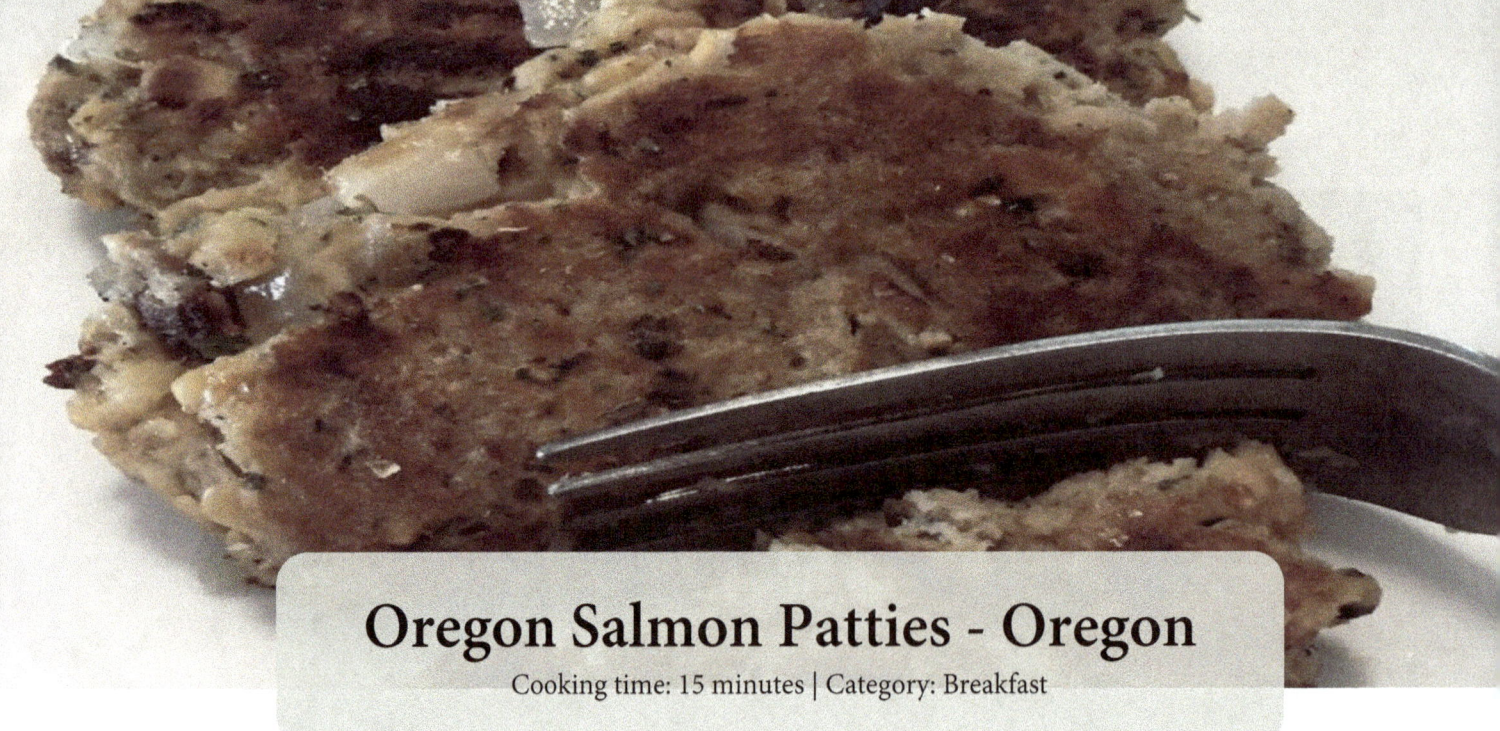

Oregon Salmon Patties - Oregon

Cooking time: 15 minutes | Category: Breakfast

Oregon Salmon Patties is a healthy choice of lunch for canned or fresh salmon patties.

This bunch of deliciousness is unique to natives of Oregon.

Ingredients

- 2 Tbsp butter
- 1 medium onion, finely chopped
- ¾ cup of crushed sourdough breadcrumbs
- 2 eggs beaten
- ¼ cup chopped parsley
- 1 tsp dry mustard
- 2 garlic cloves chopped
- 1 15 oz can of Salmon
- 3 Tbsp olive oil

Steps to Cook

1. Melt butter in a large skillet over medium heat. Add onion and cook until tender.
2. In a medium bowl, combine 1/3 of crushed breadcrumbs, eggs, parsley, mustard, and garlic.
3. Add the salmon and onions and ¾ cup of salmon juices into the bowl. Mix until well blended, then shape into six patties. Coat patties in remaining breadcrumbs.
4. Add olive oil to a large skillet over medium heat. Cook patties until brown, then carefully turn and brown on the other side.
5. Contained in each serving are 442 calories; protein 24.2g; carbohydrates 20g; fat 29g; cholesterol 123mg; sodium 634mg.

Note:

How exciting would an experience at Kahneeta Resort & Casino in Central Oregon?

Would you rather have a taste of the Native American culture, and experience the warmth at Teepee?

The choice is yours!

The state of Oregon is often overlooked due to its flamboyant neighbor-states like California and Nevada.

It shelters some of the most beautiful views in the entire United States, home to over 360 State Parks.

If adventure is what you're looking for, Oregon's got it all.

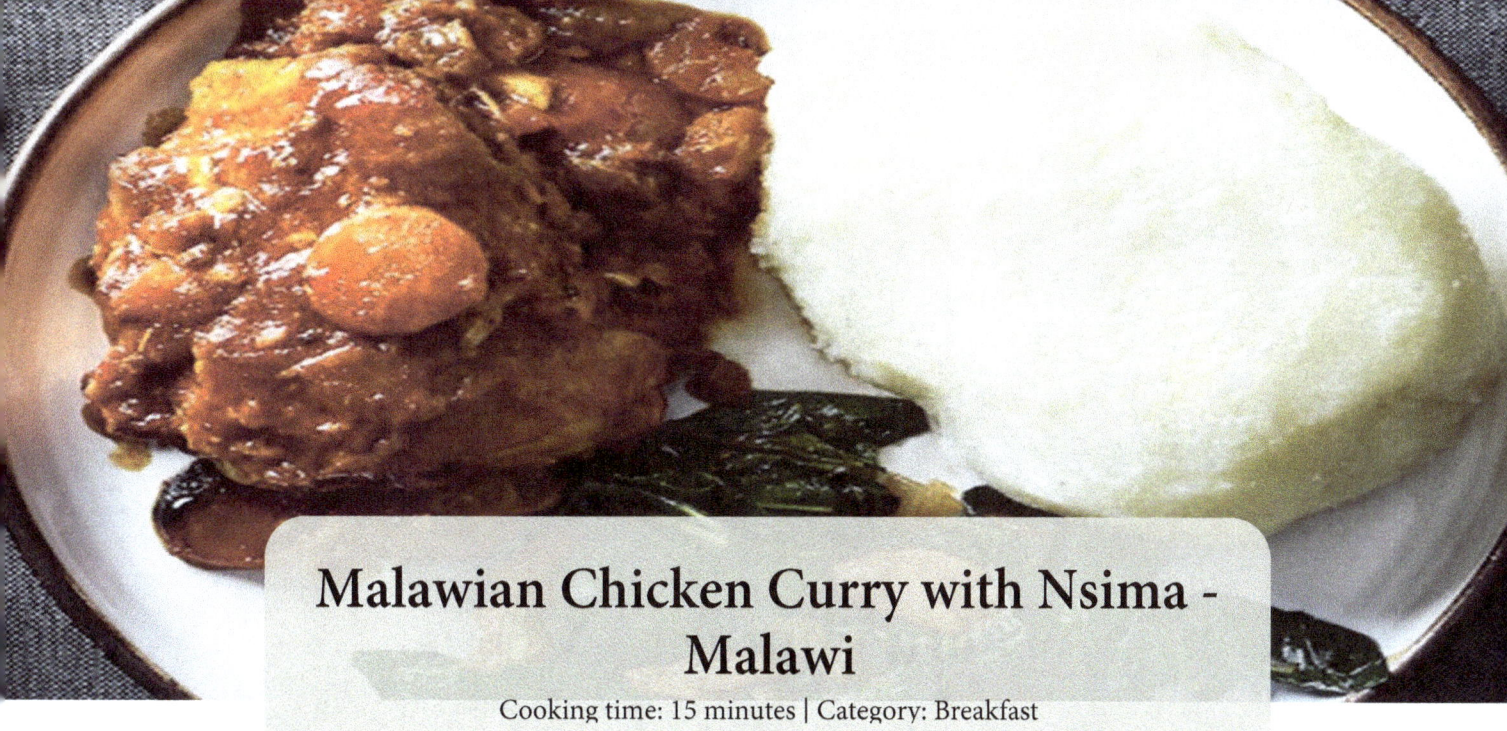

Malawian Chicken Curry with Nsima - Malawi

Cooking time: 15 minutes | Category: Breakfast

Nsima is a cornmeal made from corn flour as the starch that is deliciously paired with meat and or vegetable curry. It's better to combine both.

Ingredients

- 3 tablespoons vegetable oil, divided
- 2 medium white onions, sliced into 1/4-inch half-moons
- 3 celery stalks, sliced 1/4-inch thick
- 4 garlic cloves, minced
- Kosher salt, to taste
- Freshly ground black pepper, to taste
- 4 large carrots, sliced in 1/4-inch rounds
- 1 (12-ounce) can of tomato paste
- 1 (28-ounce) can of whole peeled tomatoes
- 1/2 cup white distilled vinegar
- 1 lemon, juiced
- 1/4 cup yellow curry powder
- 5 pounds bone-in, skin-on chicken pieces
- 1 pinch granulated sugar (optional)

Nsima

- 2 cups Ufa (fine-ground white cornmeal)
- 5 1/2 cups of water
- 2 tablespoons unsalted butter or margarine (optional)

Steps to Cook

1. Into a very large soup pot or Dutch oven, heat 2 tablespoons of the oil over medium heat. Add onions, celery, and garlic, and season with a pinch each of salt and pepper. Cook for 4 minutes, or until vegetables are translucent, stirring occasionally with a wooden spoon.
2. Add the 1 remaining tablespoon of oil and the carrots and tomato paste. Fry for about 1 to 2 minutes, then add the whole peeled tomatoes, using a wooden spoon to break them up in the pot to 1/2-inch pieces. Add vinegar, lemon juice, and curry powder together.
3. Add the chicken pieces and season generously with salt and pepper; stir together with the 'tomatoey' vegetables. Pour enough water into the pot to cover the chicken (you may need to add more as the stew reduces). Bring to a simmer, reduce heat to a low, and cover. It takes at least 1 to 1 1/2 hours for the chicken to become fully tender, but it can also stay on the stove all day. The longer it simmers, the stronger the flavors and the more tender the chicken will be.
4. Taste and season with more salt and pepper as needed, and a pinch of sugar. Serve over nsima or cooked rice.

Nsima

5. In a saucepan, heat the water until lukewarm. Slowly mix in the cornmeal while stirring, avoiding lumps. Bring to a boil while stirring continuously. Lower heat and let the porridge gently ripple for 2 minutes; the mixture should look like thin transparent porridge. Continue stirring until the mixture is smooth and cooked through.
6. If desired, butter or margarine can be added at this point. Nsima can be served in a dish or scooped onto a plate as patties. Accompany with meat, fish, or vegetables.

Note:

Although Lilongwe is the political capital of Malawi, it is not a place to keep tourists spellbound for long. There are beautiful sceneries featured in Blantyre, Mzuzu, and Zomba. Africa's warm beating heart is none other than Malawi for a reason. If you want to experience the whole of Africa, Malawi is more than enough to satiate that desire. Other than natural wonders, teeming wildlife, and picturesque highlands, Malawi's people are known to be the friendliest.

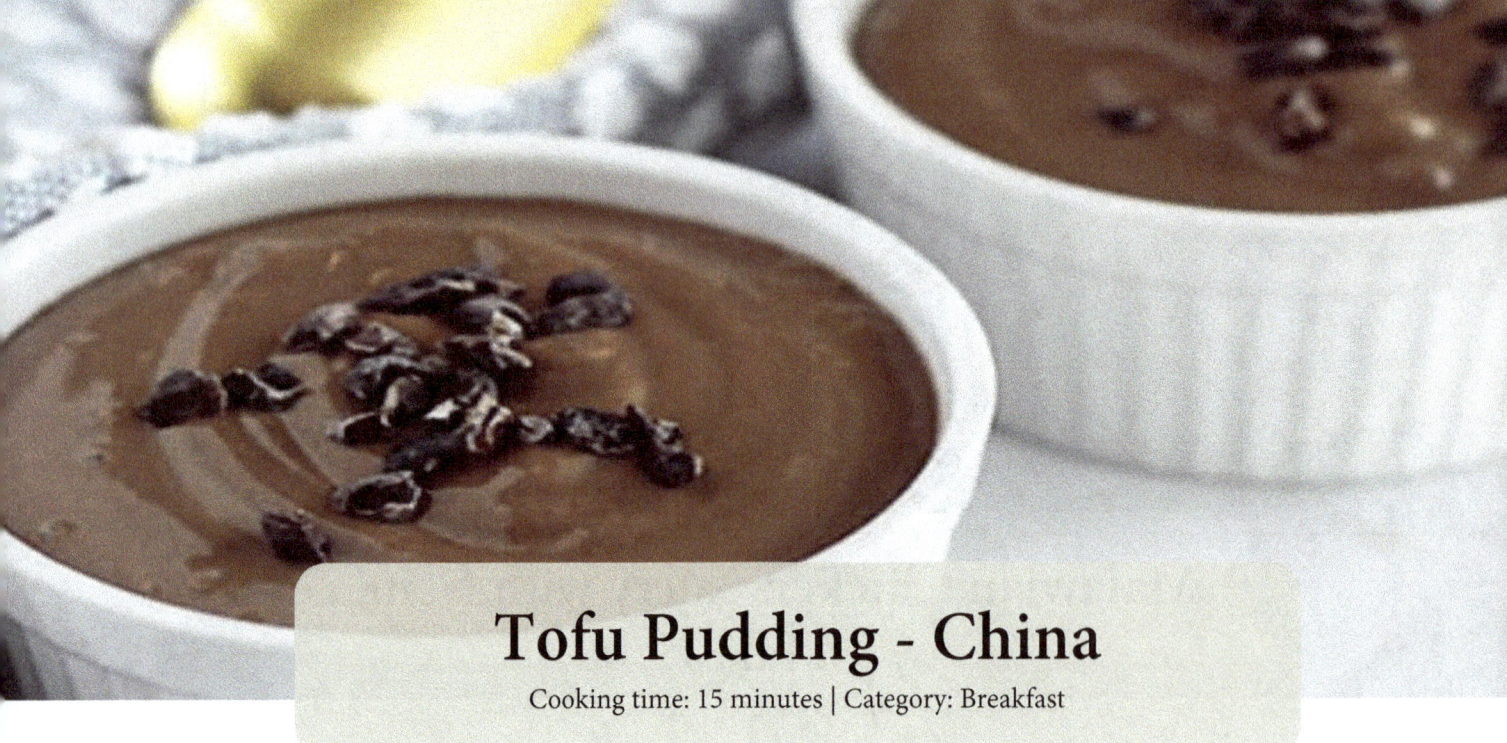

Tofu Pudding - China

Cooking time: 15 minutes | Category: Breakfast

Tofu pudding is a popular Chinese breakfast made with very soft tofu, which is made from raw beans.

Flavors of tofu pudding vary by region. In the north, people like to have salty tofu pudding with soy sauce or salt, or with meat.

However, in the south, people prefer the sweet version with ginger and brown sugar syrup.

Ingredients

- 6 ounces silken organic tofu
- ⅓ cup cacao power
- ¼ cup + 2 tablespoons maple syrup
- 1 tablespoon instant coffee
- 2 teaspoons vanilla extract

Steps to Cook

1. Add all the ingredients to a food processor and blend on high until the ingredients are combined and the texture resembles a smooth, creamy pudding.
2. Store in an airtight container in the fridge for up to four days. The pudding will get a little watery on top after the first day, but that's okay. Just mix before serving!

Note:

Each serving contains about 16 grams of protein.

On a visit to China. You will not want to miss the Chinese Tsingtao beer.

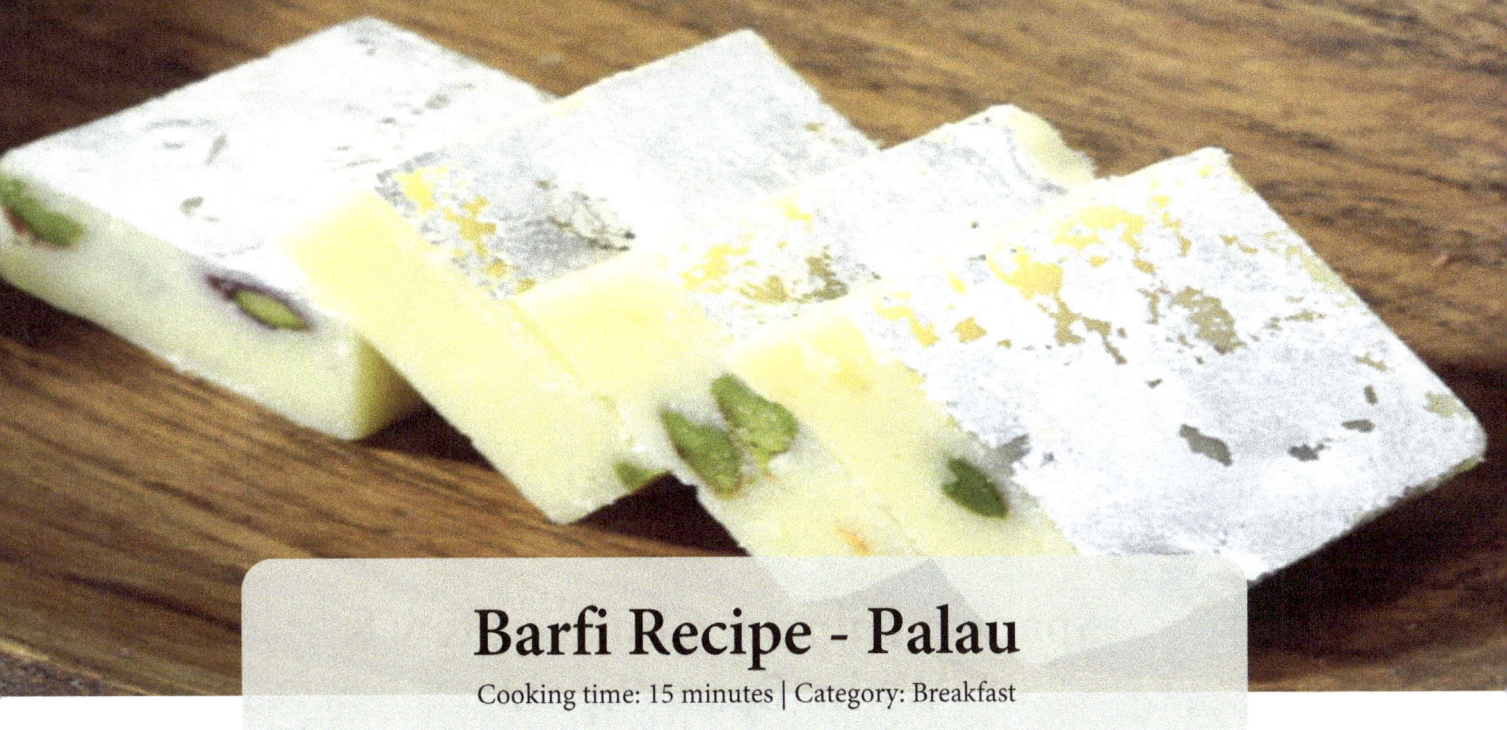

Barfi Recipe - Palau

Cooking time: 15 minutes | Category: Breakfast

This delicious Paluan lunch recipe has benefits for summer. It also promotes healing and builds immunity against diseases. More still, it is an amazing thickener for soups

Ingredients

- Palua 1/4 cup
- Milk 1litre
- Sugar 1/4 cup
- Cardamom powder 1/4tsp
- Black pepper powder a pinch
- Ghee, a little to grease the plate
- Tutti fruity for garnishing
- If you're craving for a sea adventure involving swimming with the fishes, diving under large coral reefs, and basking under the sun, then Palau is right up on your travel palate.
- This island is home to beautiful atolls, peaceful lagoons, and stunning sandbars.

Steps to Cook

1. Soak palua in water
2. After some time, it will set the bottom of the dish
3. Throw the water above and the dust particle that floats on top.
4. Again, add some water to this.
5. Repeat this cycle 2-3 times
6. Once u drain all water, you will get clean palua at the bottom.
7. Now boil milk.
8. Once boils well, add sugar.
9. Add palua and stir continuously.
10. It will become thick like custard.
11. Now add cardamom powder and black pepper powder to this.
12. Grease a plate and pour this onto the plate
13. Add tutti fruity on top.
14. Let it come to room temperature.
15. Refrigerate this
16. Cut desired shape and serve chilled.

Note:

Barfi squares can be enjoyed on the Ngardmau Falls with a soothing beverage from a Paluan local store. It has a calorie content of 190.

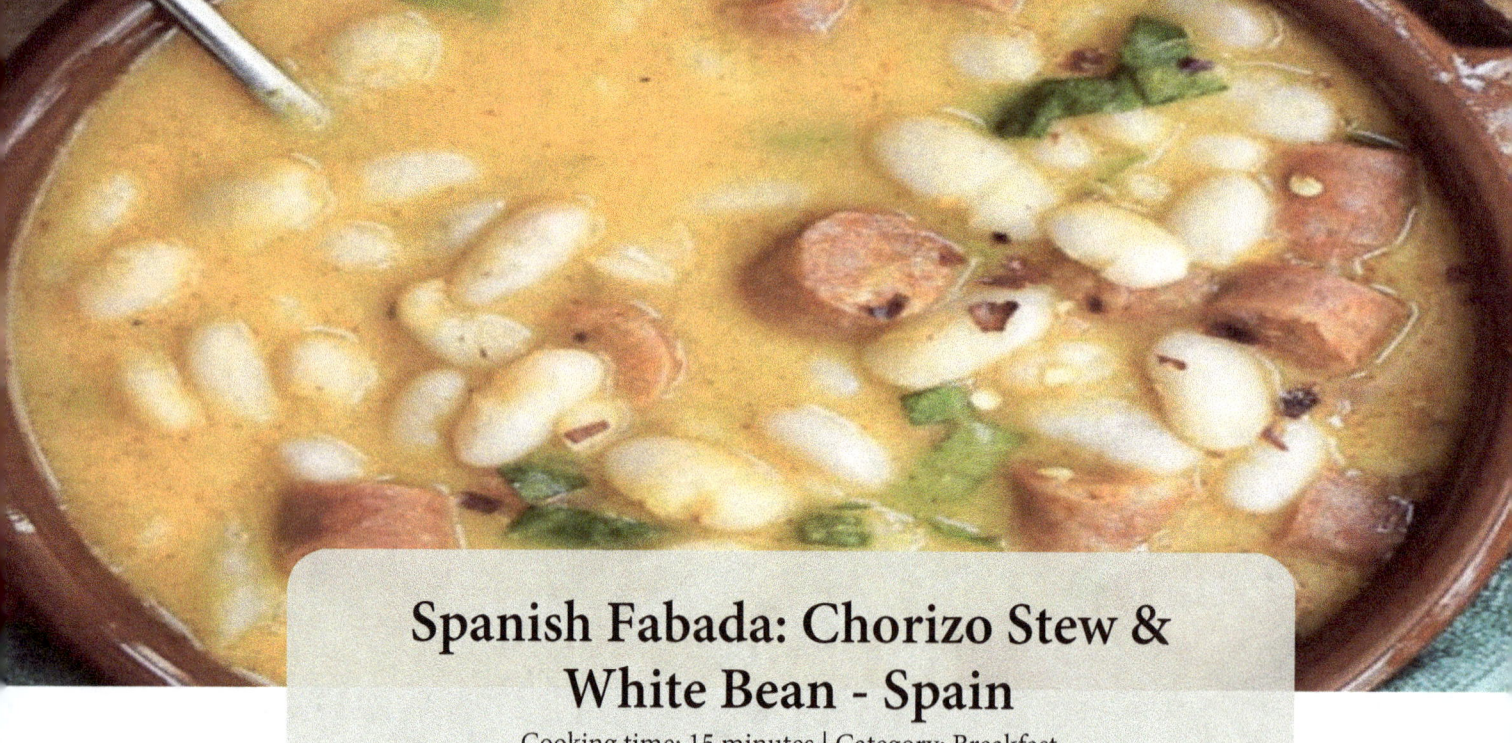

Spanish Fabada: Chorizo Stew & White Bean - Spain

Cooking time: 15 minutes | Category: Breakfast

Fabada astruiana is a rich, hearty Spanish-style stew that's perfect for cold winter months. This heavy dish of white beans, pork, chorizo, and saffron is typically served during the biggest meal of the day, which in Spain, is lunch. It can be presented as a starter but can certainly pass as a full meal. While fabada is typically cold-weather food, you can find it all over the country and in any season. You'll even see the canned version on the grocery store shelves; however, this shouldn't be your first choice!

Ingredients

- 400g 15oz of large white beans
- 1 small link of sweet semi-cured Spanish chorizo note: this is not completely raw chorizo. If that's all you can get, you'll have to sear it before using it. Also, it's only sweet, but rather made with sweet versus spicy paprika.
- 1 small link of spicy semi-cured Spanish chorizo
- 1 small link of Spanish semi-cured blood sausage morcilla
- 100 g 1/4 lb of cured pork belly (pancetta or tocino)
- 1 large carrot
- 1 small potato
- small onion
- 1 bay leaf
- 1 clove of garlic smashed (but not minced)
- 600 ml 2.5 cups of water (or ham stock if you have it!)
- Salt to taste

Steps to Cook

1. Peel and dice the onion, potato, and carrot.
2. If using completely fresh meats (ideally you can find the semi-cured ones they use in Spain), you'll have to see them on all sides.
3. If using the semi-cured meats, poke the sausages with a fork so that the casing doesn't burst once cooking.
4. Put the meats and vegetables into a large pot, along with the smashed garlic clove and bay leaf.
5. Cover the ingredients with water (or stock) and bring to a boil.
6. Lower the heat to a rapid simmer, and cook for about 15 minutes, until the vegetables are tender.
7. Drain and rinse the beans in a strainer and reserve (don't add yet).
8. Take out the meats and put them on a plate. Discard the garlic clove and bay leaf.
9. Blend the vegetables and broth to create a thick soup. Season with salt if necessary.
10. Cut up the meats into bite-sized chunks and add them back to the broth.
11. Add the beans and cook everything together over slow heat for about five minutes.

Note:

Calories: 509.72kcal To experience the true nativity of Spain, you need to visit Madrid's Parque del Buen Retiro (El Retiro Park) meaning "Park of the Pleasant Retreat" It's a majestic scenery.

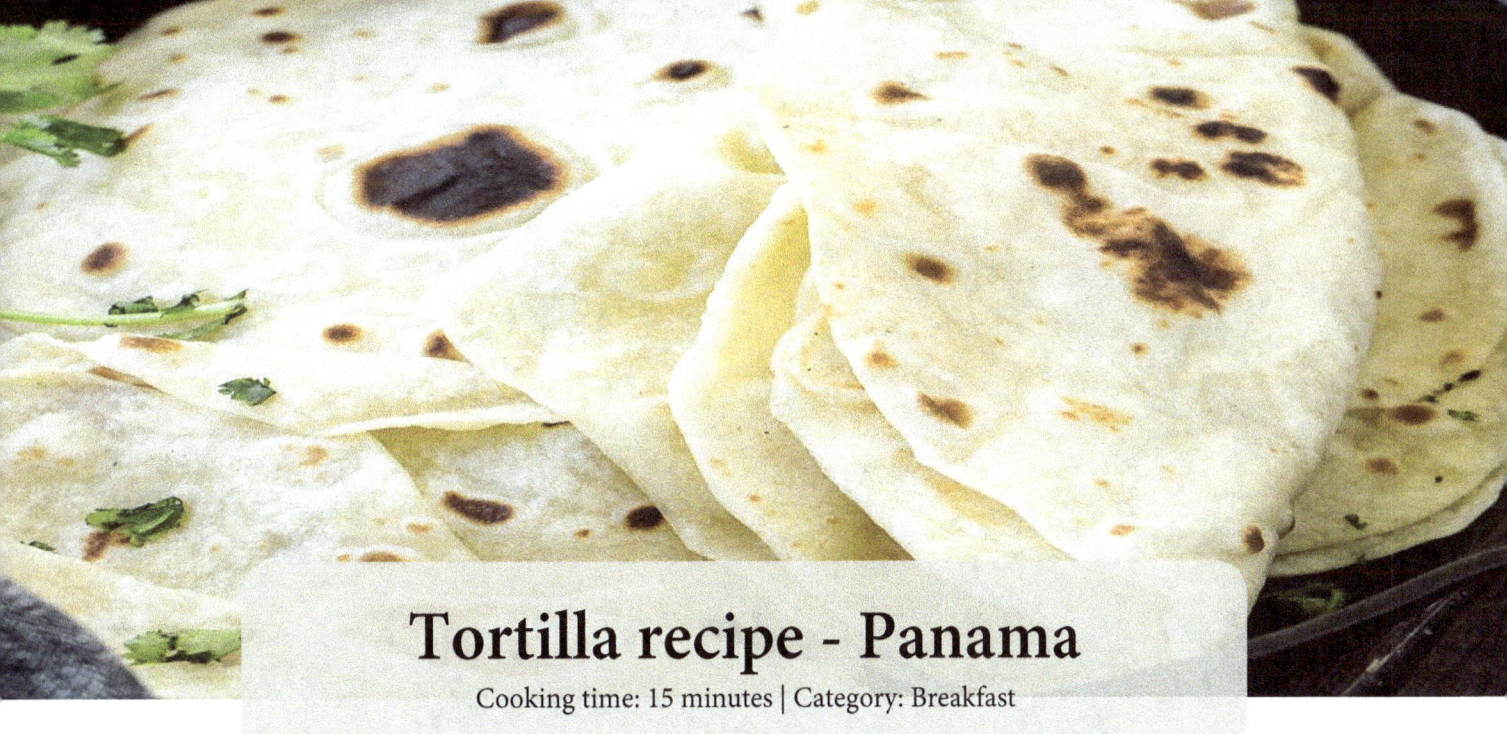

Tortilla recipe - Panama

Cooking time: 15 minutes | Category: Breakfast

Tortillas are roasted, circular corn meals ideal for breakfasts. Butter and white cheese (national cheese) can be used here, this is a delight.

It is super delicious, but many Panamanians seem to have ditched meaty breakfasts for health reasons.

Ingredients

- Cobs or corn (corn) or, hopped corn
- Salt to taste

Steps to Cook

1. Add the corn kernels to a boil until they are soft, then grind them (if you do not have the grinding machine, you can use a food processor) knead and add salt.
2. Taste that it is good, form the tortilla and ready, go you can fry or roast it.
3. To roast, use a pan, casserole, or pot, when it is very hot, add them, do not touch them and lower the temperature to the minimum, when they start to brown on the sides, you can take them off.

Note:

Each 100g serving contains 228 calories.

Your stay in Panama is certainly incomplete without sampling the scenery of the Miraflores Visitors' Center, in the man-made Panama Canal.

More still, the bus tours and day cruises around Panama Carey is the favorite spot you will want to indulge in.

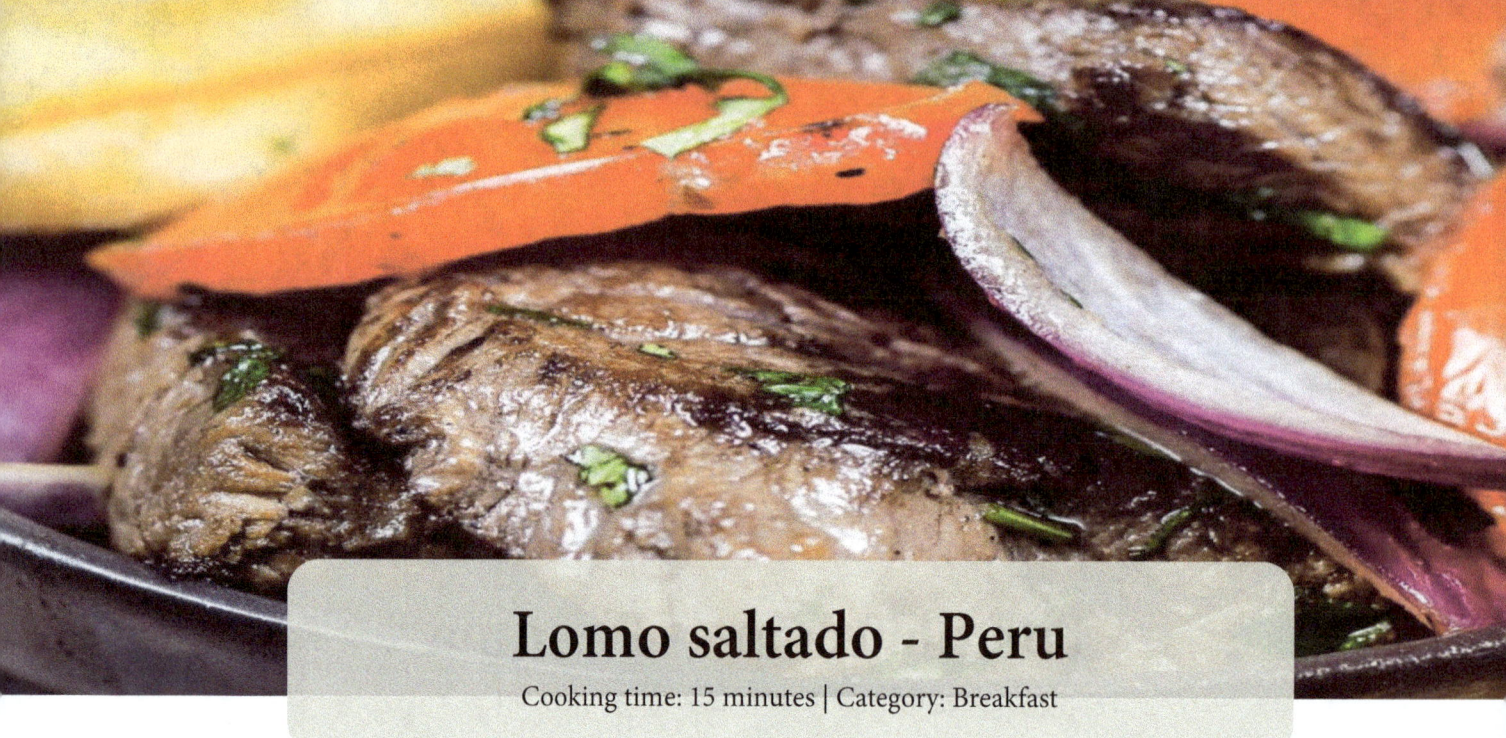

Lomo saltado - Peru

Cooking time: 15 minutes | Category: Breakfast

A well-known traditional chifa dish in Peru is Lomo saltado It is a delicious staple even in Latin America. The dish was first introduced to Peruvian eateries by the Chinese people. Later, the incorporation of beef stir-frying was introduced to Latin Americans. This Peruvian lunch recipe will satisfy completely, your lunch cravings in Peru. It can be comfortably paired with the Pisco Sour drink for a refreshing experience.

Ingredients

- 16 ounces frozen French fries
- 1 pound of sirloin steak
- 2 cloves garlic, thinly sliced
- 2 tablespoons soy sauce, divided into two portions
- 1 medium red or yellow onion
- 2 Roma or plum tomatoes
- 1 2-inch) section of ginger, grated
- 1 tablespoon white vinegar
- 1 tablespoon aji Amarillo paste (yellow hot peppers)
- 2 tablespoons vegetable oil
- Parsley or cilantro, chopped (for garnish)
- White rice, for serving (optional)

Steps to Cook

1. Add French fries to a sheet pan and bake according to the directions on the back of the package.
2. While the French fries are baking, slice the beef into thin slices. Then, place the beef into a medium-sized bowl and add the sliced garlic and one tablespoon of the soy sauce and set aside to marinate. Slice the onion into thick wedges and slice each tomato into eight wedges and remove the pulp and seeds.
3. Using a small bowl, whisk the remaining tablespoon of soy sauce, the vinegar, and aji Amarillo paste together and set aside.
4. Remove the French fries from the oven and set them aside.
5. Preheat a wok or non-stick skillet on your stove using medium heat. Next, add the oil, and once it shimmers, add the beef and cook for about two minutes until browned, stirring occasionally. Once the beef is browned on all sides, remove it from the wok and set it aside.
6. Add the onions to your wok and stir fry for about four or five minutes until soft. Then, add the grated ginger and stir fry for another minute or two.
7. Return the beef to the wok along with the tomatoes and stir-fry for two to three minutes until the tomatoes begin to break down, stirring frequently.
8. Add the soy sauce, vinegar, and aji Amarillo paste mixture to the wok and stir until combined. Next, add the French fries, stir and stir-fry for a minute or two to reheat them.
9. Serve on a plate with a formed cup of rice on the side and sprinkle everything with some of the chopped parsley or cilantro.

Note:

The current population of Peru is 33,611,307. The National Drink of Peru is called Peruvian Pisco Sour. It's a bunch of pleasantness you don't wish to forget in a hurry.

Week - 2

Reflections

- What things are you grateful for?

_____

_____

_____

- What new recipes did you try?

_____

_____

_____

- What was the taste & texture of the meal?

_____

_____

_____

- Did you add any changes to the recipes?

_____

_____

_____

- Did you make any new connections this week? _____ describe the connection?

_____

_____

_____

- What new fruit did you try this week?

_____

_____

_____

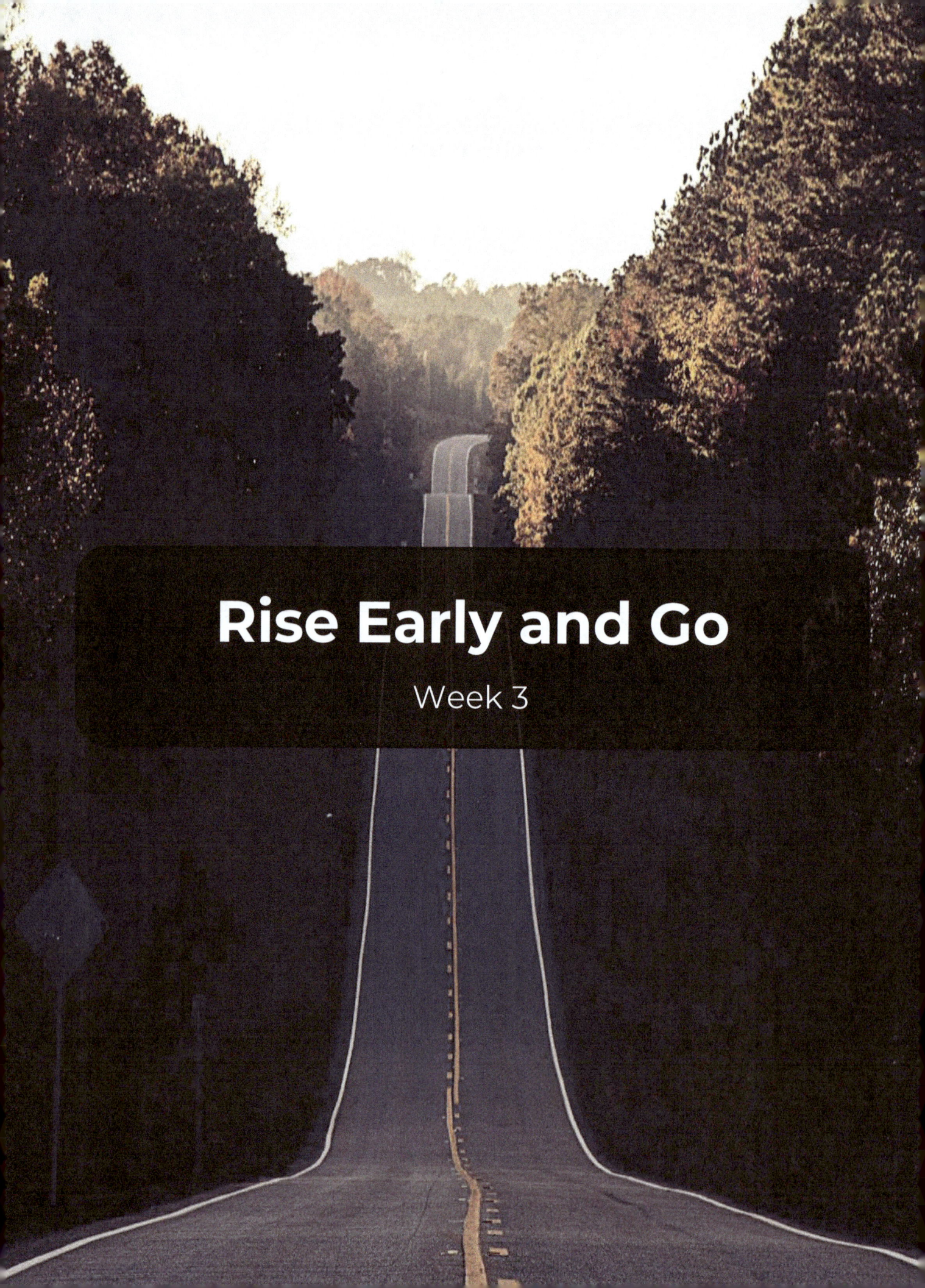

Week - 3

Take Obedient Action

- Spend 5 -10 minutes writing in your gratitude journal about giving thanks & Practice 5 minutes of meditation _____
- Select 1 Breakfast, 1 lunch & 1 Dinner recipe from week 3 & prepare them.

_____
_____
_____
_____
_____
_____

- Connect with 2 people from the 2 different countries in person or digitally.

_____
_____
_____
_____
_____
_____

- Select one new vegetable this week

_____
_____
_____
_____
_____

- Increase your cardio to 1.5 miles walk or run

_____
_____
_____
_____
_____

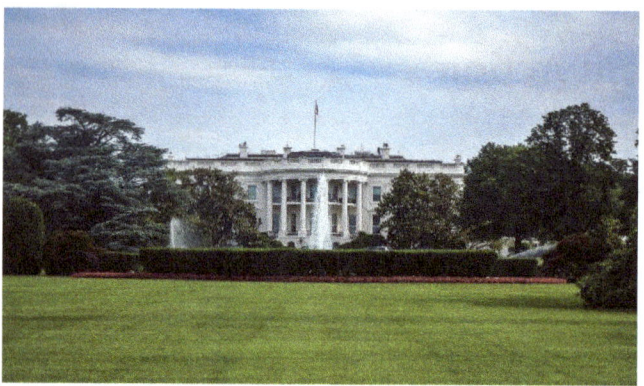

Washington DC-Dinner

It has been opined that this state capital of the United States is the only state to be named after a President.

The lush greenery of the Olympic Peninsula boasts an abundance of rainfall, making it a popular rainforest in the region.

Washington is home to the White House, and congress.

There seems to be a slight decrease in the population of residents in Washington (from 670,050 in 2021 to 657,185

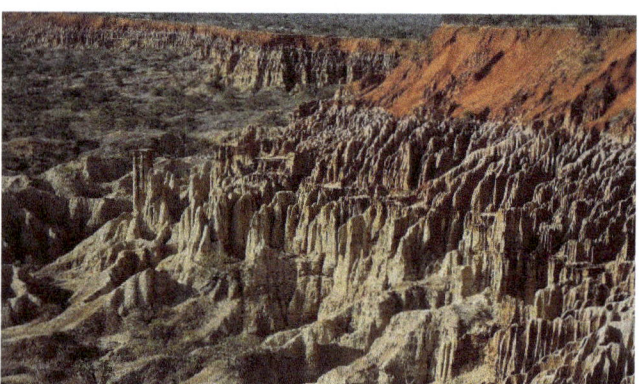

Angola-Lunch

Angola is a southwest African country with a population of over 32,000000 people. Luanda, its state capital is the center of commerce.

With the Kalandula waterfall, the semba dance and the high population of young residents therein, you are sure to have an experience of your lifetime.

Cassava is an essential staple in Angola. Your experience in Angola is incomplete without a feel of funje (a healthy staple). Coffee is a popular drink. Lunch is usually on-the-go and can include bread and cheese.

Chicken Muambaa is a household name in Central Africa and Angolans have admitted that it is their national dish. It is packed full of flavors of garlic, onions, and hot pepper. Angola is simply a land of adventure.

This part of Africa has been the center of civil war but it now quickly emerging as one of the top destinations on the continent.

You can find here one of Africa's largest and most magnificent waterfalls, the Kalandula Falls. Angola is also rich with wildlife and untouched parts of natural wonders.

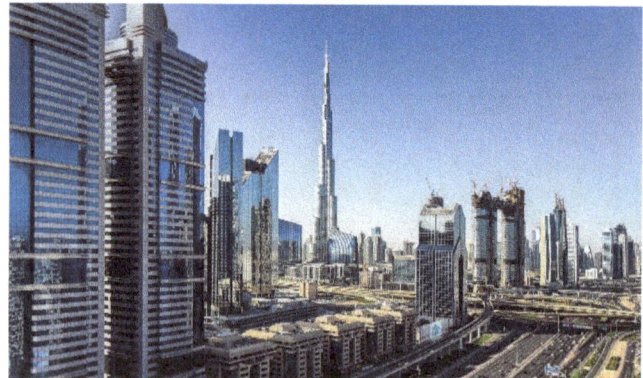

UAE-Lunch

The United Arab Emirates (UAE) is one of the easiest and most pleasant places to travel around and there are flights to UAE from all over the world.

The capital of UAE is called Abu Dhabi.

Indulge in some mouth-watering traditional drinks and food of UAE while visiting the country and satisfy your taste buds with these authentic and popular food items of UAE.

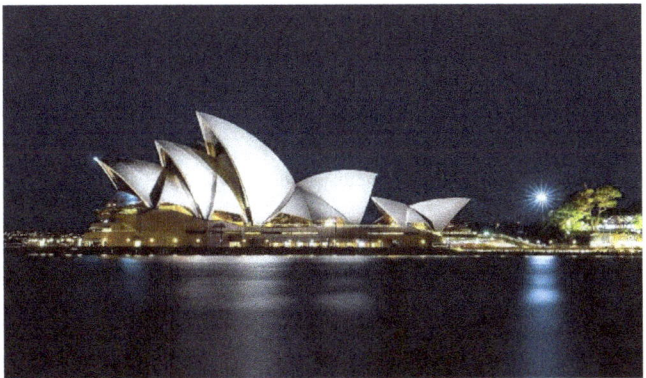

Australia-Dinner

Australia is the world's largest island and its smallest continent.

Australia's capital Canberra is slowly but surely growing into a lively and lovely place.

Affectionately (and at times derisively) nicknamed the 'bush capital',

The city lies amidst stunning nature reserves and low-lying mountain ranges in the north of the Australian Capital Territory.

Australia lies between the Pacific and Indian oceans.

It is the largest island and one of the largest countries in the world, boasting about 25,704,340 people.

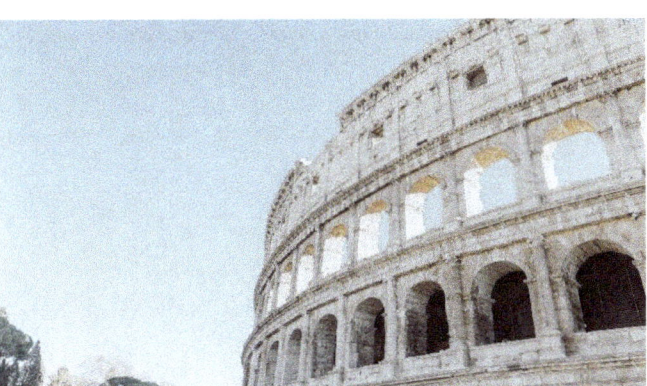

Italy-Breakfast

A favorite go-to place in Rome's capital city is called The Palatine Hill.

Rome, Florence, and Renaissance are perfect places for having a great vacation, in this European nation renowned for its western culture and cuisine.

Italy has an estimated population of over 60 million residents.

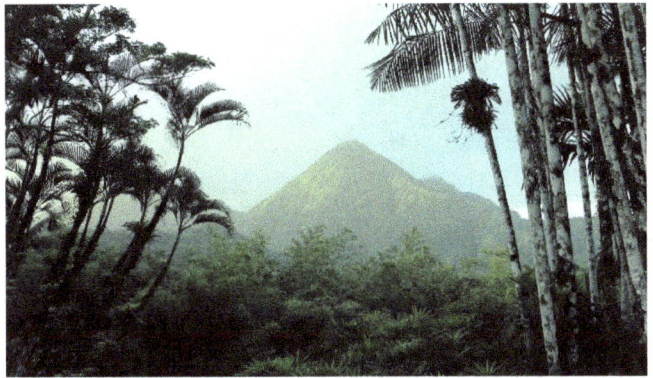

Martinique-Lunch

The Caribbean Island nation with a unique blend of French and West Indian influences. Martinique is located in North America. its capital is the sloppy Fort-de-France, with a population of 376036.

Martinican cuisine is a co-mix of African, French, Caribbean, and South Asian traditions. The recipes often reflect the complex history and varied cultural heritage of the island. Traditional dishes combine these global influences and use a range of local fruit, vegetables, fish, and meat as well as the famous piment antillais, which is hotter than any chili you have ever tried.

Colombo is an iconic Martinican dish and is a must-have to try while on your vacation. The curry-based delicacy is rooted in the island's strong Indian communities. For an excellent meal of chicken colombo, head to L'embarcadèreby the marina. It's one of the best spots on the island try the traditional meal with views of the water.

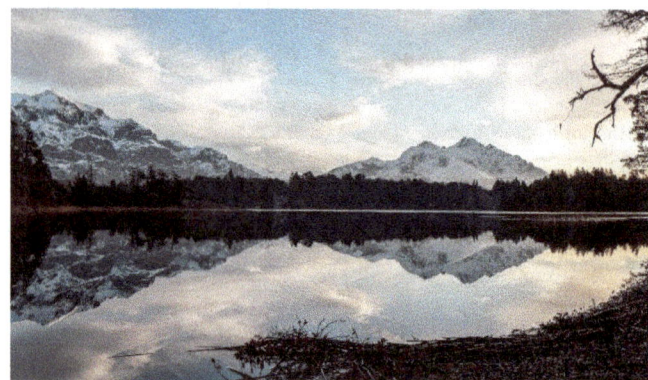

Argentina-Dinner

The world's eighth largest country.

Argentina's largest city and the capital city is Buenos Aires and borders around South America.

Argentina boasts of a teeming population of over 45,767,250 residents, with major cities as such Buenos Aires, Córdoba, Rosario, Mendoza, and Tucumán.

A taste of Argentina is a taste of palatable food and wine.

Its excellence in performing arts is a sure reason why it tops the charts amongst South American countries.

Looking forward to having dinner in Argentina? You don't want to miss vegetarian locro

Dubbed the Paris of South America, Argentina is a perfect blend of sophistication and rugged beauty.

Its culture is a blend of European and Latin America, making the cities culturally rich.

Snow-capped Andes mountains surrounding the expansive pampas (lowlands) rich in natural landscape, it is sure to take your breath away.

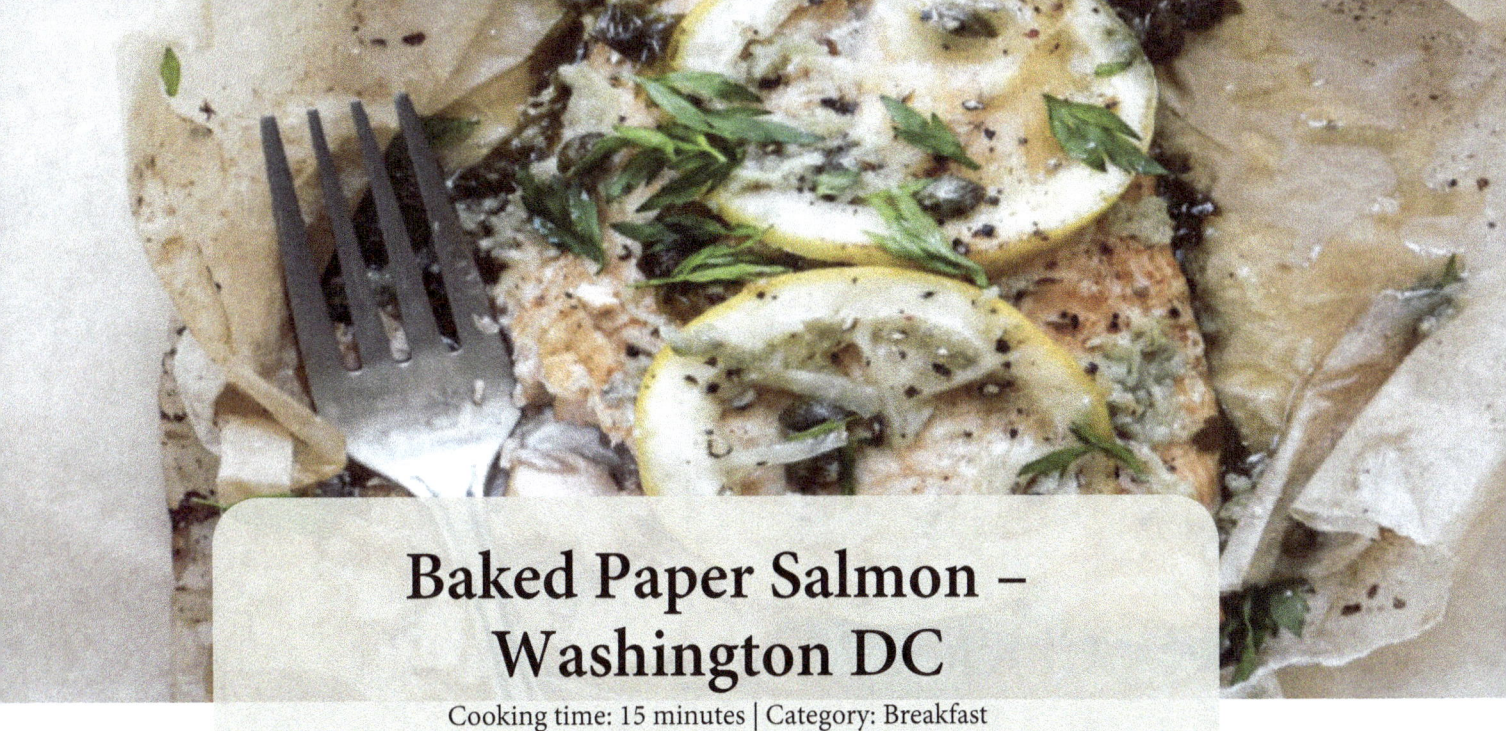

Baked Paper Salmon – Washington DC

Cooking time: 15 minutes | Category: Breakfast

A healthy protein-rich dish (29g of protein). This dish is served on paper with buttered potatoes to embrace the whole goodness therein.

Ingredients

- 141g of salmons or steaks
- 15mls of olive oil
- 30mls of frozen green peas
- 2 minced cloves of garlic
- 2 slices of lemon juice

Steps to Cook

1. Pre-heat the oven to 230oC.
2. Put each fillet on a large (12-inch) circle of parchment paper so that they are 1 inch from the center.
3. Cover each with a spoonful of peas, a clove of crushed garlic, a squeeze of lemon juice, and a drizzle of olive oil.
4. Fold the paper over into a packet and seal the edges by crimping and folding like a pasty. Place on a baking sheet.
5. Bake for 15 minutes in the preheated oven, or until it is fine to flake with a fork. To serve, place the packets onto serving plates and cut open the center in the shape of a cross.

Note:

Each serving of baked paper salmon contains 333 calories

The rich reservoir of Oysters can be attributed to the Chesapeake Bay. What's more? Washington DC is a sure bet for apple lovers. A feel of DC is a feel the DC's craft beer.

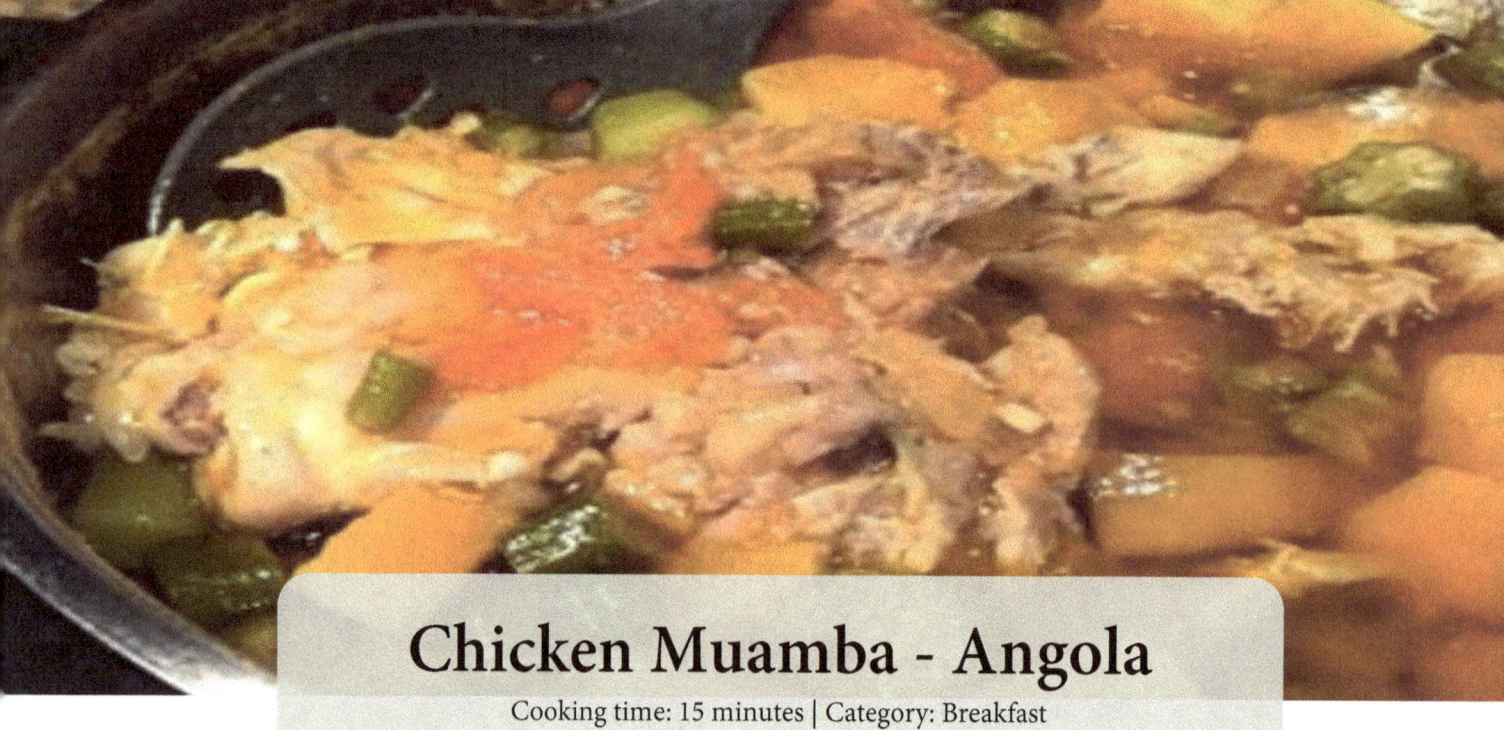

Chicken Muamba - Angola

Cooking time: 15 minutes | Category: Breakfast

Garlic, paprika and salt, and red oil are used to marinate the chicken. Then it is simmered with all the other ingredients until the chicken is thoroughly cooked and the flavors soak in. Okra could be added as a thickener, add it towards the end of the cooking for that crunchy taste. Butternut squash can be exchanged with pumpkin or sweet potatoes.

Ingredients

- 3 – 3 1/2-pound chicken cut into pieces
- ½ lemon Juice optional
- 1 teaspoon white pepper
- 1 teaspoon mince garlic
- ½ teaspoon dried thyme
- 1 teaspoon salt
- ½ teaspoon smoked paprika
- ½ teaspoon chicken bouillon powder
- ¼ cup canola oil
- ¼ cup palm oil & 4-5 garlic minced
- 2-3 onions sliced & 2 tomatoes diced
- 1 teaspoon white pepper
- 1 teaspoon smoked paprika
- Whole hot pepper pierced chili, Scotch bonnet
- ½-1 pound butternut squash cut into large cubes
- 18-20 Okra sliced in half
- 2 cups or more chicken broth or water
- Salt to taste

Steps to Cook

1. Place chicken in a large bowl or saucepan and rub with lemon juice.
2. Then add salt, garlic, thyme, white pepper, and chicken bouillon.
3. Mix chicken with a spoon or with hands until they are well coated, set aside.
4. When ready to cook, heat a large saucepan with palm and canola oil, and then add chicken, and brown both sides for about 4-5 minutes.
5. Add garlic, chili pepper, and smoked paprika, stir for about a minute then add onions and tomatoes, and for sauté 2-3 minutes until onions are translucent.
6. Add chicken stock, if necessary, to prevent any burns
7. Next add chicken stock or water (about 2 cups or enough to cover the chicken. Add chicken bouillotte on, and squash. Bring to a boil and let it simmer until the sauce thickens, it might take about 20 or more depending on the type of chicken used. Throw and n okra, continue cooking until desired texture is reached about 5 minutes or more
8. Adjust for salt, pepper, and stew consistency.
9. Serve warm with Cornmeal mash or rice.

Note:

Take a ride to Porto de Luanda to get a first-hand experience of the Angolan culture, visit the exotic Dala Waterfalls and settle for the Maiombe forest to finally immerse yourself in Angolan wildlife nature. If you are a natural drinks-enthusiast, you drool for Kissangua, an Angola non-alcoholic drink believed to have some healing importance.

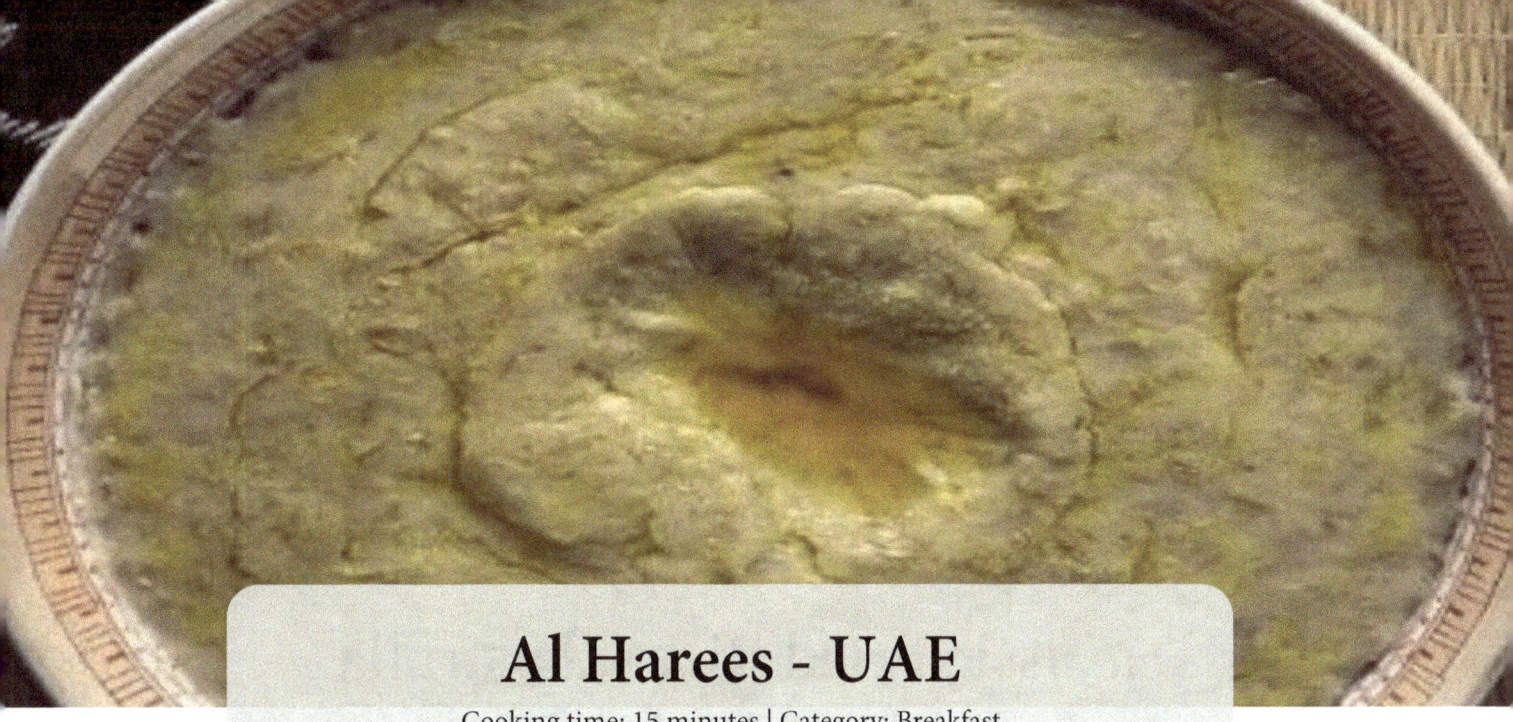

Al Harees - UAE

Cooking time: 15 minutes | Category: Breakfast

One of the most traditional dishes of the UAE, Al Harees is usually served during weddings and other religious festivals, especially during the month of Ramadan. This porridge-like dish is cooked with simple ingredients and takes a couple of hours to prepare. The usual method to make Al Harees is by mixing meat and wheat in a pot, along with water and salt, and then cooking for a long time. Another method of preparing it is by cooking wheat in slightly salted water for several hours, then adding meat and letting it cook for approximately four more hours. Even though the preparation time is slightly longer, the result is quite worth it.

Ingredients

- 475g harees (wheatberries)
- 1kg lamb
- 1 tsp black pepper powder
- 2-3 tsp salt
- 2-3 cinnamon sticks
- Water, for soaking the wheat
- Samen (local clarified butter) or melted butter or ghee

Steps to Cook

1. Soak the wheat overnight in plenty of water and then drain. In a large, heavy-bottomed pot (or special harees pot), place the wheat with the lamb, salt, pepper, and cinnamon sticks. Add enough hot water so that it is about 5cm above the wheat and meat mixture.
2. Place a damp cloth or aluminum foil over the pot and cover with a tight lid. Bring to a boil, reduce the heat and cook on a very low heat for 2-3 hrs, stirring occasionally to skim off the froth or fat from the surface.
3. Once the wheat is soft and most of the water has been absorbed, remove from heat and allow to cool (If all the water has been absorbed add about 1 cup of boiling water; if there is too much water but the wheat is cooked, ladle out the excess water).
4. Remove the bones of the lamb and shred any large pieces of meat. Mix the wheat and tender meat until it reaches a slightly elastic, paste-like consistency using a blender, adding a little salted boiling water to thin it down if required (a large wooden spoon is traditionally used for this). Check the seasoning and add more if desired. Transfer to a serving dish or tray.
5. Place the samen in a pan and gently warm until it melts. Pour the melted butter over the harees and serve hot.

Note:

Enjoy sun, sand, and surf at Al Bateen Beach and Qurm Beach. Arabic Coffee is one beverage you must try in Abu Dhabi.

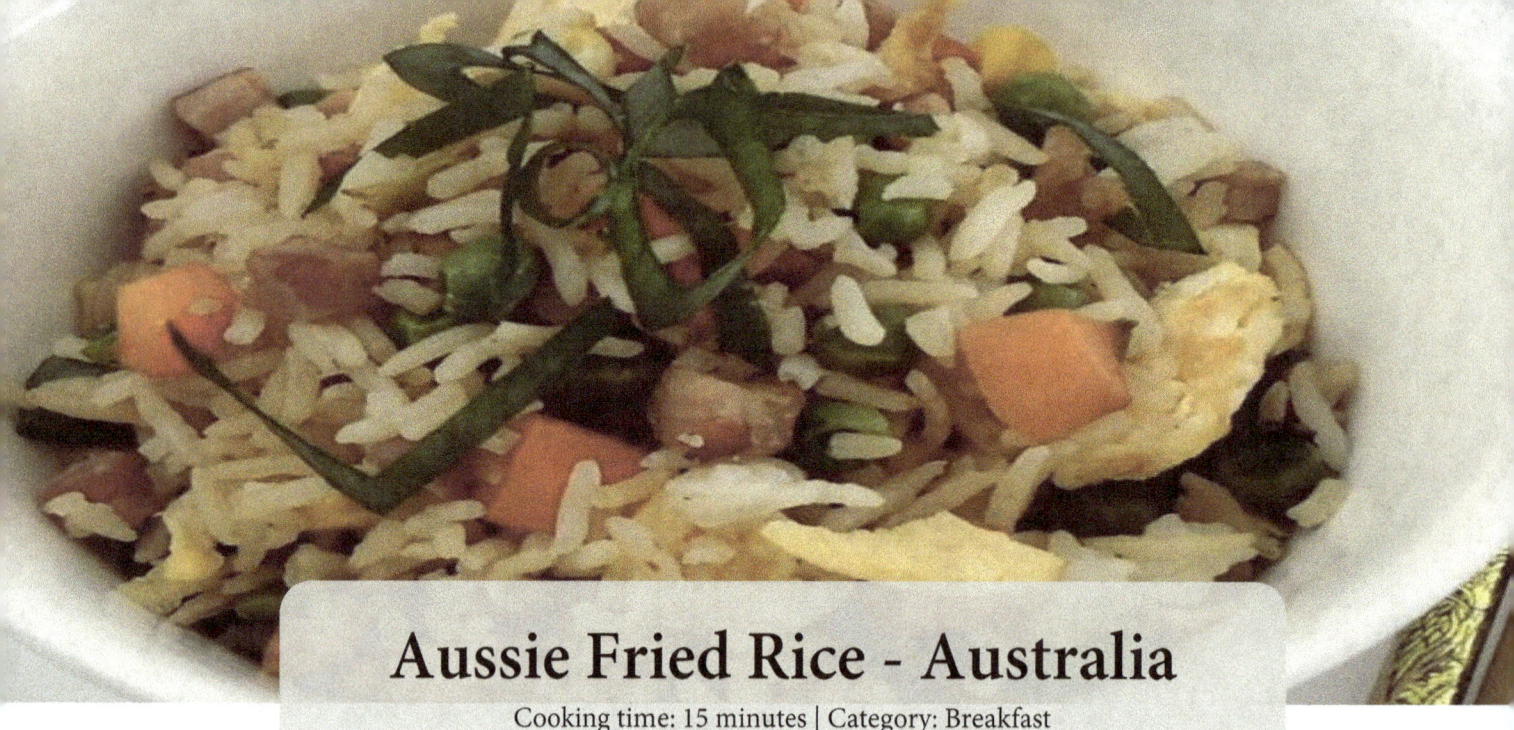

Aussie Fried Rice - Australia

Cooking time: 15 minutes | Category: Breakfast

A very tasty homemade fried rice, that will perfectly satisfy your lunch cravings in Australia

Ingredients

- 400g long-grain white rice
- 3 eggs lightly beaten
- 3 celery sticks finely chopped
- 1 red capsicum finely chopped
- 8 spring onions finely chopped
- 4 bacon rashers diced
- 300g cooked pork
- 300g cooked chicken
- 300g cooked prawns
- 2 tbs oil
- 2 tsp soy sauce
- 1 pinch of salt and pepper to taste

Steps to Cook

1. Cook rice in boiling, salted water for 10-12 minutes. Do not overcook. Drain well and rinse under cold running water.
2. Spread rice evenly over 2 shallow trays to dry out completely overnight.
3. Beat eggs lightly with a fork. Season with salt and pepper.
4. Heat 1 tablespoon of oil in a pan and pour in the egg mixture. Remove from pan and slice into thin strips then dice.
5. Heat the remaining oil in a pan or wok and fry the bacon until crispy.
6. Add celery and capsicum, and fry together.
7. Add rice and stir for 5 minutes.
8. Add meat, egg, spring onions, and prawns. Mix lightly.
9. When completely heated through, add soy sauce, salt, and pepper. Mix well.

Note:

Catch the excitement at the pinnacles or the Karijini National Park or the Bryon Bay. Cable Beach is one of the most beautiful beaches in Australia. More active holidaymakers can visit the fantastic rock formations at the Entrance point and the red cliffs and dinosaur footprints at Gantheaume point; both of which lie nearby. Melbourne is Australia's second most populated city

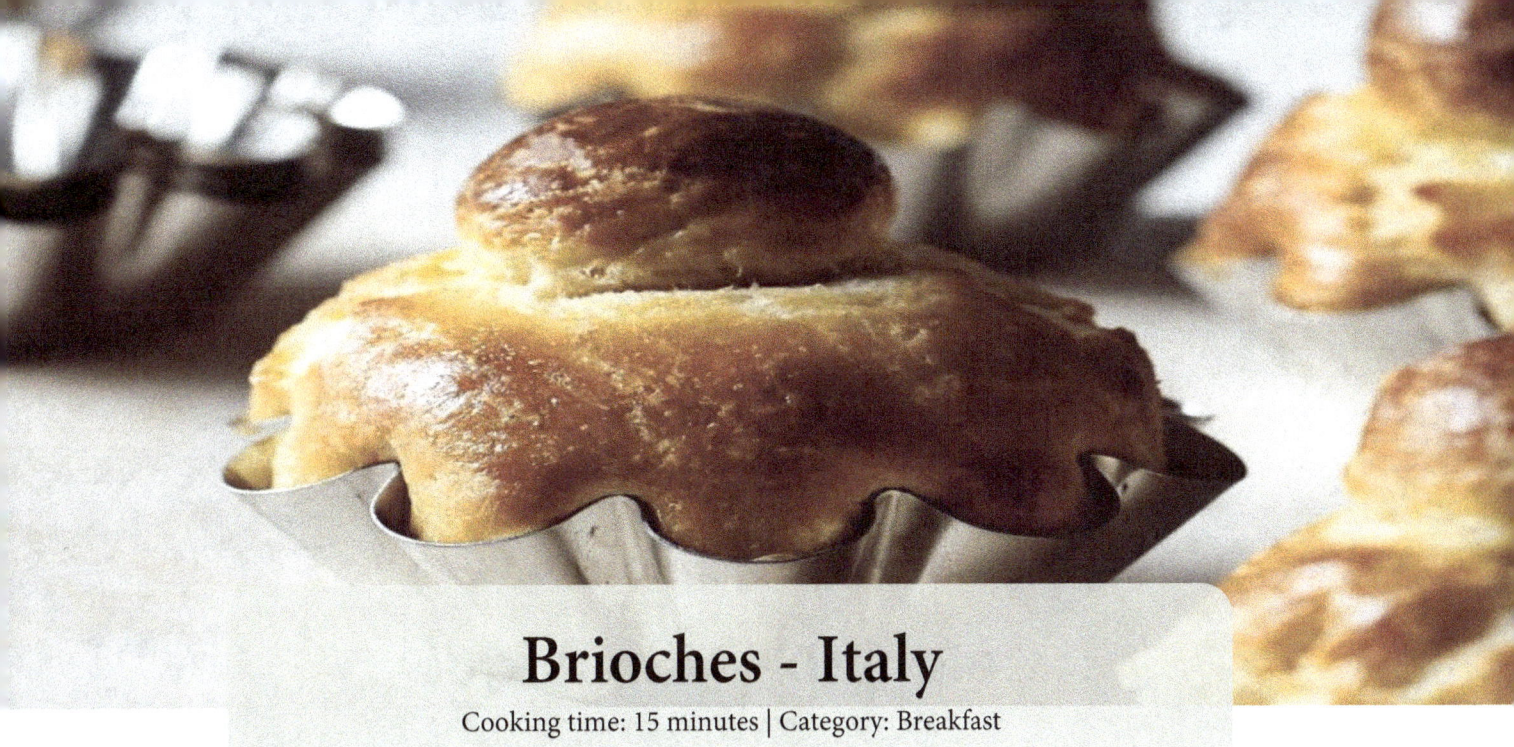

Brioches - Italy

Cooking time: 15 minutes | Category: Breakfast

Brioches are an Italian pastry made of sweet dough. They are found in Italian pastry shops and cafes usually served with coffee. There are many ways to eat brioche, but they are filled with vanilla cream, jam, or almond paste.

Ingredients

- 450g strong white flour
- 2 tsp fine sea salt
- 50g caster sugar
- 7g dried active yeast
- 100ml whole milk
- 4 eggs at room temperature, beaten, plus 1 for egg wash
- 190g salted butter, cubed and softened

Steps to Cook

1. Put the flour in a bowl of a stand mixer with a dough hook. Add the salt to one side and sugar to the other. Pour in the yeast to the side with the sugar. Mix each side into the flour with your hands, then mix it all with the dough hook.
2. Heat the milk until warm to the touch, but not hot. Mix into the flour mixture until combined. With the dough hook on medium, gradually add the eggs and mix for 10 mins.
3. Gradually add the softened butter, one or two cubes at a time, until combined. This will take 5-8 mins. Scrape down the sides, the dough will be very soft.
4. Scrape the dough into a large bowl, cover with a tea towel and leave for 1 hr 30 mins-2 hrs until doubled in size and well-risen. Once risen, put in the fridge for 1 hr.
5. Line the bottom and sides of a 900g loaf tin with baking parchment. Portion the dough into seven equal pieces (the easiest way to do this accurately is to weigh it). Lightly dust a work surface with flour, take a piece of dough and pull each corner into the middle to form a circular shape. With a bit of pressure, push down and roll into the ball. Repeat with the six remaining pieces.
6. Put the balls into the tin, four on one side and three in the gaps on the other side. Cover with a tea towel and leave to prove for 30-35 mins until almost doubled in size. Heat the oven to 180C/160C fan/gas
7. Lightly brush the dough with the egg wash and bake for 30-35 mins until golden and risen. Leave to cool in the tin for 20 mins, then remove and cool completely.

Note:

A 45g serving of yummy brioches contains 240 calories. Brioches pair well with cuppa cappuccino or coffee as a beverage.Biscotti is a healthy choice for whoever prefers it crunchy or nutty. Do well to stop by the Vatican City to pray if you would!

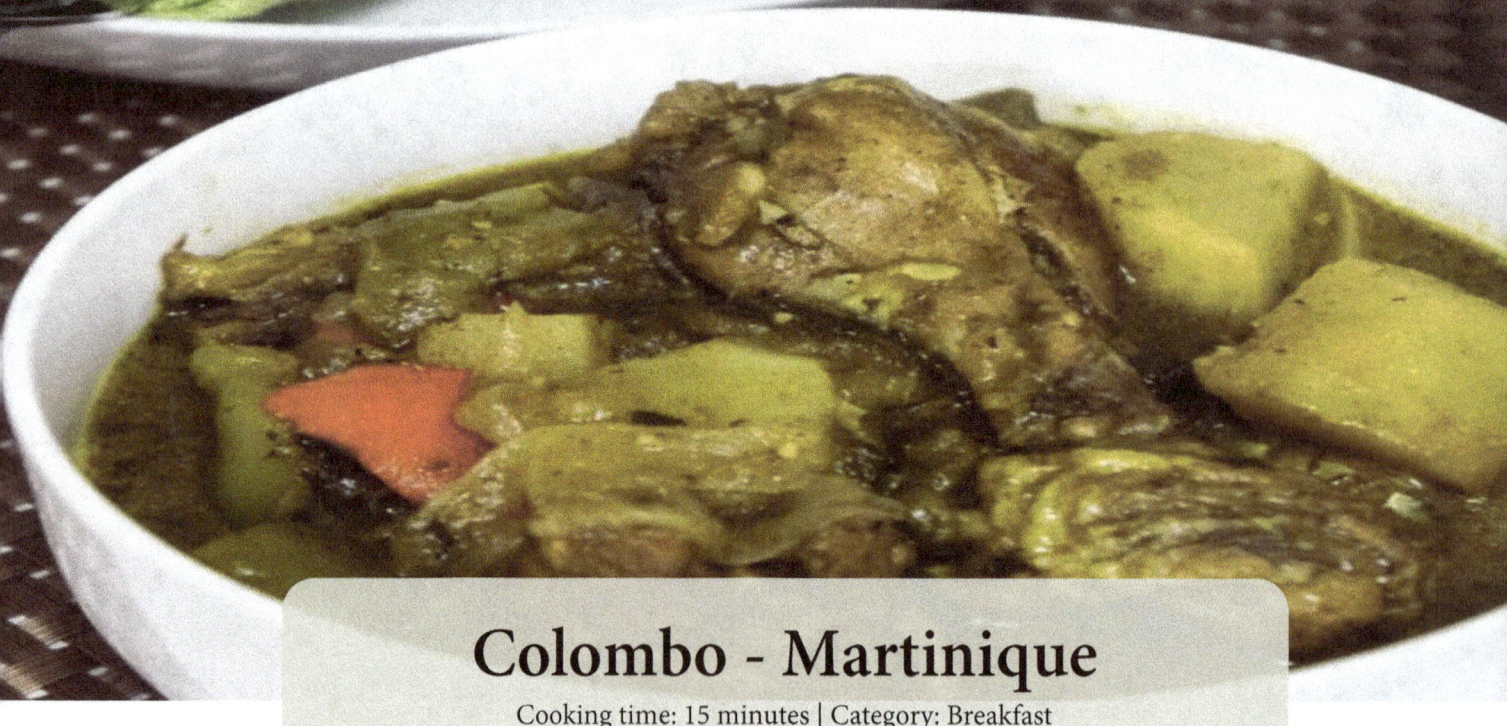

Colombo - Martinique

Cooking time: 15 minutes | Category: Breakfast

This dish is a taste of the Caribbean! It can be made with different meats, with chicken, pork, or lamb Colombo being the most common. The meat is typically served with rice, stewed beans, lentils, plantains, and vegetables in a curry sauce.

Ingredients

- 4 boneless skinless chicken breasts & Juice of 1 1/2 limes about 2 oz.
- 3 garlic cloves peeled & a pinch of crushed dried red chili peppers
- 1 1/2 medium onions peeled
- a few sprigs of thyme leaves stripped
- 3 tablespoons chopped parsley
- 4 tablespoons extra virgin olive oil
- 8 tablespoons colombo spice blend, divided see recipe below
- 1-1/2 cups water & 1- 14 oz. can of coconut milk
- 3-4 medium zucchini & salt and white pepper

Steps to Cook

1. Put the chicken breasts in a large glass dish just large enough to hold the chicken in a single layer. Sprinkle with half of the lime juice. Mince one garlic clove and sprinkle over the chicken. Slice half of an onion into thin slivers and distribute evenly over chicken. Add thyme leaves, 2 tablespoons of parsley, a crushed dried chili pepper, add drizzle tablespoon of extra virgin olive oil. Season with salt and pepper. Turn the chicken breasts to coat them and refrigerate for 2 hours.
2. Cut the whole onion into thin wedges. In a large sauté pan, that will hold the chicken breasts in a single layer, heat 3 tablespoons of extra virgin olive oil. Add the onion wedges and sauté for about 5- 8 minutes over medium heat. Add 5 tablespoons of the colombon spice blend and two minced garlic cloves and sauté for another 1-2 minutes.
3. Add the chicken breasts in a single layer and the marinade from the chicken. Stir 3 tablespoons of colombo spice blend into 1-1/2 cups of water and pour into a sauté pan with chicken. Add the 14 oz. can of coconut milk and stir to mix. Bring to a boil and then lower heat and simmer covered for about 15 minutes.
4. Cut the zucchini into 1-1/2-inch pieces and add to the sauté pan. Make sure they are immersed in the liquid. Simmer covered for another 30 minutes or until chicken is cooked through.
5. Serve with rice and garnish with parsley and remaining lime juice.

Note:

The calories per serving of Colombo dish is 300 calories

A taste of Martinique is a taste of Ti Punch; a traditional Martinican drink that is an inherent part of the cultural and historical landscape. Ti punch drink blends well with chicken Colombo. There are eye-popping gardens and beautiful scenery that will keep a tourist spellbound. The sloppy scenery and beaches are must-go spots to have a taste of Martinique Rich in biodiversity and full of unspoiled beaches, Martinique is every nature-lovers dream. You got the idyllic coastline, sprawling rainforests, well-tended botanical garden and the majestic Mont Pelee as the backdrop.

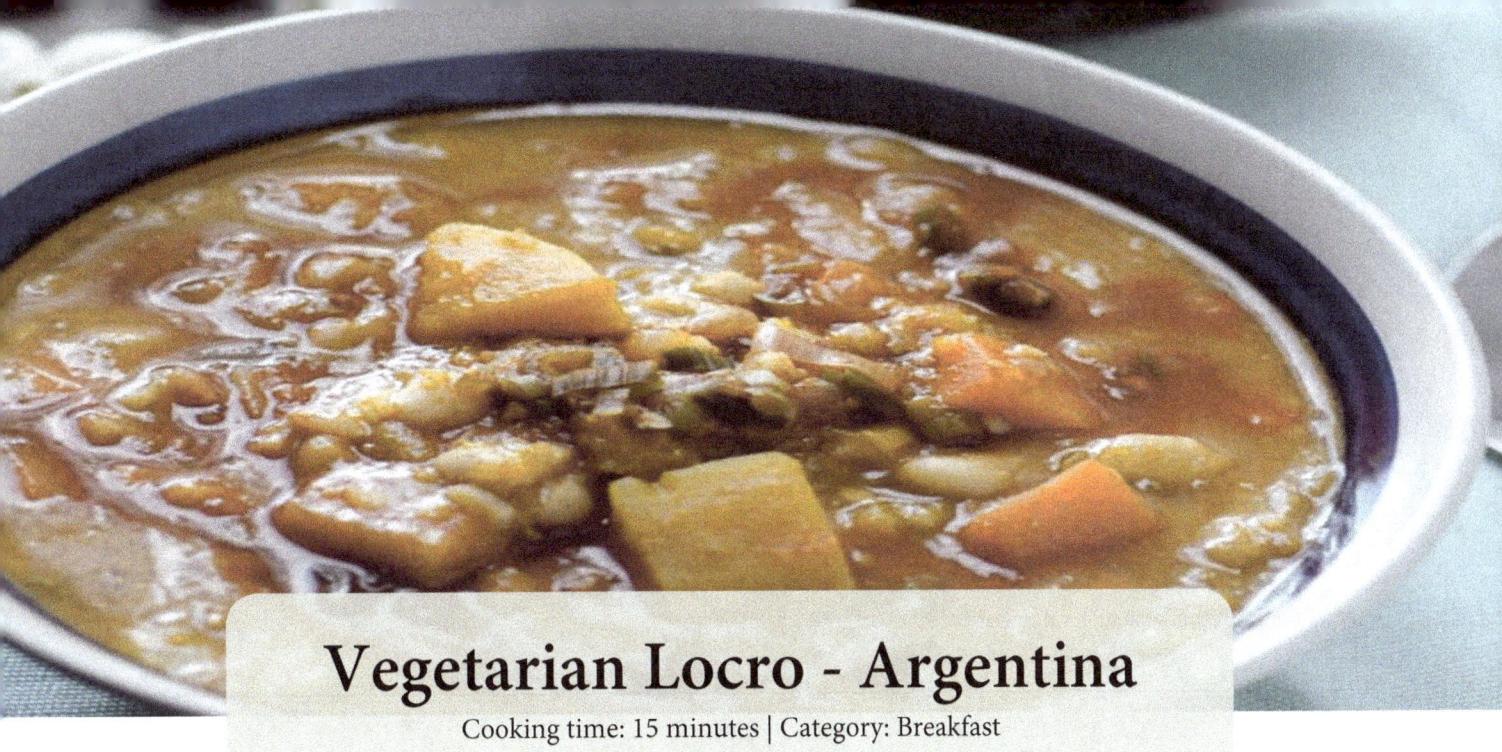

Vegetarian Locro - Argentina

Cooking time: 15 minutes | Category: Breakfast

A sweet blend of veggies, cooked beans, and then corn. It's delicious, yet very healthy. To make a sumptuous stew for locro, carrots and potatoes should be added.

Ingredients

- 1 Onion
- 2 Leeks
- 2 Garlic cloves
- 1 green Bell Pepper
- 1 red Bell Pepper
- 1 cup of cooked Beans
- 1 Butternut Squash
- 2 Yams
- 2 Corns on the cob
- 1 jar of Tomato sauce
- 1 bunch of Green Onion
- 1 tbsp. Cayenne Pepper
- 1 tsp. Paprika
- Salt and pepper
- Water

Steps to Cook

1. Chop the vegetables.
2. Sauté the onion, the leeks, the green, and red pepper, add the tomato sauce and cook for a few minutes.
3. Cut squash and yams into cubes. Add the yams and the squash to the stew.
4. When the vegetables are tender, add the corn kernels and season with salt, pepper, and paprika.
5. Add cooked beans.
6. Let it boil and stir now and then. Add water if necessary.
7. To make the hot sauce, quickly sauté the sliced green onion in olive oil.
8. Add paprika and cayenne pepper.
9. Finish stew with hot sauce

Note:

The vegetarian locrodish contains 107 calories per 100g serving

Your stay is incomplete in Argentina with visiting the Perito Moreno located in Los Glaciares National Park. Glacier is one of the most important attractions in all of Argentina's Patagonia. Recommended healthy rum for your relaxation is chilled corn ulpada or mate.

Week - 3

Reflections

- On a scale of 1-10 how was your practice of meditation?

_____
_____
_____

- What things are you grateful for this week?

_____
_____
_____

- What new recipes did you try?

_____
_____
_____

- What people & countries did you connect with this week?

_____
_____
_____

- What new Vegetable did you try this week?

_____
_____
_____

- What are you observing about yourself?

_____
_____
_____

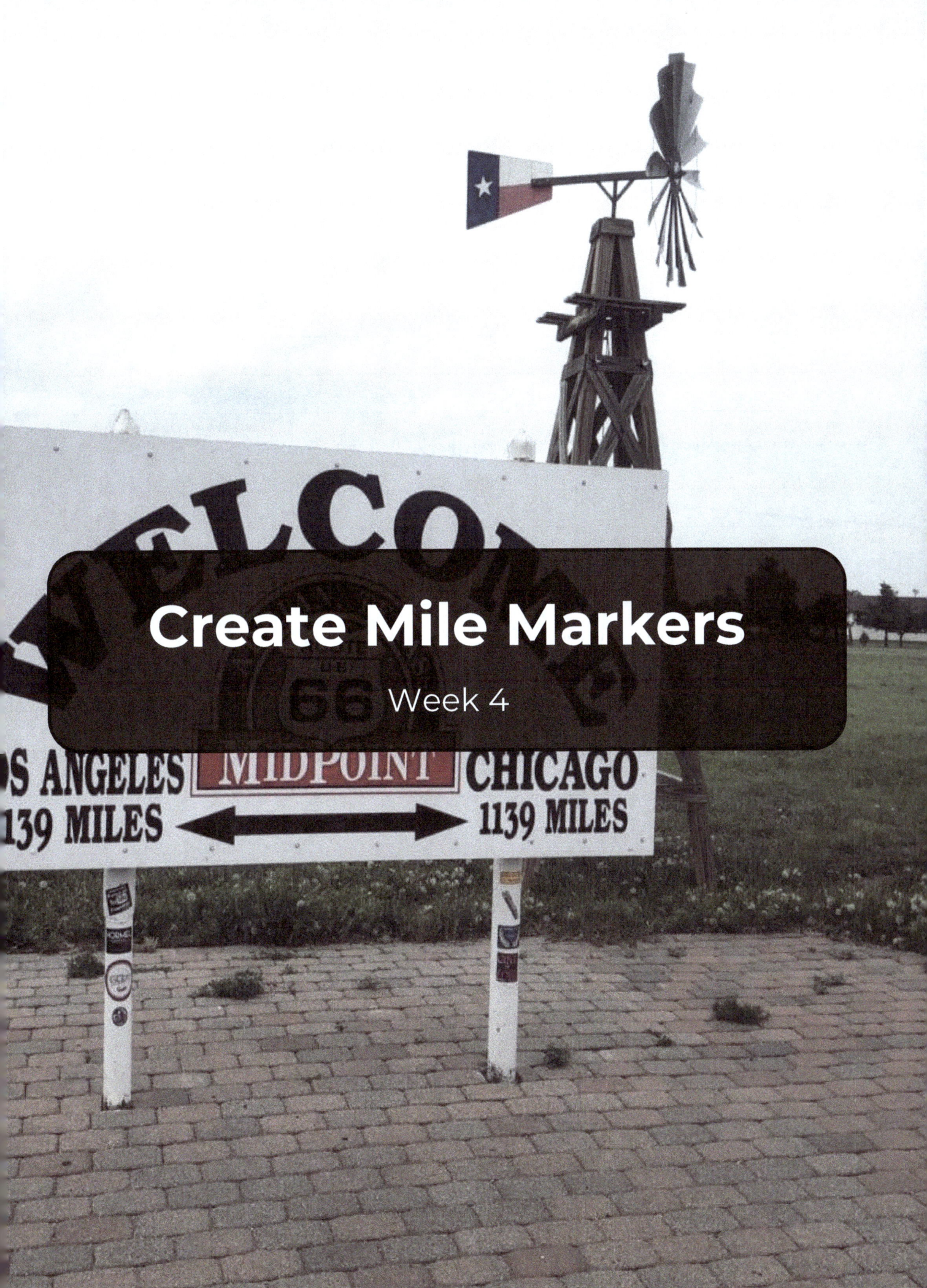

Create Mile Markers

Week 4

Week - 4

Take Obedient Action

- Spend 5 -10 minutes writing in your journal about gratitude & Practice 5 minutes of meditation_____
- Select 2 lunch recipes from week 4 & prepare them.

_____
_____
_____
_____

- Connect with 4 people from 4 different countries digitally or in person

_____
_____
_____
_____

- Share a meal with someone from one of the countries

_____
_____
_____
_____

- Visit a new supermarket this week

_____
_____
_____
_____

- Increase your cardio to 1.5 miles of walking or running add 10 minutes of stretching

_____
_____
_____

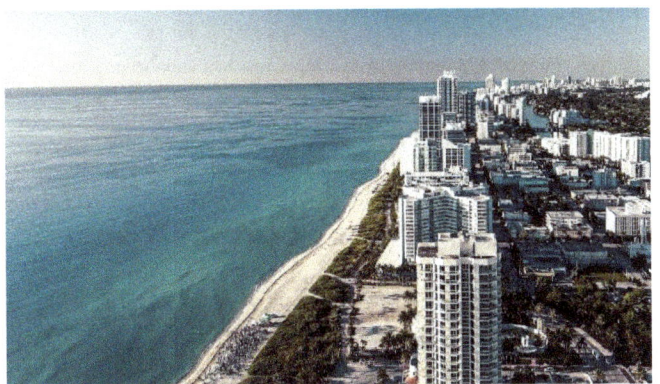

Miami-Breakfast

Would you ever visit Miami without catching the excitement ae Miami Beach?

This official capital of Florida boasts of white-sand beaches, Cuban coffee, exotic cuisine, and more. My favorite go-to places are Zoo Miami, Bayside Marketplace, Little Havana, and Ocean Drive.

Miami is in south-eastern Florida, United States, with Latin-American influences. Its current population of residents is 2,721,110.

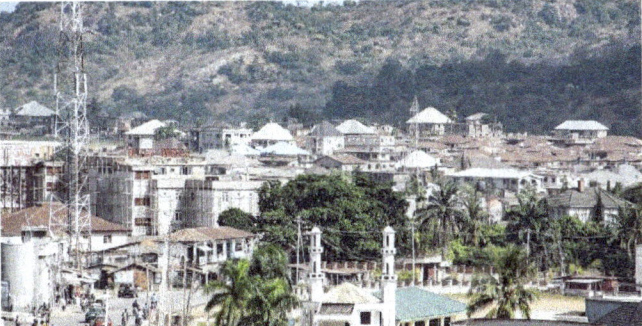

Nigeria-Lunch

Popularly known as The Giant of Africa with a current population of 213,257,126 residents, and Abuja, as its capital city.

The are many sites of attraction such as Erin-Ijesha Waterfalls, Ikogosi warm springs, Yankari game reserve, Obuducattle ranch, and many more to satisfy your viewing pleasure.

Nigeria has one of the best cuisines in the world, which comprises dishes or food items obtained from the numerous ethnic group that makes up the country.

Nigerian cuisine like those of other West African countries such as Ghana and the Benin Republic contains spices and herbs alongside palm or groundnut oil to produce deeply flavored sauces and soups with an enticing aroma.

Healthy Jollof rice is a population dish found on many Nigerian tables.

It can be beautifully paired with pork, chicken, or goat meat. Vegetable salads or coleslaw is perfect vegan dressings to suit this dish.

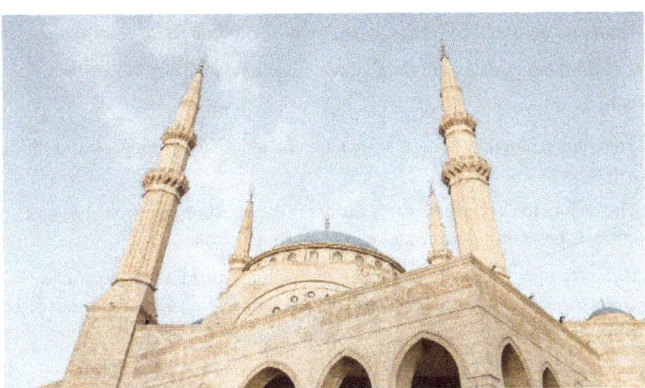

Lebanon-Dinner

The capital city of Lebanon is Beirut.

Officially it is recognized as the Republic of Lebanon, with a population of over 6,00000 people.

Lebanon has an amazing history of archaeological heritage.

The country's major archaeological museum is a big go-to place.

Lebanese cuisine involves a lot of whole grains, fruits, vegetable, fresh fish, and seafood.

Poultry is eaten more often than red meat, and when red meat is eaten, it is usually lamb and goat meat.

It also includes copious amounts of garlic and olive oil, often seasoned with lemon juice.

Chickpeas and parsley are also staples of the Lebanese diet.

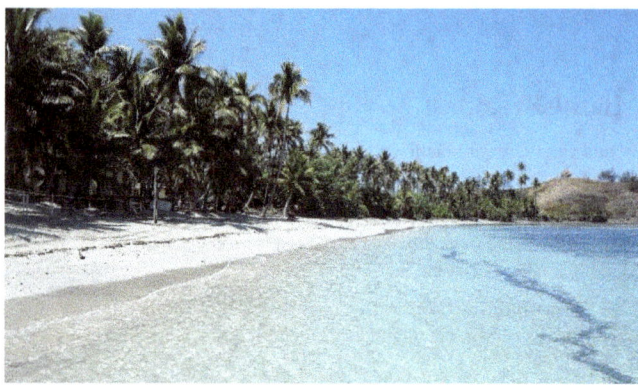

Fiji-Breakfast

With an abundance of islands, palm-fringed beaches, and thriving coral reefs.

Fiji has become a plug for adventure and relaxation.

Traditional Fijian food consists of fresh fish, coconut, root crops, and steamed greens.

A choice dish, roro, is made from steamed taro leaves, onion, garlic, oil, and coconut milk.

The result is comfort food that goes well with just about any Fijian dish.

It tastes like a tropical version of creamed spinach

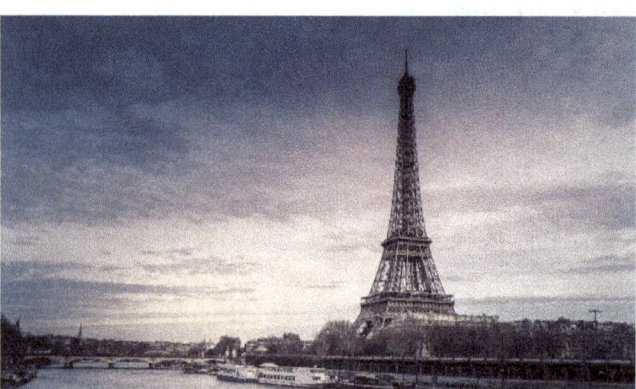

France-Lunch

France, in Western Europe, encompasses medieval cities, alpine villages, and Mediterranean beaches.

Paris, its capital, is famed for its fashion houses, classical art museums including the Louvre, and monuments like the Eiffel Tower.

The country is also renowned for its wines and sophisticated cuisine.

From soufflés to croissants to crêpes, fancy French recipes will add something new to your table, and, oftentimes, are easy to make.

There are lovely French recipes that will make lunchtime an exciting experience.

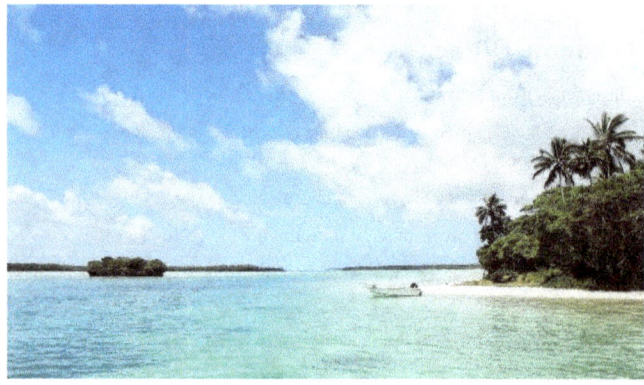

Jamaica-Dinner

Rastafarian movement, reggae, red stripe beer, blue mountain sprite, jerk sauce, and Jamaican rum are very familiar words in this island country of the West Indies.

Jamaica is an island country situated in the Caribbean Sea.

The third largest Island in the Caribbean has its capital city in Kingston.

Jamaicans love spicy food!

Pretty much anything can be spiced up with jerk sauce, from pork and ribs to fish tacos and chicken.

The recipes for jerk sauces vary, as does the application to meats, fish, and other dishes, but the name and effect remain the same.

If you try a good jerk spot in Jamaica, it is almost guaranteed that you're going to want to take some jerk sauce back home with you to try to recreate your meal!

Ackee and salt fish (fish and sauce dish) —is Jamaica's national dish.

It was ranked by National Geographic as the second-best national dish in the world,

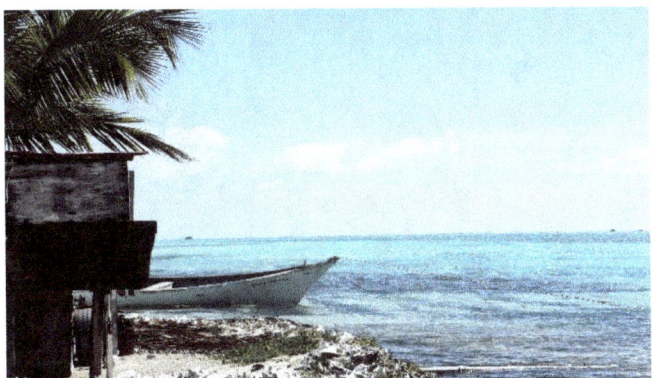

Venezuela-Breakfast

Isla de Margarita and the Los Roques archipelago will sure ring a bell in this South American country.

Venezuela's capital city is Caracas. The country has an estimated population of over 29,000000 residents.

Venezuela is home to The Angel Falls, the world's highest uninterrupted waterfall, has the world's largest known oil reserves and has been one of the world's leading exporters of oil.

Arepas is the national dish of Venezuelans and a famous drink from Venezuela is called Chi Cha Andina, made from rice or corn flour.

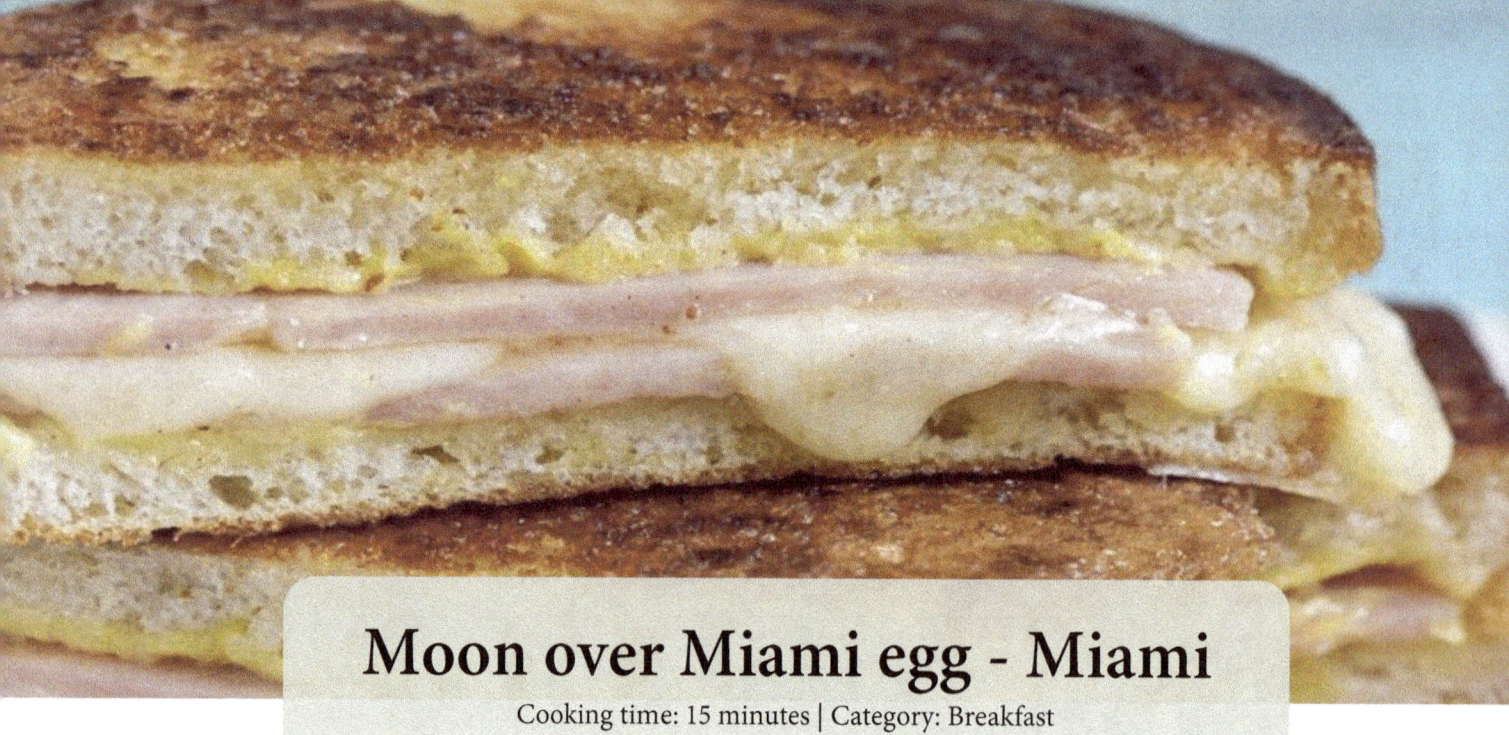

Moon over Miami egg - Miami

Cooking time: 15 minutes | Category: Breakfast

A classic protein-rich diet is unique to Miami residents. This is a classic fried egg breakfast! Also known as Toad in a Hole or Bird in a Nest, It's a cage-free egg that's cooked inside of the grain.

Ingredients

- 1 slice whole grain bread (I used Pepperidge Farm Harvest Blend)
- 1 teaspoon oil (avocado coconut, or olive)
- 1 large egg cage-free organic, if possible
- Sea salt (tiny pinch)
- Garnish options
- 1 sprig parsley finely chopped
- 1 squash blossom finely chopped
- hot sauce

Steps to Cook

1. Preheat a medium skillet over medium heat.
2. Use a cookie cutter or your fingers to make a hole in the center of the bread. Make the hole just large enough for the yolk to fit into.
3. Use a pastry brush or oil spritzer to apply oil to one side of the bread. (You could also just pour the oil directly into the pan but applying it directly to the bread will help it get nice and golden brown.)
4. Place the bread oiled side down into the pan. Cook for 1 minute, then carefully open the egg over the bread so that the yolk falls into the hole in the center. Sprinkle salt over the egg.
5. Cook for 1 more minute to allow the bread to toast, then use a large spatula to gently flip the bread and egg over. Continue to cook until the egg is cooked to your liking. (About 2 minutes for a runny yolk and 3-4 minutes for a hard yolk.
6. Remove the egg from the rom pan and transfer it to a serving plate with the yolk side up. If desired, apply any/all the garnish options before serving.

Note:

Number of Calories: 190kcal

Satisfy your healthy wine cravings at Margot Natural Wine in Miami beach, whilst sampling the beauty of aquatics nature.

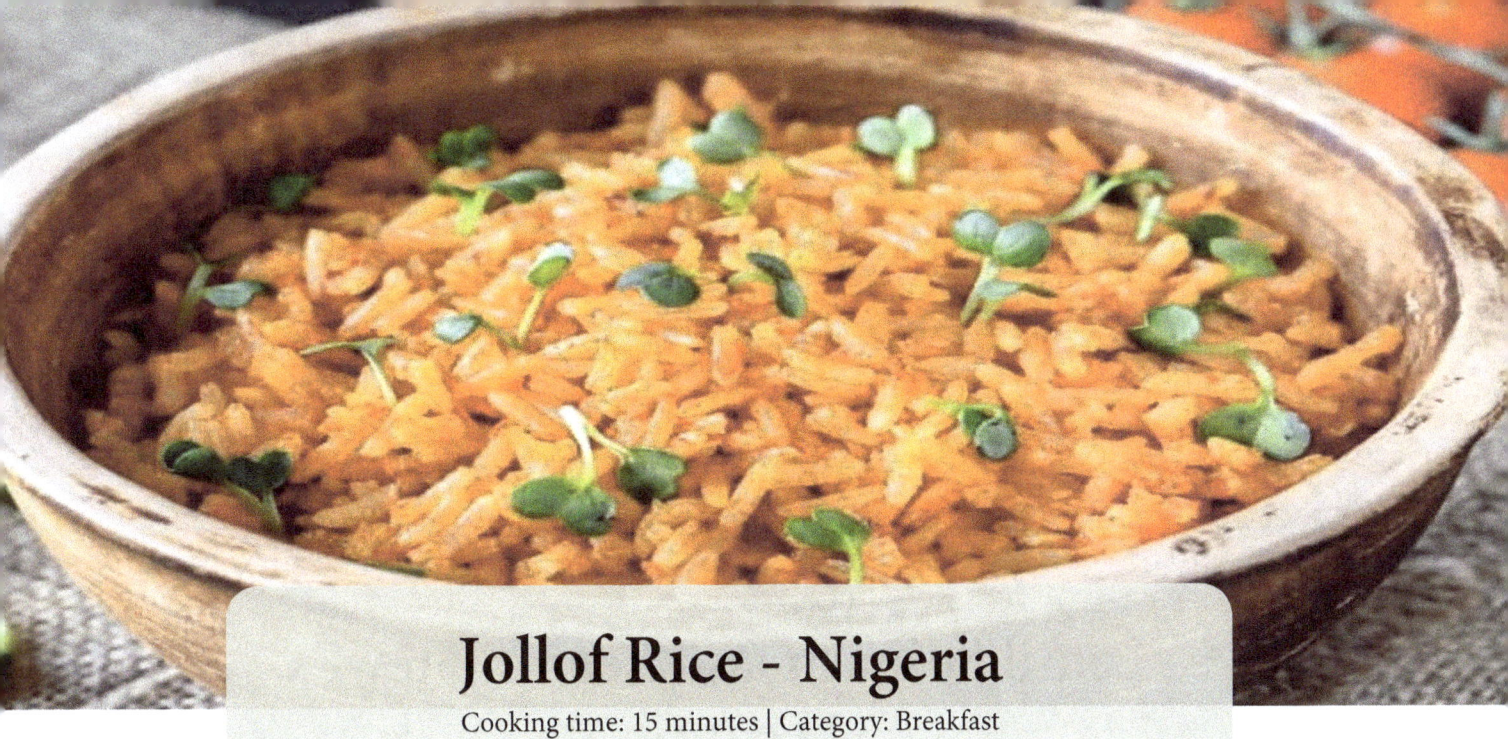

Jollof Rice - Nigeria

Cooking time: 15 minutes | Category: Breakfast

Notes: Normally, the bay leaves should be removed once the rice is done. However, if you can't find the bay leaves after the rice is done, don't be tempted to dig through it since over-stirring will cause the rice to break. Just leave it and remove it whenever you find it.

If you choose not to use butter, you will need to add an extra tbsp of Oil

Ingredients

- 6 Cups Rice Long grain & 3/4 Cup Olive Oil
- 5 Tbsp Tomato paste & 4 Cups Chicken stock
- 1 Tbsp Curry Powder & 1 Tbsp Thyme
- 4 cloves Garlic & 2 bay leaves
- 1 Tbsp Ginger Grated
- 1 Tsp Salt or to taste
- 1 Onion Medium-sized (sliced)
- 1 Tomato sliced (Large size)
- 1 Tbsp seasoning powder or seasoning cubes
- 1 Onion Sliced
- White Pepper or black pepper to taste
- For the sauce, blend:
- 3 Red Bell Pepper & 3 Tomatoes Plum
- 2 Scotch bonnet
- 1 Onion Diced

Steps to Cook

1. In a large pan, preheat the cooking oil. Once the oil is hot, add the diced onions and fry for about 3 to 5 minutes or till the onions become soft.
2. Add the Tomato Paste. Fry for about 5 minutes, then add the garlic, ginger, and bay leaves and let it cook in the tomato paste for about 2 minutes.
3. Add the blended pepper and allow the pepper to cook until the water is reduced entirely, and the oil is seen floating on the fried pepper.
4. Season with thyme, curry powder, salt to taste, and seasoning cubes. Leave to cook for another 2 to 5 minutes.
5. Stir in the rice until it is well coated with the sauce. Add the Chicken stock and cover it with a tight-fitting lid, then allow it to come to a boil.
6. Once it starts boiling - about 3 to 5 minutes after placing it on the stove, reduce the heat immediately to medium-low and steam until the rice is done.
7. Turn off the heat and add the sliced tomato and onions and stir together briefly. Then, cover it up immediately so that the heat remaining in the rice can steam up the vegetables a little bit.
8. You can serve with Plantains, Chicken, and Vegetables or as desired. ENJOY!

Note:

Calories: 418kcal per serving Soybean milk and fresh palm wine are healthy options of beverage in this tropical rainforest nation called Nigeria. Catch the Nigerian excitement on your next trip to Jabi lake located in Abuja capital city.

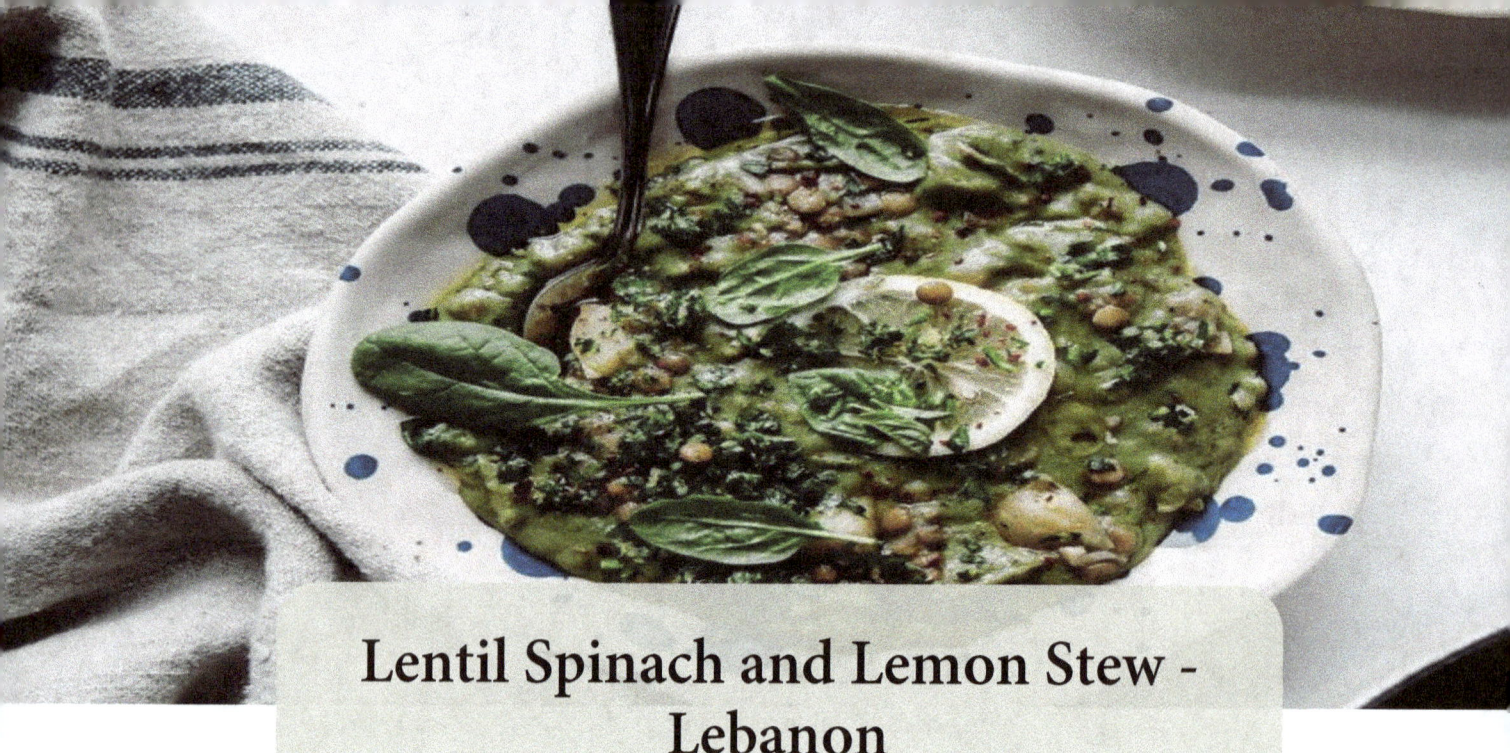

Lentil Spinach and Lemon Stew - Lebanon

Cooking time: 15 minutes | Category: Breakfast

A warming combination of brown lentils, fresh spinach, and potatoes in a zesty broth, perfect on its own or with your grain of choice. This is a perfect dinner recipe that is common with the locals. Cumin and lemon provide a dash of bright flavor to this lentil soup.

Ingredients

- 1 large yellow onion, diced
- 2 cloves of garlic, crushed
- 1 tbsp coconut oil (you can use olive or canola oil if you prefer a more neutral taste)
- 3 cups organic vegetable stock (highly recommend the Kallo brand)
- 1 tbsp lemon juice + ½ tbsp finely grated lemon zest
- 1 cup brown lentils, uncooked
- 3 cups of fresh spinach, roughly chopped
- 1 medium potato, peeled and cubed
- Sea salt and black pepper to taste

Steps to Cook

1. Start by sautéing the chopped onion and garlic in your oil of choice on medium heat for 3-5 minutes until the onions are translucent.
2. Add in the lentils and stir thoroughly before adding in the vegetable stock and lemon. Cover and let cook on low heat for about 15-20 minutes until the lentils are about three-quarters of the way cooked.
3. Taste the broth and adjust seasonings as needed with salt, pepper, and additional lemon if you like things extra tangy.
4. Add in potato cubes and spinach then cover and cook until lentils are tender, and the potato can be pierced with a knife easily, about another 15 minutes.

Note:

Aryan and Jallab are 2 beverages you don't intend to miss in Beirut, whilst catching the excitement at Zaitunay Bay

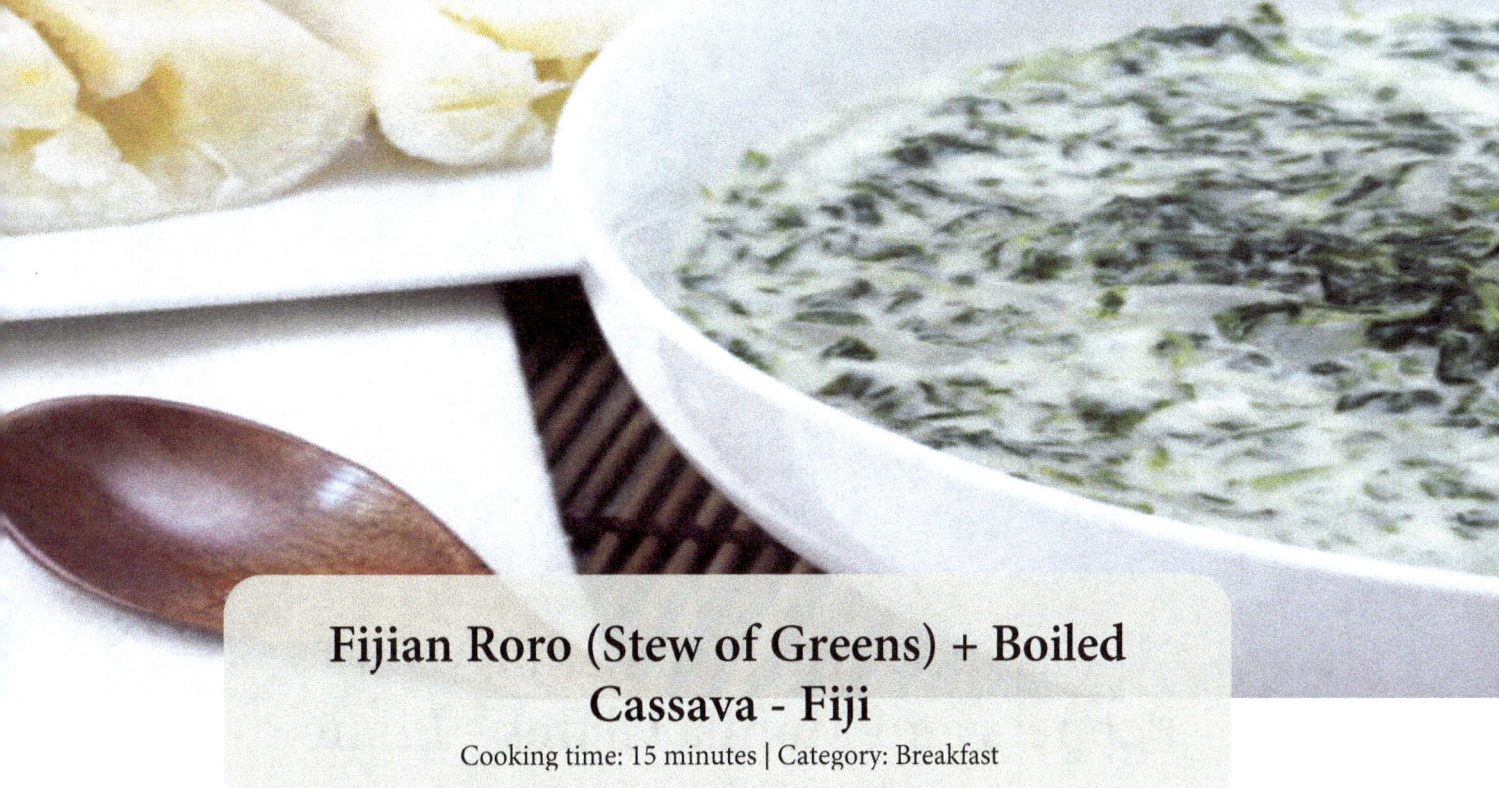

Fijian Roro (Stew of Greens) + Boiled Cassava - Fiji

Cooking time: 15 minutes | Category: Breakfast

Every culture has its comfort foods.

For Fijians, this Roro recipe is warm and hearty and embodies the wonderful flavors of the island using creamy coconut milk and greens.

And although this Roro recipe looks exotic, it's low-carb/keto, paleo, vegan, and gluten-free ingredients

Ingredients

- 10 oz (280 g) frozen chopped spinach
- 14 oz can of coconut milk
- 2 cups of water
- ½ cup (30 g) onions, chopped
- 1 tsp garlic paste, or 4 small cloves chopped
- ½ lime, to taste
- 2-3 Thai chilis, or to taste
- 1 tsp salt, or to taste
- *Optional frozen cassava or taro for serving

Steps to Cook

1. Remove the frozen chopped spinach out of the wrapper, place on a microwave safe plate, and heat for 1½ minutes on high in your microwave oven, until it has mostly thawed.
2. In a medium saucepan, bring one cup of water to a boil; add in the chopped onion, garlic paste, chilis, and salt, and simmer with the lid closed until tender (about 4 minutes).
3. Add the spinach to the pot, adding more water if needed (it should be just covering the spinach). Let the spinach cook for an additional 4-5 minutes, until everything is tender.
4. Reduce the heat to medium and add the entire can of coconut milk and stir. Let this boil for an additional 4-5 minutes, until the milk thickens and absorbs all of the flavors.
5. Add a cup of water at this stage, to prevent the coconut milk from burning; boil until you reach the desired consistency (similar to a Thai curry).
6. Season with the juice of half a lime, adding more lime and salt per your taste.
7. If serving with cassava or taro, thaw the frozen root crop properly before boiling (countertop or microwave), otherwise find fresh root crop at your local ethnic grocer.
8. Bring a quart of water to a boil and cook the cassava or taro the same way you would a potato, by boiling until tender in the center when poked with a fork or a knife.
9. strain and let rest before serving

Note:

Catch the Fijian fever at the the Mamanuca Islands, for a taste of the rich Fijian culture. Enjoy your favorite dessert with the Kava drink to calm your nerves

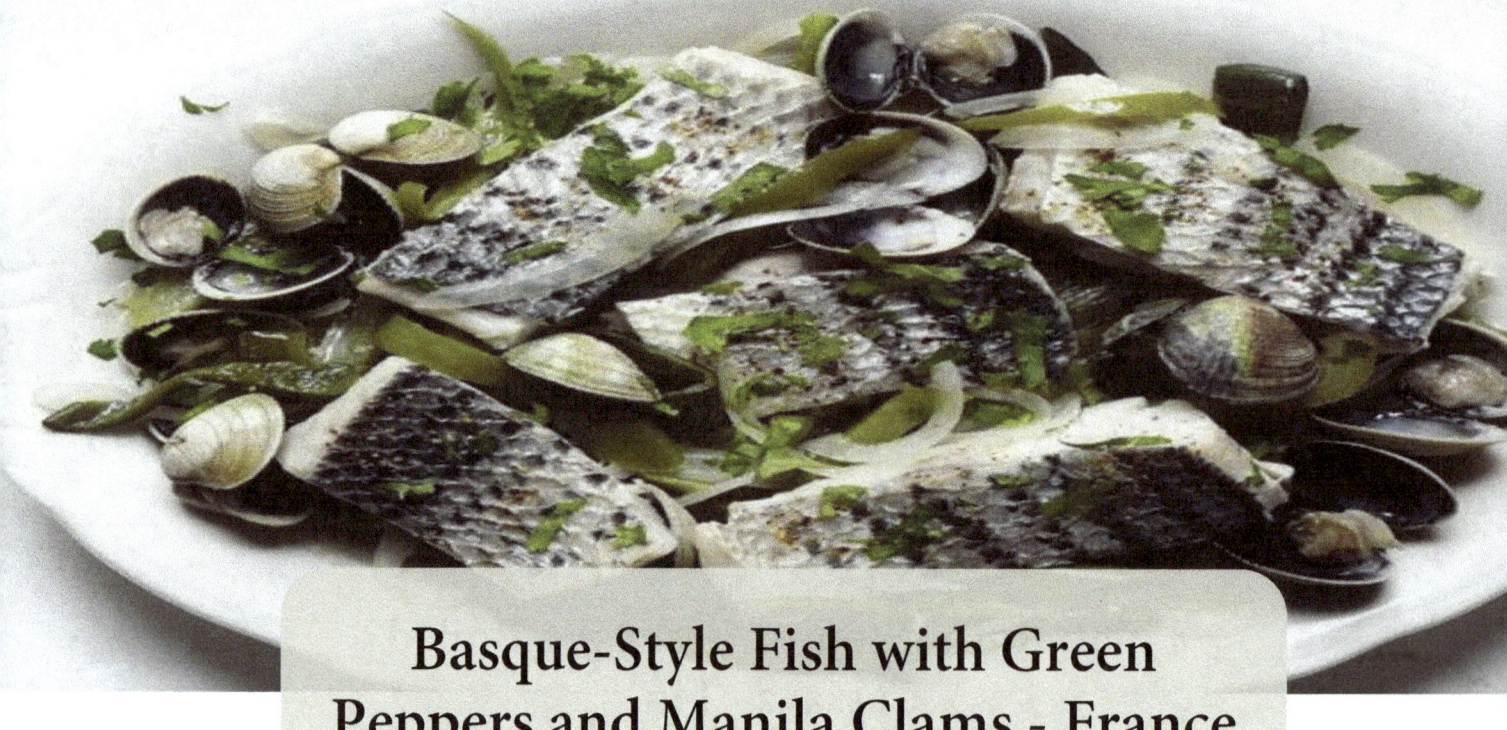

Basque-Style Fish with Green Peppers and Manila Clams - France

Cooking time: 15 minutes | Category: Breakfast

This riff on Basque pipérade, a classic dish of stewed peppers, incorporates seafood from the region. Hake is traditional, but mild, white-fleshed fish like striped bass or haddock make fine substitutes. Fresh clams offer a briny sweetness. Any assortment of mild peppers will work here.

Ingredients

- 1/3 cup extra-virgin olive oil
- 2 cloves garlic, finely chopped (1 Tbsp.)
- 1 tbsp. all-purpose flour
- 1/2 cup dry white wine
- 2 cups fish stock or clam broth
- 3/4 tsp. kosher salt, plus more to taste
- 1 lb. assorted mild green peppers, cut into 1/4-inch strips (3 1/2 cups)
- 1 medium Spanish onion, thinly sliced
- 2 tbsp. coarsely chopped Italian parsley, plus more for garnish
- 2 lb. skin-on, hake fillets cut into 8 equal portions
- 12 small, fresh clams, scrubbed
- 1-2 tsp piment d'Espelette (optional)

Steps to Cook

1. In a large skillet, heat the olive oil over medium-high heat. Add the garlic and cook, stirring occasionally, until just beginning to brown, 1 minute.
2. Sprinkle the flour over the garlic and stir to combine. Add the wine and cook, stirring rapidly, until the mixture thickens and reduces slightly about 2 minutes.
3. Add the fish stock and salt, then bring the mixture back to a boil. Add the peppers, onion, and parsley, and spread into an even layer on the bottom of the pan.
4. Raise the heat to high, cover the pan, and simmer until the vegetables are softened about 5 minutes.
5. Uncover the pan and place the hake pieces skin-side up in a single layer atop the vegetables.
6. Nestle the clams between the fillets and season the fish with salt to taste.
7. Cover and cook until the fillets are just opaque at the center and the clams have opened 5–7 minutes. (Discard unopened clams.)
8. On a deep serving platter, scatter the vegetables, then place the fish and clams on top.
9. Spoon the remaining broth over the fish and garnish with chopped parsley and Espelette pepper, if using; serve immediately

Note:

The historical region of Burgundy (Bourgogne in French) produces some of the best French wines and some of the best in the world, and the most expensive. With over 67million residents in France and the legendary Paris as the state capital, it tells a lot about the France culture. You will love the Fishing Villages, Historic Ports & Beaches in Brittany Just hearing the word France evokes images of the Eiffel Tower, glamorous and posh Paris, The romantic Seine River, quaint villages that came straight out of fairy tale books, and a cuisine that has a classification of its own by how diverse and intangible it is from France's cultural legacy. France remains one of the most-visited countries in the world and will do so for a long time.

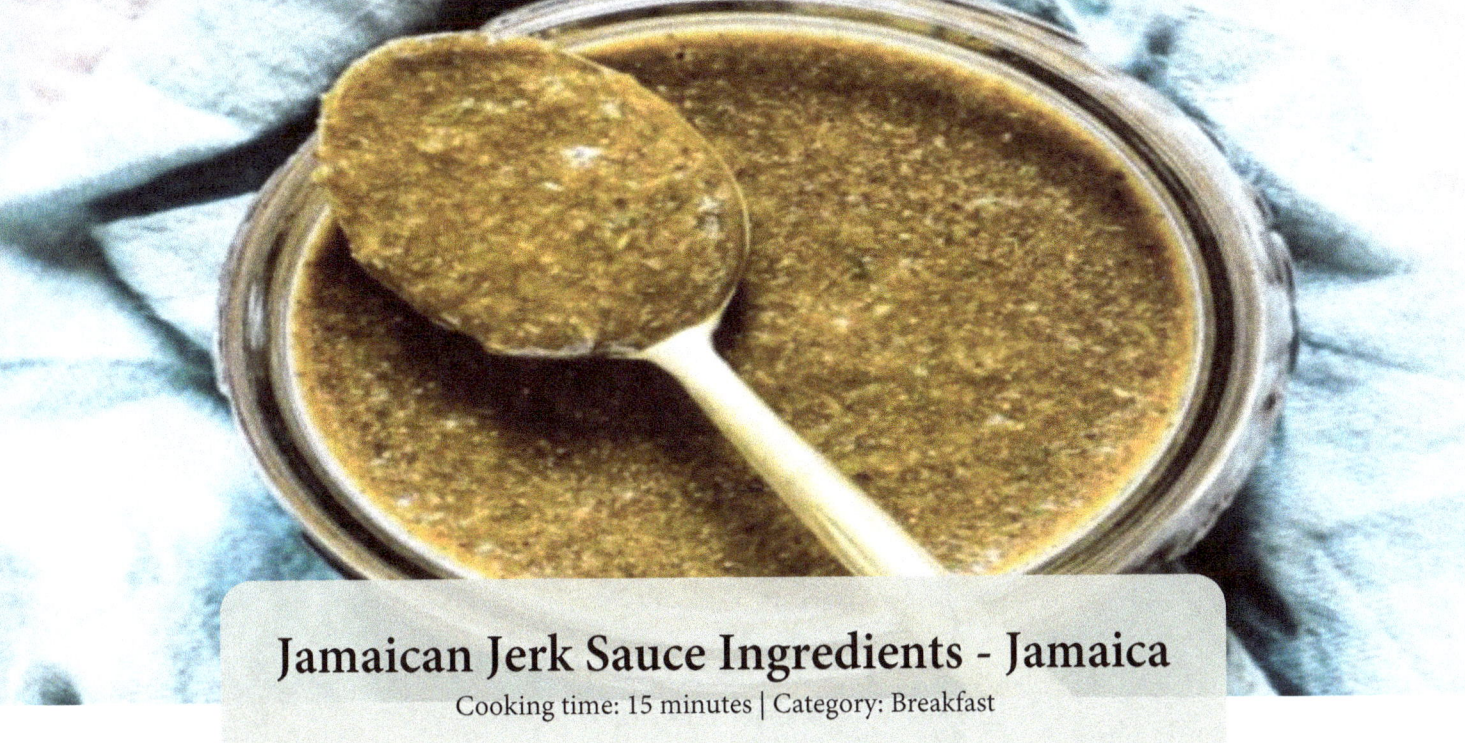

Jamaican Jerk Sauce Ingredients - Jamaica

Cooking time: 15 minutes | Category: Breakfast

Jerk is a style of cooking that originated in Jamaica where a wet sauce or dry rub is applied to the meat of choice and then cooked. Jerk marinade or sauce tends to be spicy due to the classic use of scotch bonnet (a very spicy pepper option). Authentic versions should also include the use of allspice and thyme, as those ingredients bring the right Jamaican flavors.

Ingredients

- 4 organic scotch bonnet peppers* 3 ¼ oz
- ½ large red onion or 1 medium yellow onion chopped
- 6 cloves of garlic
- 5 stalks of scallion
- 1/4 cup white vinegar
- 1/4 cup soy sauce
- 1 ½ teaspoons sea salt
- 1 tablespoon ground black pepper
- 1 tablespoon grated fresh ginger
- 2 tablespoons fresh pimento seeds
- 2 tablespoons brown sugar I used organic
- 1 teaspoon of freshly grated nutmeg
- 2 tablespoons oil
- 7 sprigs of fresh thyme
- Squeeze lime

Steps to Cook

1. Add all the ingredients to a high-speed blender and blend until completely incorporated.
2. Pour into a sanitized jar and place it in your fridge.
3. You can enjoy it immediately or let flavors meld together for as long as you like! Enjoy with friends!

Note:

Each serving contains 45kcal. Don't be afraid to try out the local Jerk Shacks along the road but know that every beach and Sandals Resort has a Jerk Shack as well - and it's all included. Be sure to have a taste of sorrel and Jamaican rum for an experience of Jamaica. A kaleidoscope of island experiences brimming with life and color. This is what this Caribbean Island has in store for you.

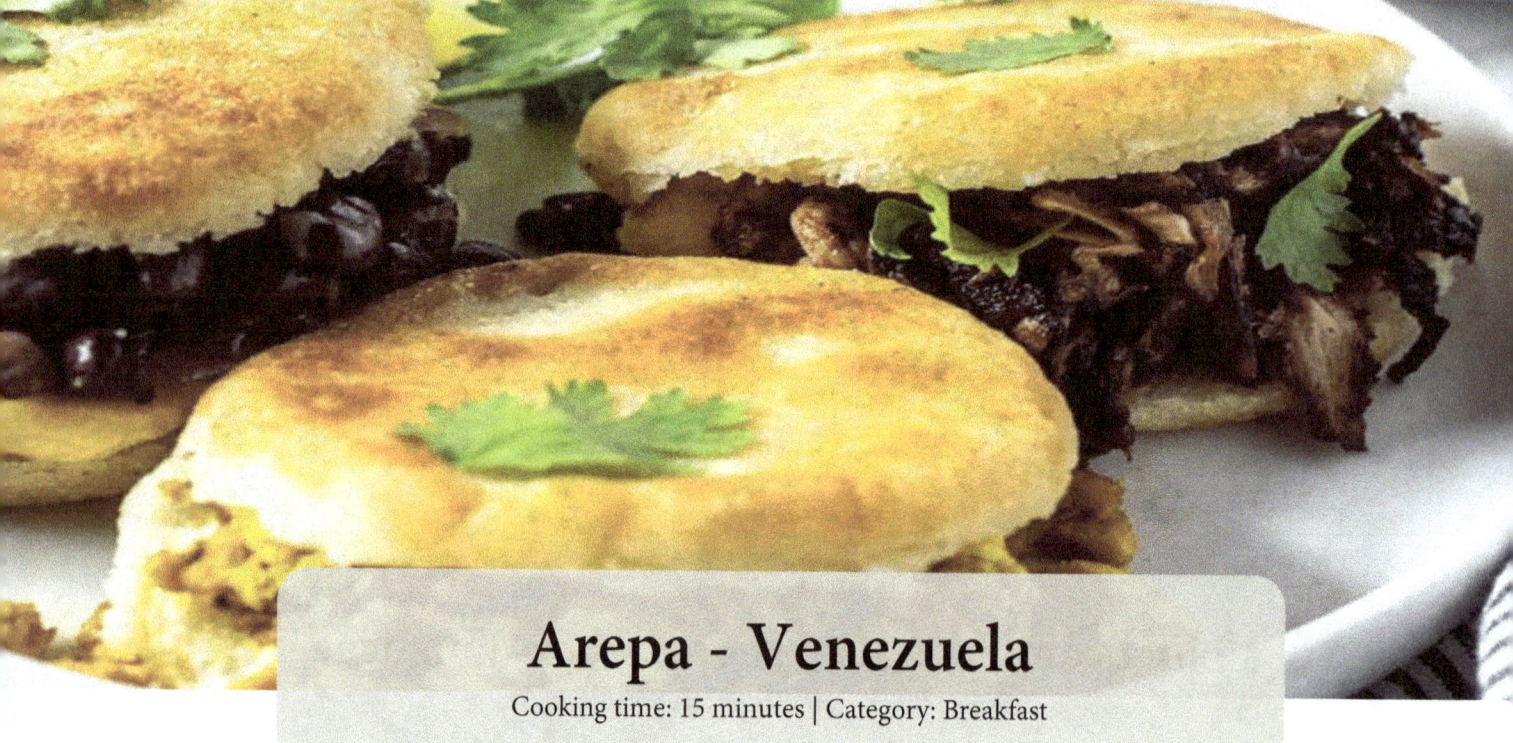

Arepa - Venezuela

Cooking time: 15 minutes | Category: Breakfast

In Venezuela, the eating area is not exclusive to the economic class, city, or time of the day. It is lavishly enjoyed by all. Arepa is a very popular corn meal made from ground corn dough or precooked corn flour. It is well eaten in Venezuela, Colombia, Panama, and Puerto Rico. The nutritious golden disks are commonly packed with all or some of these, beans, cheese, avocado, shredded beef, and onions.

The chicken or pork is first shredded and then cooked with little spice. For Venezuelan breakfasts, arepas are traditionally paired with a cup of strong coffee and hot dipping chocolate. Areperas are restaurants where arepas are usually served.

Ingredients

- 2 cups fresh corn flour or white precooked cornmeal
- 2 teaspoons salt (kosher salt)
- 2 tablespoons neutral vegetable oil
- Choice fillings (chicken or pork, stewed black beans with cheese and lime, corn salad with onion and fresh herbs; for serving)
- lime wedges

Steps to Cook

1. Into a bowl, mix arena flour, and salt. Create a depression in the center and add 2½ cups of warm water.
2. Gradually add your dry ingredients, and stir continuously using a wooden spoon
3. Ensure there are no lumps. Allow resting for a little while.
4. Work on the dough in the bowl by kneading smoothly a few times, then divide it into 8 pieces. Roll each piece on the work surface into a ball, and then gently flatten.
5. Heat 1 tbsp of vegetable oil in a large non-stick skillet over medium heat. Depending on the size of the bowl, add some arepas, allowing for enough cooking space, cover, and fry until golden brown. Flip sideways until another side is golden brown, 6–8 minutes. Transfer arepas to a wire rack.
6. Repeat with the remaining 1 Tbsp. oil and dough.
7. Split arepas and stuff with choice fillings; serve with lime wedges.

Note:

Arepas contain 219 calories per 100g of serving.
Do well to partake in the beauty of the tropical resort islands along its Caribbean coast and enjoy its natural drink (the cocada). Venezuela is a gem in South America, hiding a plethora of beautiful sights from coastal towns to beaches to stunning mountain tops. They say a path is that east taken often leads to breathtaking experiences, and Venezuela is a perfect example of that. You can find here Angel falls, the tallest waterfall in the world standing at 979 meters, a personal encounter with the Andes peaks, and the great rivers of the Orinoco Delta. Due to the recent political unrest and high inflation, safety remains a top concern but seasoned travelers all over the world look forward to coming back.

Week - 4

Reflections

- How was your practice of meditation & gratitude this week?

_____

_____

_____

- What new recipes did you try?

_____

_____

_____

- What new people & countries did you connect with this week?

_____

_____

_____

- Who did you share a meal with this week?

_____

_____

_____

- What are you observing about yourself?

_____

_____

_____

- What is your time for a 1.5miles run or walk?

_____

_____

_____

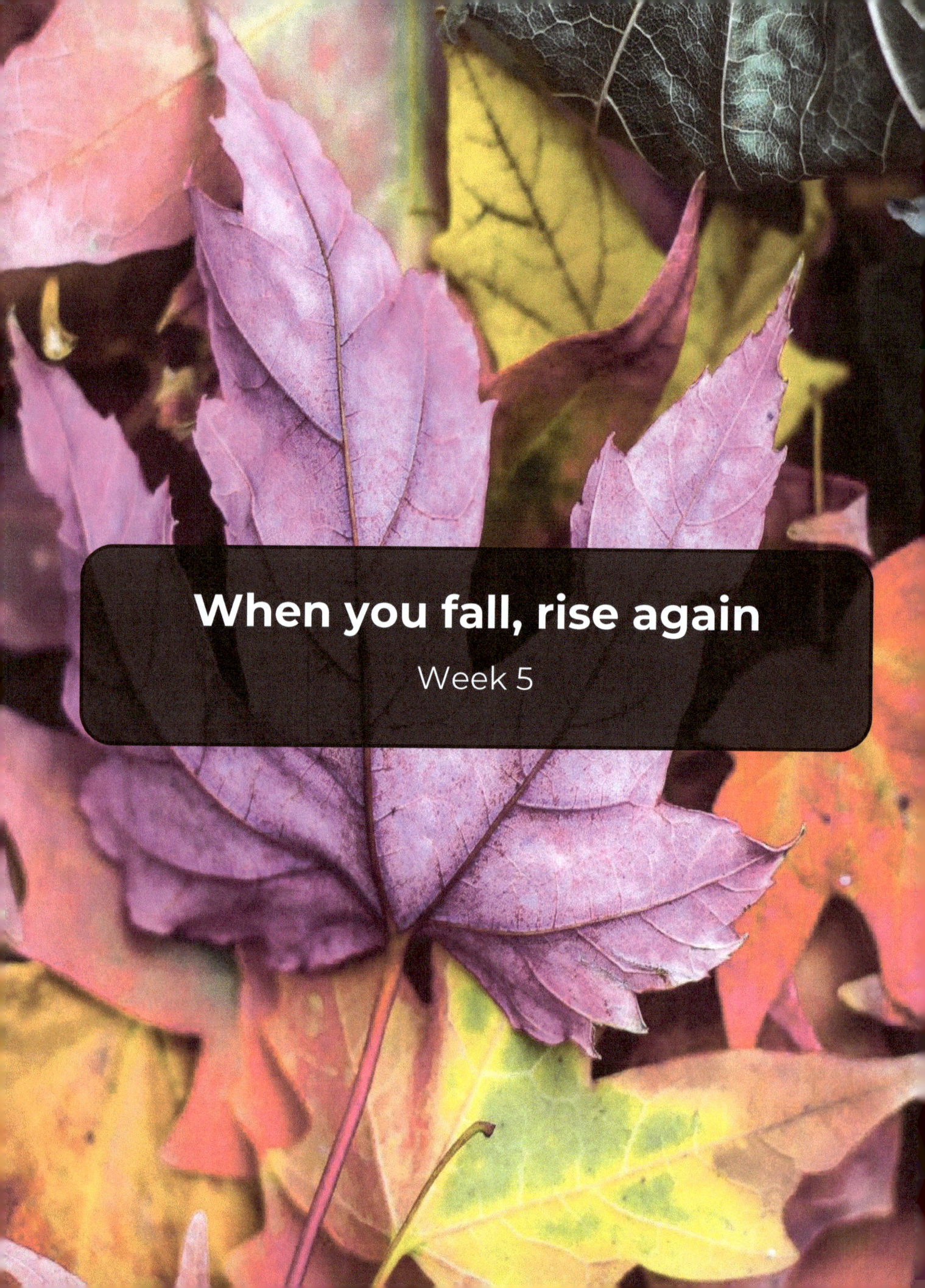

Week - 5

Take Obedient Action

- Spend 5 -10 minutes writing in your gratitude journal about giving thanks & Practice 5 minutes of meditation
- Select 2 Dinner & 1 lunch recipes from week 4 & prepare them.

- Connect with 4 people from the 4 different countries digitally or in person

- Share a meal with someone from one of countries

- Visit a new supermarket this week
- Increase your cardio to 1.5 miles walk or run add 10 minutes of stretching

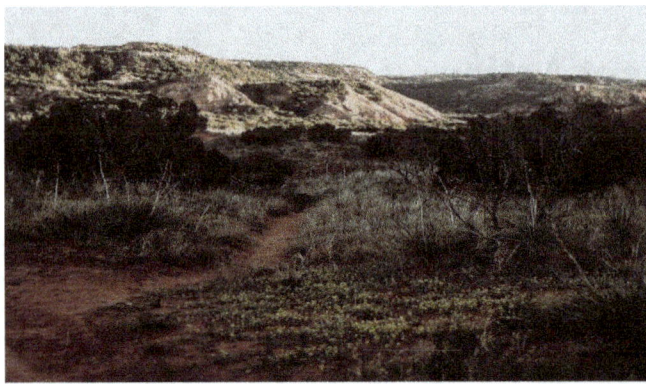

Texas-Lunch

Texas is the second-largest U.S. state by both geography and population, with more than 29.1 million residents.

The bustling American state is also known as the 'Lone Star State and is famous for its BBQ, live music, hot temperatures, etc.

Tourists should visit The Texas State Capitol in Austin, whilst lovers of heights will love Bend National Park.

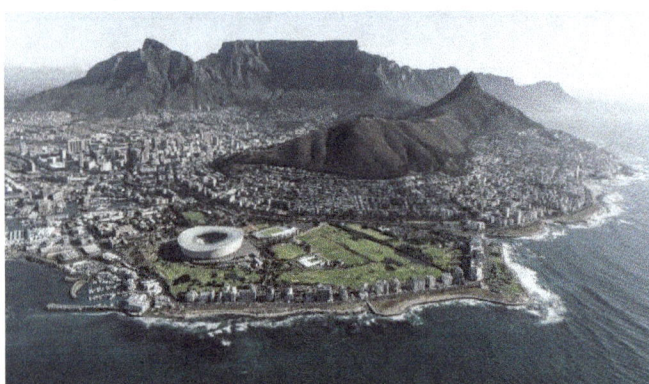

South Africa-Dinner

The current south African population is over 60,041,994with its capitals as Cape Town, Pretoria, Bloemfontein. It will interest meat lovers to know that South Africa is the largest producer of meat in Africa.

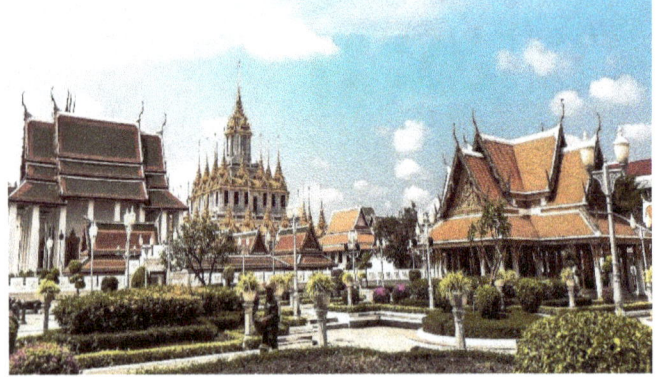

Thailand-Breakfast

The Southeast Asian country is known for tropical beaches, opulent royal palaces, ancient ruins and ornate temples displaying figures of Buddha.

In Bangkok, the capital, and the country's major urban hub, this engrossing city is a visual feast of gold-tipped temples, shining skyscrapers, and streets busy with food stalls, tuk-tuks, and the occasional, orange-robed monk.

Thai food is, for many, the world's number one cuisine.

It balances spice with fragrance, offers complexity without fussiness, and manages to always leave you wanting a second helping.

Even more extraordinary is that whether you're purchasing food from a stall in the haze of the Bangkok streets or at a shack beside the crystalline Andaman Sea, the quality seems to be of a piece.

Naturally, specialism varies, with the northeast known for heat and sticky rice while the south prefers seafood marinating in fresh coconut milk sauces.

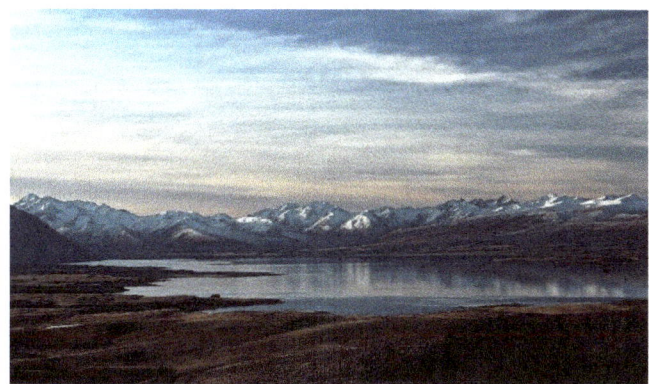

New Zealand-Lunch

New Zealand is an island country in the southwestern Pacific Ocean.

It consists of two main landmasses—the North Island and the South Island. Its capital is Wellington.

You can visit natural reserves, volcanoes, and glaciers across several islands. You can walk alongside kiwi birds, sheep, and penguins.

New Zealand food is largely driven by local ingredients and seasonal variations.

An island nation with a primarily agricultural economy, New Zealand yields produce from the land and sea.

Similar to the cuisine of Australia, the cuisine of New Zealand is a diverse British-based cuisine, with the Mediterranean and Pacific Rim.

New Zealand is home to some amazing seafood.

Roast lamb is common too because of the abundance of sheep.

Dairy product silk and cheese) are also popular and abundant in New Zealand.

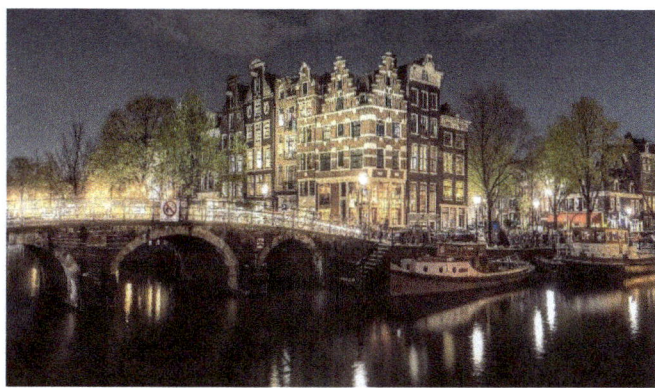

The Netherlands-Dinner

The four largest cities in the Netherlands are Amsterdam, Rotterdam, The Hague, and Utrecht. Amsterdam is the country's most populous city and nominal capital.

The Netherlands may be a small country, but it is known for many things.

The country is most known for its cheese, wooden shoes, windmills, tulips, coffee shops, and canals of Amsterdam.

The Netherlands has the highest population density in Europe (over 17,140,098).

In the Oxfam Food Index of 125 countries, they rank number one for having the most plentiful, nutritious, healthy, and affordable food: above France and Switzerland"

This is interesting information for foodies!

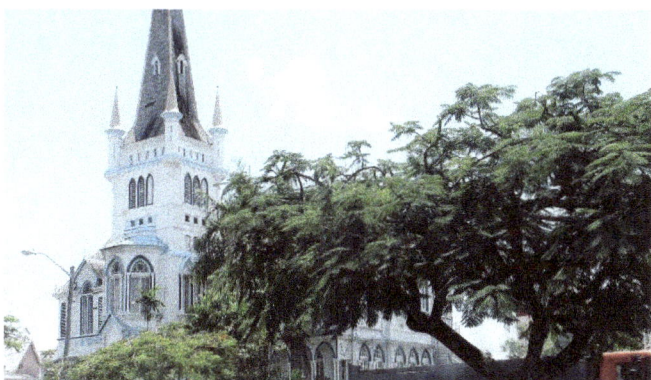

Guyana-Breakfast

Guyana is also called the Co-operative Republic of Guyana, and the capital city is Georgetown.
Its virgin rainforest, lovely waterfalls, and St. George's Anglican Cathedral are all important markers.
Guyana is also home to the world's large single-drop waterfall – the Kaieteur Falls.
Guyana is predominantly dominated by rainforests. Hence, a majority of inhabitants live in the state capital.
Surama is the perfect place to explore the cultures and traditions of the country.
Experience the traditional dances and daily chores such as the production of cassava of the Macushi tribe.
This richly spiced dish is traditionally served on Christmas morning and many other special occasion meals in Guyana.

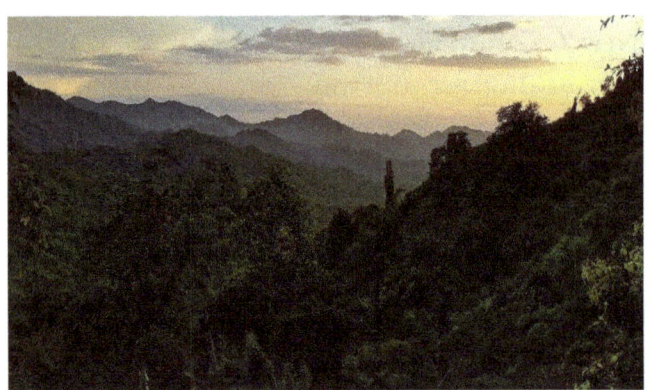

Colombia-Lunch

The capital of Colombia is Bogotá, and a current population of over 51,641,190

The South American country is famous for its arepas and specialty coffee, as well as the kindness of its people.

It's known for its diverse landscapes and culturally rich heritage where art, music, and theater mix.

It also has its share of famous people like Shakira and Sofia Vergara.

Other cities in Colombia include Cartagena, and Medellin, their inhabitants are very hospitable.

Colombian coffee is 100% arabica, which is sweeter and lighter than the robusta variety.

Another reason Colombian coffee is so good is that it is all picked by hand.

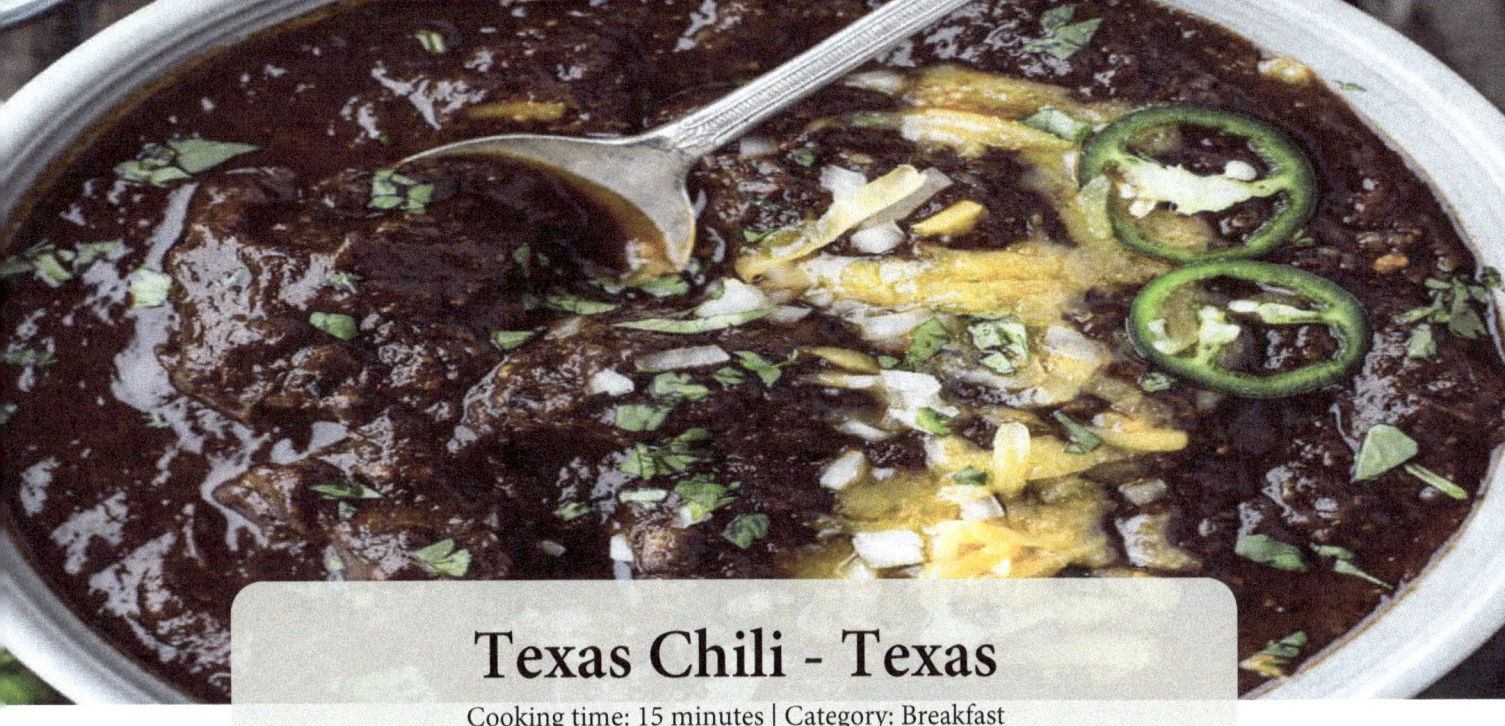

Texas Chili - Texas

Cooking time: 15 minutes | Category: Breakfast

There is nothing more satisfying than a big bowl of the Texan National dish on a chilly day! Texas Chili has a lot of goodness to offer, from its fleshy consistency, utmost satiety, time conserving bunch of deliciousness.

Ingredients

- 2 pounds coarse ground beef, 80/20 or chuck also called chili grind
- Vegetable oil as needed
- 2 cups yellow onions chopped
- 2 tablespoons garlic, minced
- 3 tablespoons chili powder
- 2 tablespoons ground cumin
- 1 tablespoon smoked paprika
- 1 tablespoon oregano
- 2 teaspoons salt
- 2 teaspoons black pepper
- 2 bay leaves
- 1 can of crushed tomatoes
- 3 tablespoons tomato paste
- 1 heaping tablespoon better than Bouillon - beef flavor
- 1 (12-ounce) bottle of amber ale beer
- 1 cup of water
- 2 tablespoons masa
- Toppings:
- cheddar cheese shredded
- sour cream
- red onions chopped
- jalapeno sliced

Steps to Cook

1. In a 6-quart saucepan, over medium-high heat, brown the beef crumbling as it browns, in batches so as not to crowd the pan.
2. Remove the browned meat to a paper towel-lined plate.
3. Remove all but 1/4 cup of the fat in the pan, if there's not 1/4 cup fat, add vegetable oil, as needed.
4. Add the onion and cook, on medium, stirring occasionally, until browned and soft, about 10-12 minutes.
5. Stir in garlic, chili powder, cumin, smoked paprika, and oregano and cook, stirring constantly so as not to burn the spices, until the spices are fragrant, about 1-2 minutes.
6. Return the browned beef to the saucepan and add the salt, pepper, bay leaves, crushed tomatoes, tomato paste, Better than Bouillon, 3/4 cup of the amber ale beer, and 1/3 a cup of water and simmer for 20 minutes.
7. Add the remaining 3/4 cup of beer, another 2/3 cup of water, and masa and simmer for 30-40 minutes, stirring occasionally, until chili is thick.
8. Serve with any toppings you like.

Note:

The number of Calories in Texas Style Chili is 267. Immerse yourself completely in the Texan style by having a glass of the Texan ranch water. Nature addicts will certainly drool. They say everything is bigger in Texas and yes, it is. It is one of the biggest states in the US, sprawling land of rugged terrain, desert Badlands and prairies that would remind you of those cowboy flicks where the sheriff chases the masked rider onwards to the sunset

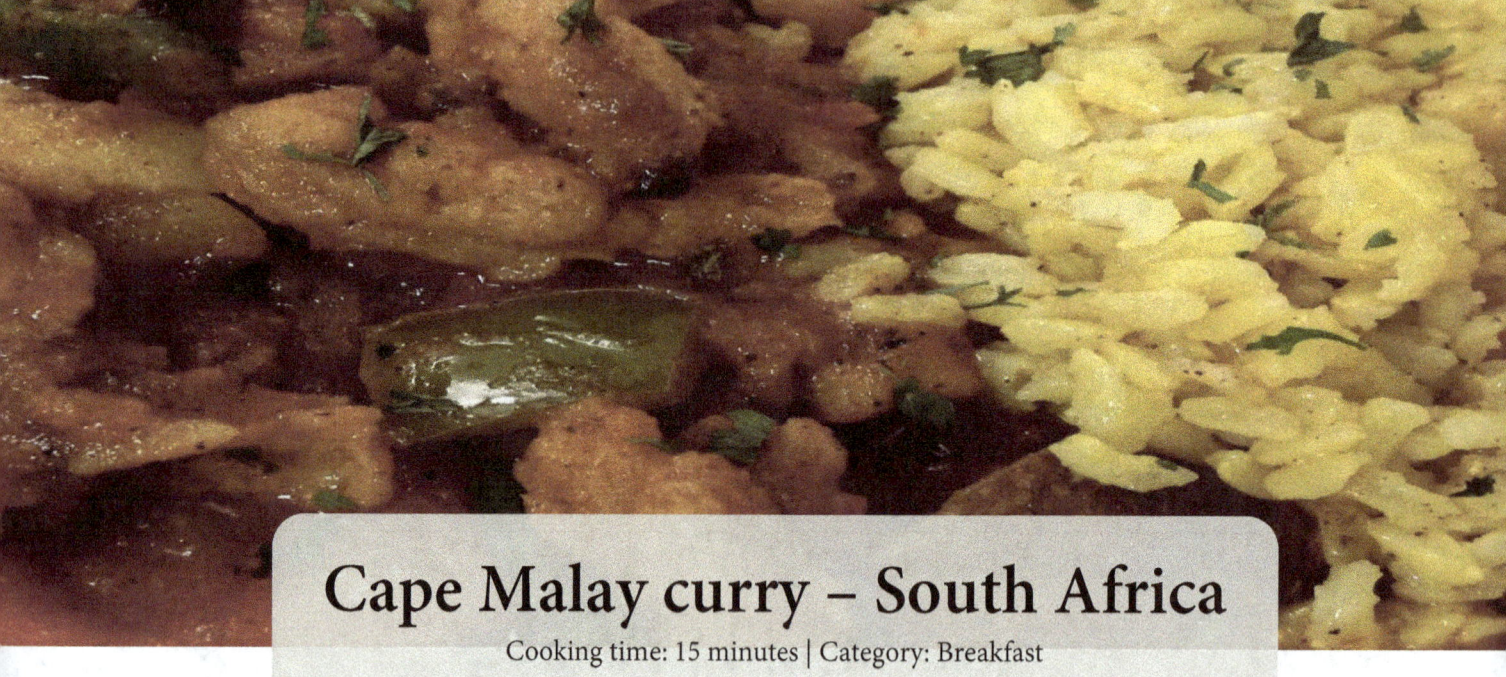

Cape Malay curry – South Africa

Cooking time: 15 minutes | Category: Breakfast

In the 17th century, the Dutch and French landed and settled in Cape Town, bringing slaves from Indonesia, India, and Malaysia, along with their spices and traditional cooking methods. When combined with local produce, the aromatic spices such as cinnamon, saffron, turmeric, and chili created fragrant curries and stews, which are still popular in the area today.

Ingredients

- 2 tbsp sunflower or rapeseed oil
- 1 large onion, finely chopped
- 4 large garlic cloves, finely grated
- 2 tbsp finely grated ginger
- 5 cloves
- 2 tsp turmeric
- 1 tsp ground white pepper
- 1 tsp coriander & 1 tsp cumin
- seeds from 8 cardamom pods, lightly crushed
- 1 cinnamon stick, snapped in half
- 1 large red chili, halved, deseeded, and sliced
- 400g can of chopped tomatoes
- 2 tbsp mango chutney
- 1 chicken stock cube, crumbled
- 12 bone-in chicken thighs, skin removed
- 500g potato, cut into chunks
- small pack of coriander, chopped

For the yellow rice

- 50g butter
- 350g basmati rice & 50g raisins
- 1 tsp golden caster sugar
- 1 tsp ground turmeric
- ¼ tsp ground white pepper
- 1 cinnamon stick, snapped in half
- 8 cardamom pods, lightly crushed.

Steps to Cook

1. Heat the oil in a large, wide pan. Add the onion and fry for 5 mins until softened, stirring every now and then. Stir in the garlic, ginger, and cloves, and cook for 5 mins more, stirring frequently to stop it sticking.

2. Add all the remaining spices and the fresh chili, stir briefly, then tip in the tomatoes with 2 cans of water, plus the chutney and crumbled stock cube.

3. Add the chicken thighs, pushing them under the liquid, then cover the pan and leave to cook for 35 mins. Stir well, add the potatoes and cook uncovered for 15-20 mins more until they are tender. Stir in the coriander.

4. About 10 mins before you want to serve, make the rice. Put the butter, rice, raisins, sugar, and spices in a large pan with 550ml water and 0.5 tsp salt. Bring to the boil and, when the butter has melted, stir, cover and cook for 10 mins. Turn off the heat and leave it undisturbed for 5 mins. Fluff up and serve with the curry.

Note:

South Africa is full of record-breaking animals. Wildlife enthusiasts will be drawn to the sights. It's where you'll find the largest land mammal (elephant), the largest bird (ostrich), the tallest animal (giraffe), the largest fish (whale shark), the largest reptile (leatherback turtle), the fastest land mammal (cheetah) and the largest antelope (eland) I am very sure maize loves will love Umqombothi, made from corn, and enjoyed amongst the locals.

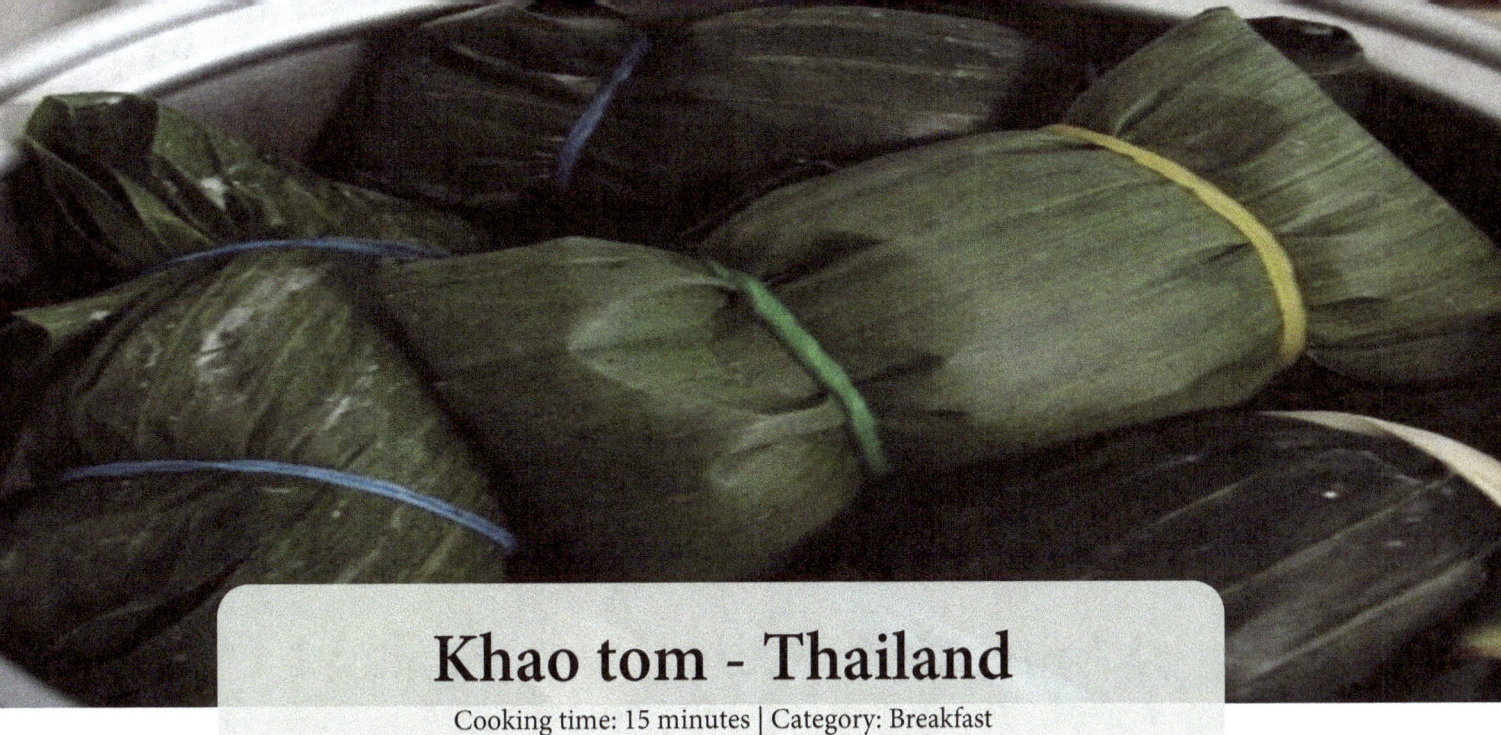

Khao tom - Thailand

Cooking time: 15 minutes | Category: Breakfast

Khao tom is very popular and breakfast in Thailand.

It is made up of boiled rice with desired protein which is slightly like thin porridge or oatmeal.

Ingredients

- 2 cups cooked rice (white or brown)
- 1/4-pound ground turkey or pork
- 1 tablespoon fish sauce (more to taste)
- 2 eggs
- 1 green onion, chopped for garnish
- 1 handful of cilantro, for garnish
- 1 pinch ground black pepper, to taste
-

Steps to Cook

1. Bring 1 cup of water to a boil. Lower to medium heat and cook the ground meat in the water for about 5 minutes, separating the meat into chunks.
2. Drain the meat from the boiling water and wash the pot. Add the meat and rice to the pot.
3. Add enough water to just cover the rice by an inch and heat to boil. Lower the heat to a simmer for another 10 minutes for the rice to soften.
4. While the rice and meat are cooking, add fish sauce to taste. Start with 1 tablespoon and add more for more flavor.
5. Poach the eggs in the porridge for at least 2 minutes depending on how runny you like your eggs.
6. Divide into bowls and top with pepper, cilantro, and chopped green onion.

Note:

Do not leave Thailand and miss the enthralling feel of Cha yen, or Thai tea. Exquisite island breaks are what Thailand is known for the world over. While there is a galaxy of well over 1,000 islands.

This dizzying number can be swiftly reduced into manageable east and west coast groupings that excel in the kind of palm tree, jasmine-scented breeze experience that Thailand consistently delivers

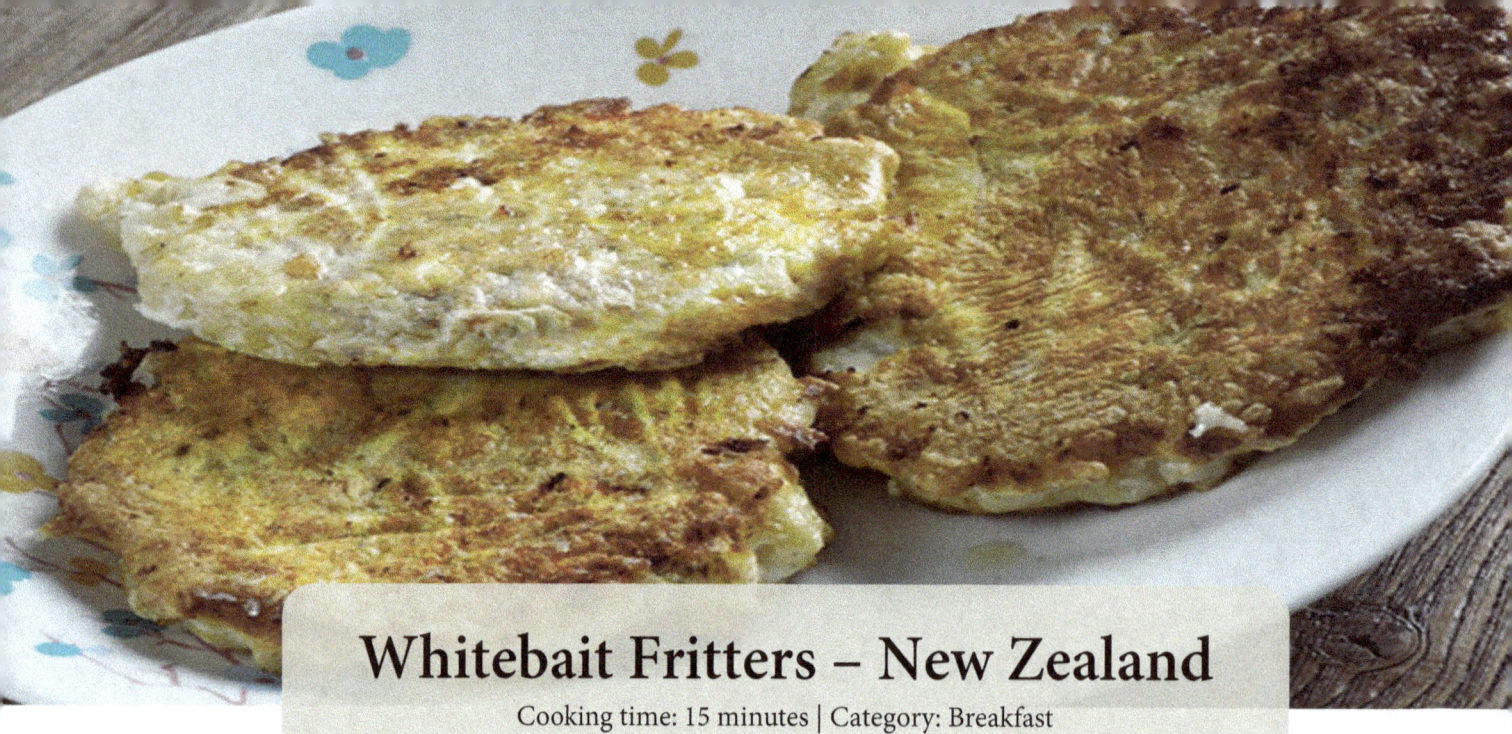

Whitebait Fritters – New Zealand

Cooking time: 15 minutes | Category: Breakfast

Mention whitebait fritters and suddenly everyone is in the kitchen eating them straight from the pan with a squeeze of lemon.

Make a little go a long way by making mini fritters. All you need are eggs to bind the whitebait together, parsley, salt, and pepper to season and butter to cook these delicate delights. The flavor speaks for itself.

Ingredients

- 200g whitebait
- ½ tsp salt
- Freshly ground pepper
- 1 Tbsp chopped parsley
- Knob butter for cooking
- Lime or lemon to squeeze

Steps to Cook

1. Place the whitebait in a bowl. Add the eggs, salt, pepper, and parsley and combine well.
2. Heat a knob of butter in a frying pan. Cook a tablespoon of mixture to test the heat. Cook for 1-2 minutes on each side until just cooked through. Continue to cook the remainder of the fritters.
3. Serve warm with a squeeze of lemon or lime.

Note:

Perhaps you could take a trip to Blue Lake, which is in Nelson Lake National Park in the Southern Alps. It is said to be the clearest water body in the world. You could virtually see its bottom on a closer look. Breath-taking birds, untouched beech forests, a treasure trove of outdoor adventures both land and sea. These are just a few of what's in store for you in New Zealand. This small country has served as a backdrop for many fantasy films but the effects you see on TV in the cinemas don't give it justice. You'll just have to experience it yourself.

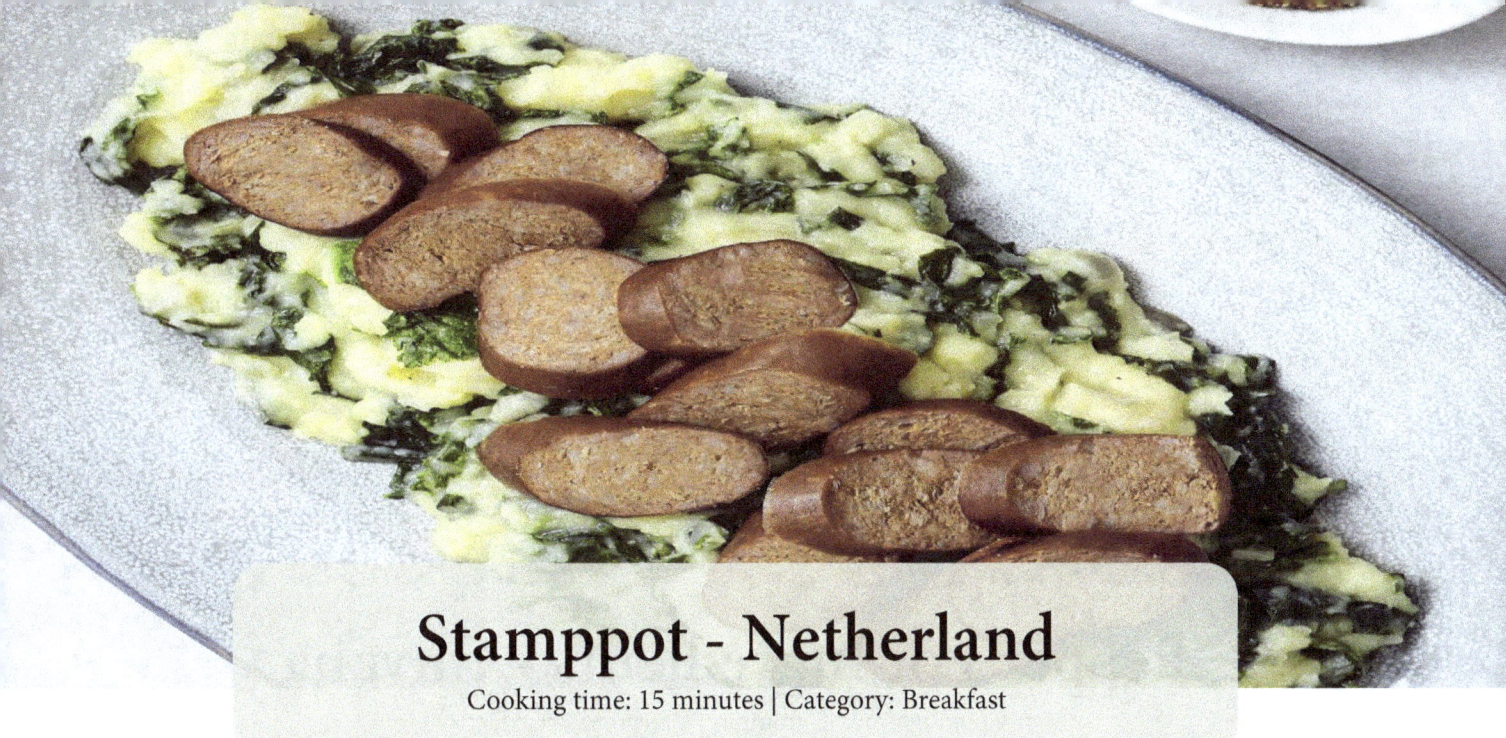

Stamppot - Netherland

Cooking time: 15 minutes | Category: Breakfast

Stamppot, also known as a hotspot, is the national dish of the Netherlands and a great choice for dinner after a tiring day. It is a hearty dish made of mashed potato, vegetables, and smoked sausages such as Dutch Rookworst, Spanish Chorizo, or Polish Kielbasa. There are different versions of this dish depending on whether kale, sauerkraut, or endives are used.

Ingredients

- 5 large Idaho russet potatoes, peeled and cut into 1-inch pieces (4 pounds)
- 4 teaspoons kosher salt, divided (plus more for seasoning)
- 2 tablespoons unsalted butter
- ½ cup 2% milk (or whole milk)
- ½ teaspoons freshly ground black pepper (plus more for seasoning)
- 3 tablespoons extra virgin olive oil, divided
- 1 medium onion, peeled and finely chopped
- 2 large cloves of garlic, peeled and minced (1 tablespoon)
- 1 bunch of curly kale, stemmed and chopped into ½-inch pieces (about 12 ounces)
- ¼ cup water & ½ teaspoon white wine vinegar
- 1 pound fully cooked, smoked pork sausage such as Dutch Rookworst (or substitute Spanish Chorizo or Polish Kielbasa), cut crosswise into thin slices
- 4-5 teaspoons olive oil, optional garnish
- 4 green onions trimmed and chopped, optional garnish.

Steps to Cook

1. Put potatoes and 2 teaspoons salt in a large pot. Cover with cold water. Bring to a boil over high heat.
2. Reduce to a simmer and cook until potatoes are tender, 10-15 minutes. Scoop out a cup of potato cooking water and set aside. Drain potatoes and return them to the pot.
3. Add butter, milk, 2 teaspoons salt, and ½ teaspoon pepper. Mash potatoes with a potato-masher. For creamier potatoes add potato cooking water, a little at a time, stirring, until you get the desired texture.
4. In a large heavy skillet or pot with a lid, heat 2 tablespoons of oil over medium-low heat.
5. Add onion and cook, stirring occasionally, for 6-7 minutes, until translucent.
6. Add garlic and cook for 30 seconds. Raise heat to medium.
7. Add kale, ¼ cup water, and ½ teaspoon vinegar. Cover pot and wait 2-3 minutes for the kale to wilt.
8. Remove cover and cook, stirring occasionally, for 3-4 minutes longer or until the kale is tender.
9. Sprinkle with a pinch of salt and a few grinds of black pepper. Add kale mixture to potatoes and mash until thoroughly combined.
10. In the same heavy skillet used for the kale, heat 1 tablespoon olive oil over medium-high heat.
11. Cook the sausages for 4-5 minutes, until nicely browned on both sides and heated through.
12. Divide the kale-potato mash between 4 or 5 bowls. Arrange sausages on top. Drizzle on a teaspoon of olive oil per bowl and sprinkle with chopped scallions, if you like. Enjoy!

Note:

Each 100g serving contains 148 calories. The Netherlands is famous for many Dutch brews, which include many well-known brands such as Heineken, Grolsch, and Amstel. When it comes to traveling to Europe, it's best to go DUTCH…. because the Netherlands is a destination you do not want to miss. See for yourself the sprawling rows of colorful tulips bordered by windmills, the amazing castle gardens, and fairy-tale-like the setting of Amsterdam's picturesque neighborhood and canals. rue, Netherlands may be small, but it is one of the happiest places in world to live in. With its efficient healthcare, excellent transportation, and inclusive society, you might just be tempted to stay.

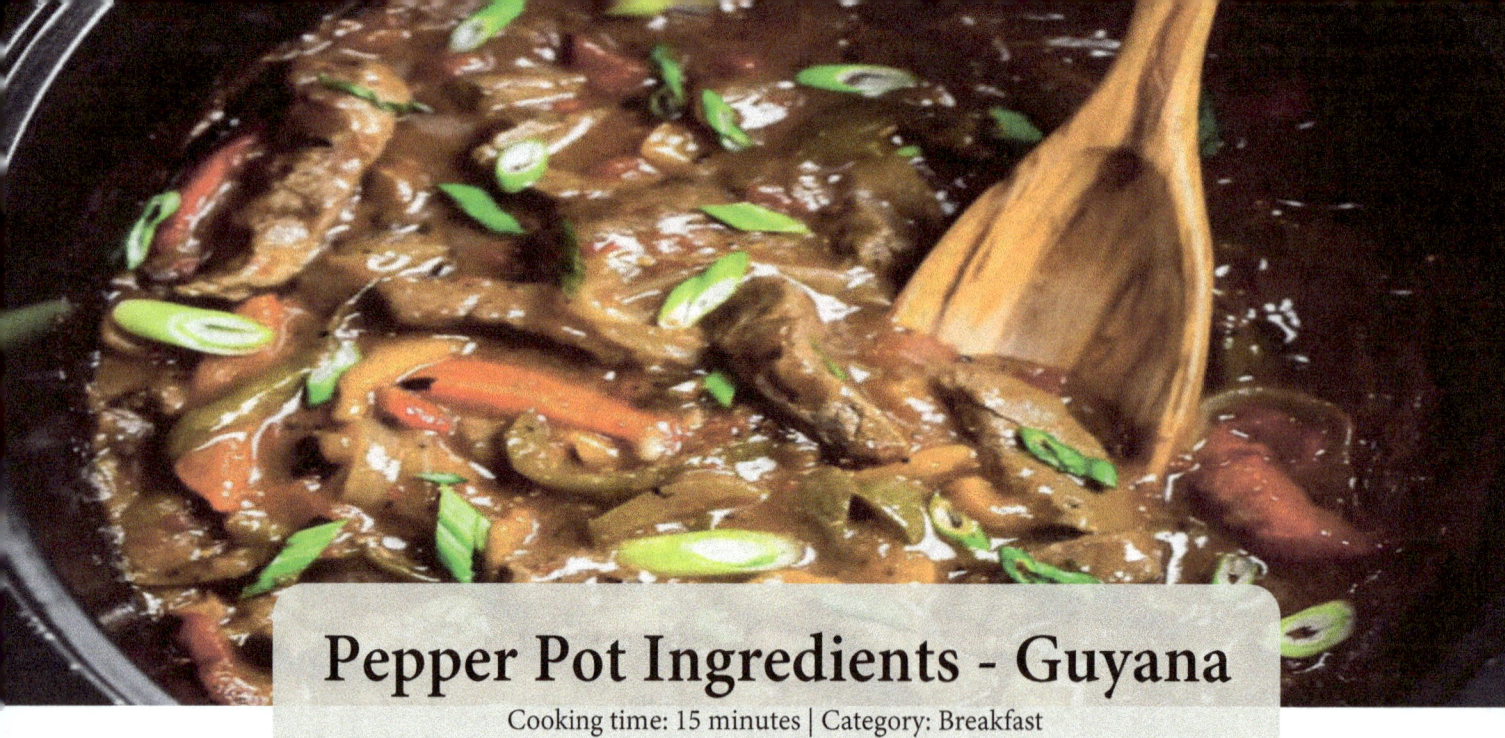

Pepper Pot Ingredients - Guyana

Cooking time: 15 minutes | Category: Breakfast

Cassareep is a thick, dark, heavily seasoned, molasses-like syrup made from yucca. Though scarce in North America, it is worth seeking out for the irresistible flavor it adds to this stew.

Ingredients

- 3 lbs. boneless stewing beef cubes, such as chuck, brisket, or bottom round
- 1 tsp salt
- 1/2 tsp black pepper
- 1 tbsp vegetable oil
- 1 large onion, chopped
- 4 garlic cloves, chopped
- 1/2 cup cassareep, (see tips)
- 2 habanero peppers, or 3 to 4 wiri wiri peppers, left whole or seeded and chopped
- 2-in. piece ginger, peeled and minced
- 3 tbsp brown sugar
- 2 3-inch strips of orange and e, zest, removed with a vegetable peeler
- 4 sprigs thyme
- 1 2-to 3-in. cinnamon sticks
- 1/4 tsp allspice, (optional)
- 3 whole cloves

Steps to Cook

1. 1. Pat beef dry and cut into 1 ½-inch pieces. Season with salt and pepper.
2. 2. Heat oil in a large pot or Dutch oven over medium heat.
3. 3. Add the meat in batches and brown on all sides. Transfer to a plate. Drain all but 1 tablespoon of fat from the pot (if necessary, add more fat) and add onion and garlic. Cook, stirring, until softened, about 6 minutes.
4. 4. Return the meat to the pot along with cassareep, habaneros, or wiri wiri peppers, ginger, brown sugar, orange zest, thyme, cinnamon stick, allspice, and cloves.
5. 5. Add enough water to the pot to just cover the meat. Bring to a boil, then reduce the heat, cover, and simmer gently over medium-low heat until the meat is completely tender about 3 hours. Remove the cinnamon stick, herb sprigs, and orange zest (and peppers, if left whole).
6. 6. Serve as a stew with crusty white bread. Or, to serve over rice, transfer the meat to a plate with a slotted spoon. Reduce the liquid in the pot over medium-high heat until it has thickened into a sauce.
7. Return the meat to the pot, let stand for a few minutes, and serve with cooked rice, Coconut Rice, Garnish with chopped cilantro.

Note:

Tips: Order cassareep online or find it at well-stocked Caribbean markets. If you cannot find it, substitute 1/3 cup molasses, 1 tablespoon soy sauce, and 1 tablespoon Worcestershire sauce. Guyana is quite famous for its rums as well. XM Supreme 15-year-old is a rum brand produced by the Banks DIH Limited. A taste of this rum is a feel of Guyana.

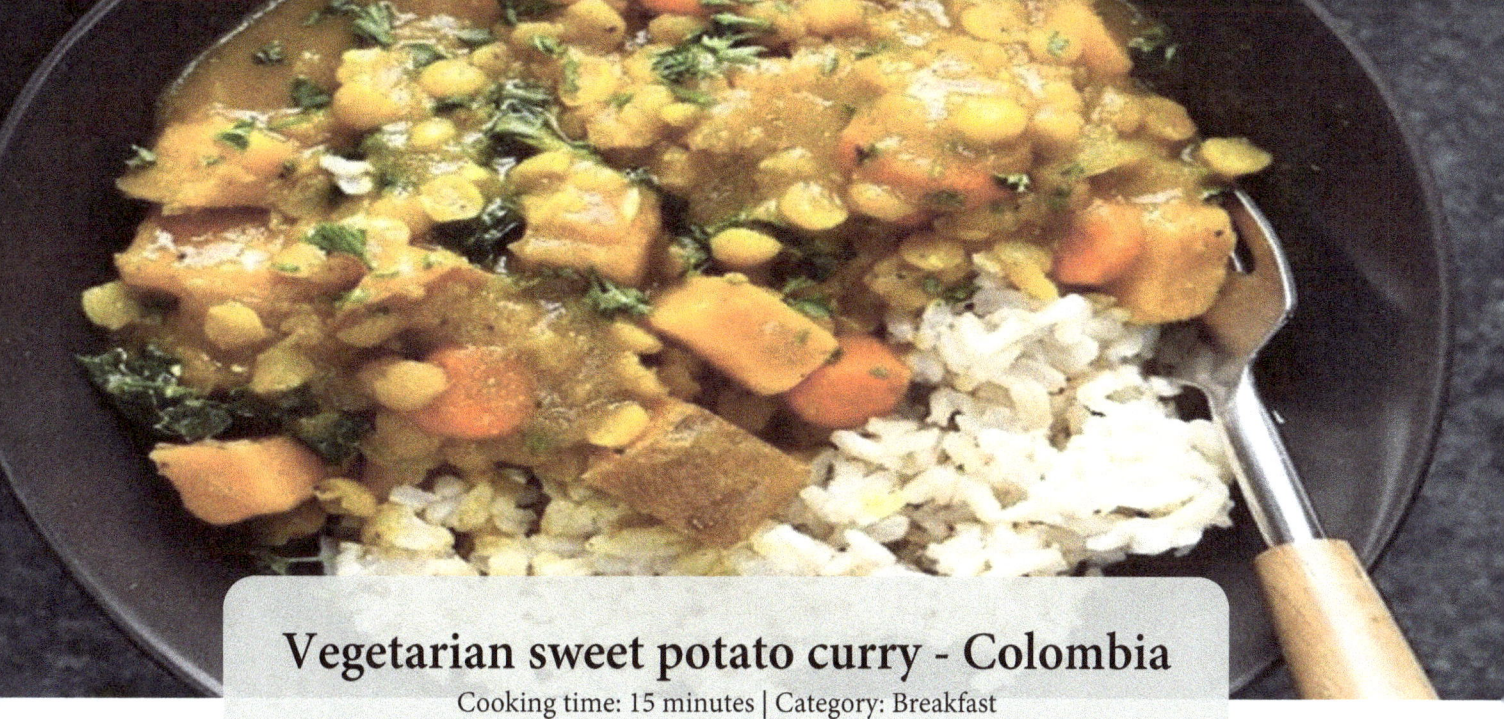

Vegetarian sweet potato curry - Colombia

Cooking time: 15 minutes | Category: Breakfast

This Easy Sweet Potato Curry is made in one pot (perfect for a weeknight meal) & makes the ultimate hearty meal. It is the perfect blend of flavors and is excellent for meal prep!

Ingredients

- 2 1/2 cups sweet potato (diced, about 1 medium)
- 2 1/2 cups eggplant (diced, about 1 small)
- 2 cups zucchini (diced, about 1 medium)
- 2 cups green beans (chopped, 1-inch long)
- 2 cups broccoli florets (chopped)
- 1 tablespoon coconut oil
- 2 large garlic cloves (minced)
- 29 ounces diced tomatoes (I used fire roasted)
- 27 ounces full-fat coconut milk
- 2 tablespoons soy sauce (or wheat-free tamari)
- 1 tablespoon ginger (freshly grated)
- 1 teaspoon red pepper flakes (optional)
- 1 cup of water (optional)
- fresh herbs (For serving, or grains, optional)
-

Steps to Cook

1. Ready all veggies, cutting them into bite-sized pieces. Set aside.
2. Turn Multi-Cooker onto the "Sauté" setting. Once preheated, add coconut oil, garlic, and sweet potatoes. Cook until sweet potatoes have started to brown, 2-3 minutes.
3. Pour in tomatoes and coconut milk and stir to combine.

Note:

Bird lovers and florists are sure to have a field day in this country. An adventure in the Andes, with the Aguardiente drink with some of the friendliest people ever will not be a bad idea

Week - 5

Reflections

- How was your practice of meditation & gratitude this week?
_____
_____
_____

- What new recipes did you try?
_____
_____
_____

- What new people & countries have you connected with this week?
_____
_____
_____

- Who did you share a meal with this week?
_____
_____
_____

- What are you observing about yourself?
_____
_____
_____

- What is your time for 1.5 miles run or walk?
_____
_____
_____

Seek out Accountability

Week 6

Week - 6

Take Obedient Action

- Spend 20 minutes writing in your gratitude journal about giving thanks & Practice meditation and prayer

_____

_____

_____

- Select 1 Dinner, 1 Lunch & 2 Breakfast recipes from week 6 & prepare them.

_____

_____

_____

- Connect with 4 people from 4 different countries digitally or in person

_____

_____

_____

- Visit a new supermarket this week
- Increase your cardio to 1.5 miles walk or run add 10 minutes of stretching

_____

_____

_____

- Record your assessment of health
    Blood Pressure_____

    Heart Rate_____

    Total Weight _____

    Body fat _____

    Girth measurement- waist, hip, chest _____

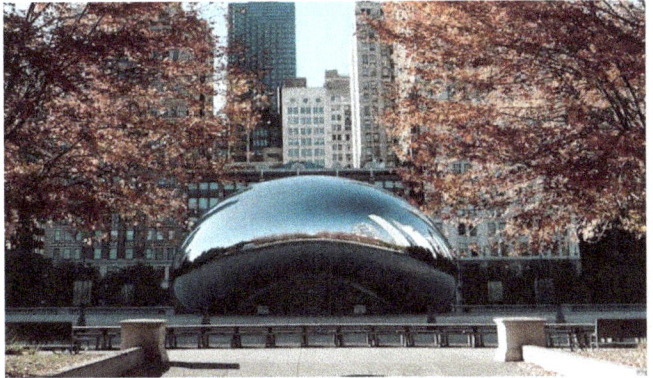

Illinois-Dinner

The Prairie State' (as nicknamed) is marked by farmland, forests, rolling hills, and wetlands.

Chicago, one of the largest cities in the U.S, is in the northeast on the shores of Lake Michigan.

It's famous for its skyscrapers and distinct deep-dish pizza and hot dogs.

Illinois is home to 'The Sears Tower in Chicago, the tallest building in America.

Chicago is the largest city in Illinois with a population of 2,720,546 people and ranks third in the country.

Illinois' state snack is popcorn

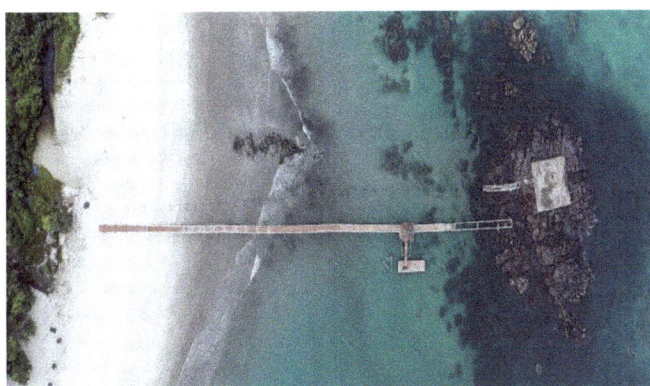

Sierra Leone-Breakfast

This western African country owes its name to the 15th-century Portuguese explorer.

The original Portuguese name, Serra Leone ('Lion Mountains'), referred to the range of hills that surrounds the harbor.

Sierra Leone's many waterways are the home to many varieties of fish, such as Bonga (a type of shad), butterfish, snapper, and sole.

The coastal waters contain such shellfish as shrimp, lobster, and oysters.

Freetown is Sierra Leone's capital city, largest city, and major commercial hub

Rice, the main food crop, is widely cultivated on swampland and upland farms.

The abundance of rice makes any meal with rice, incomplete. Rice lovers are in for a treat here!

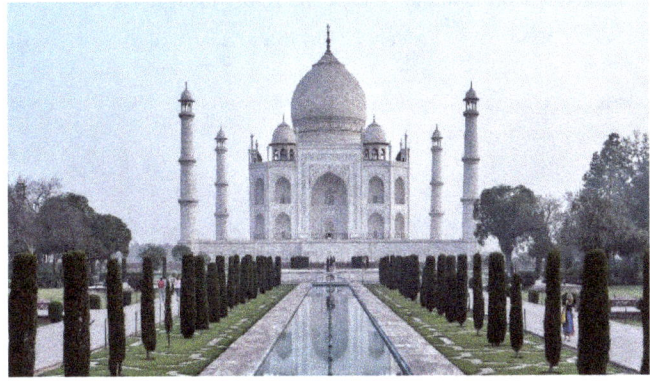

India-Lunch

India is officially called the Republic of India. The South Asian country boasts a very large expanse of land, that is densely populated with residents. It is the seventh-largest country by area, and the second-most populous country (1.37 billion people).

The multi-lingual (22 languages) home of Bollywood is the birthplace of yoga and Siddha medicine

There is a noticeable difference in the flavors of food cooked in the neighboring states of Tamil Nadu and Kerala. Similarly, the staple food in Goa is different from the food consumed in Maharashtra.

Each State is famous for its unique cuisine, and each State has lip-smacking good food — Butter Chicken, Fish-Curry Rice, Appam and Chicken Stew, Naan, Prawns Fry, Poha.

The capital city of India is New Delhi. A feel of India is a feel of these major cities: Mumbai, New Delhi, and Bangalore. India has the highest population of vegetarians on a global scale.

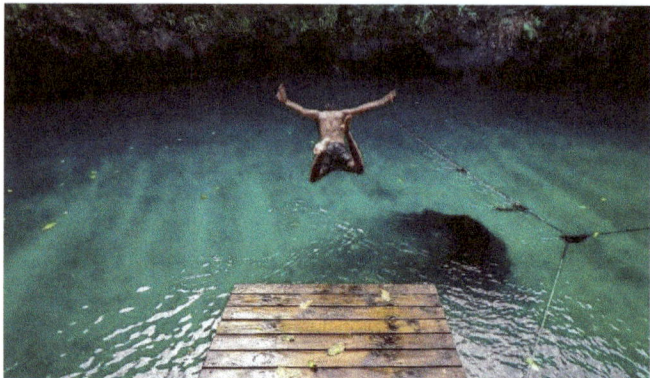

Samoa-Dinner

Also called the Cradle of Polynesia.

The current population of this Polynesian Island country is home to a variety of Islands of which some are currently inhabited.

Polynesia culture is reflected in the music, lifestyle, and visual art.

Samoans are beneficiaries of lush natural scenery, eye-popping beaches, mountain tops, as well as a boisterous aquatic life.

Cacao trees are very common in many families in Samoa.

The ingredients for Samoan staples are sourced from the land and seas.

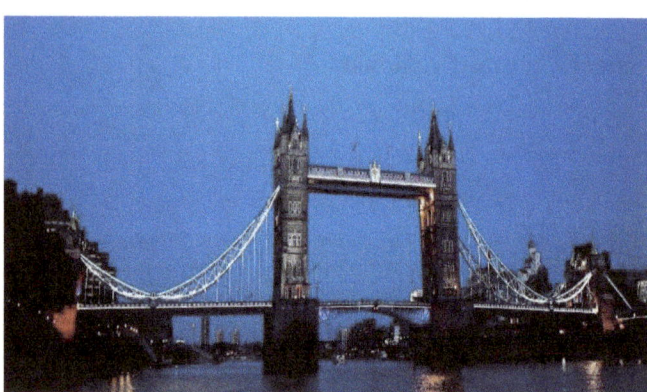

The United Kingdom-Breakfast

The United Kingdom made up of England, Scotland, Wales, and Northern Ireland is an island nation in north-western Europe.

England – the birthplace of Shakespeare and The Beatles – is home to the capital, London, a globally influential center of finance and culture.

The Clyde waterfront in Glasgow, Buckingham palace in London, and many more are must-go places

---

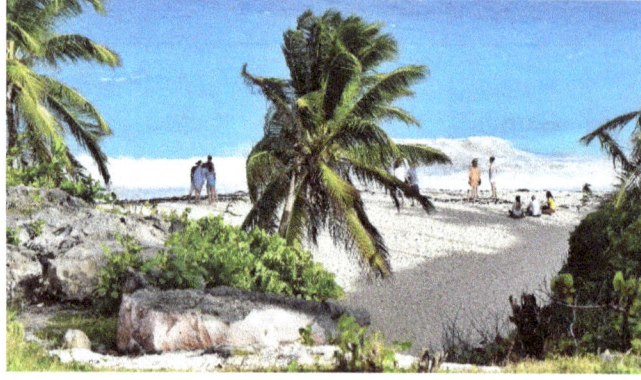

Barbados-Lunch

Barbados is a small island country in the south-eastern Caribbean Sea.

Its neighbors include Saint Lucia, to the north, Saint Vincent and the Grenadines, to the west, and Trinidad and Tobago to the south.

It is a flat island, but with Mount Hillaby rising via terraced tablelands to 336 meters.

Barbados is surrounded by coral reefs.

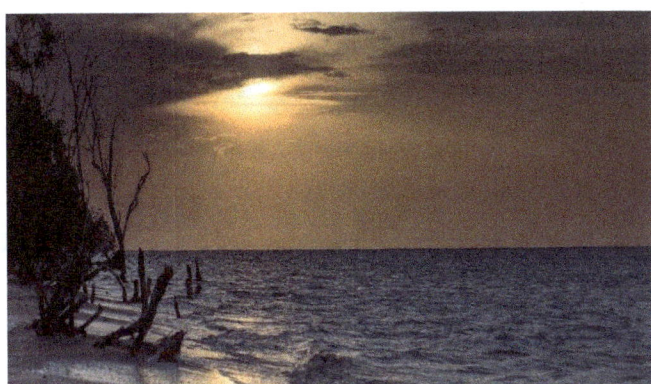

Suriname-Dinner

Suriname is the smallest country in South America.

It's defined by vast swaths of tropical rainforest, Dutch colonial architecture, and a melting-pot culture.

It has a population of 586,634 with its capital city in Paramaribo.

From party dishes to everyday meals, Suriname's cuisine features several colorful recipes.

The country's only true national dish is chicken and rice.

Pom (locally called pomtajer) was introduced by Portuguese-Jewish enslaved people and landowners as a potato casserole.

Potatoes needed to be imported, this ingredient was replaced with the tayer root.

The tayer root comes from the native plant Xanthosoma sagittifolium, also called the arrow leaf elephant ear.

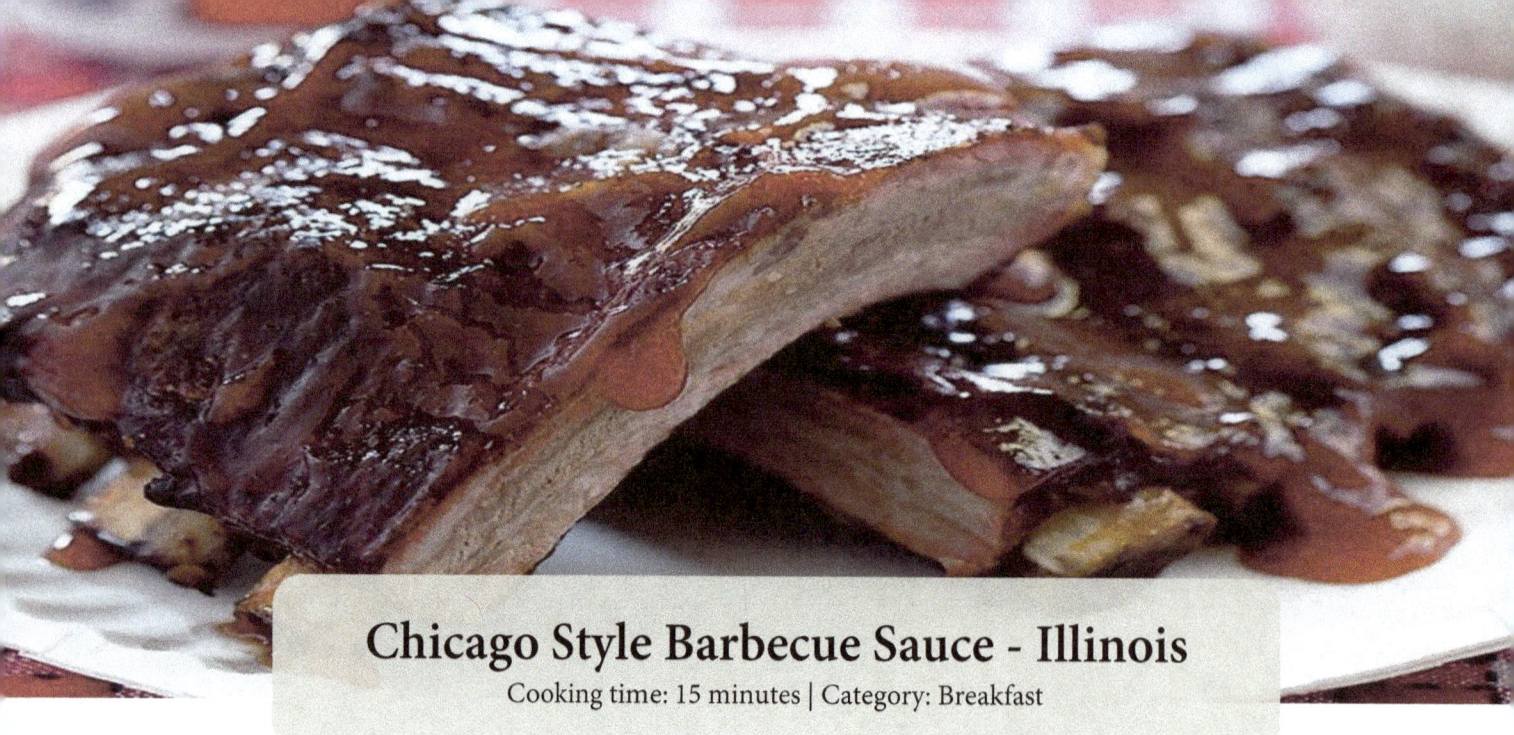

Chicago Style Barbecue Sauce - Illinois
Cooking time: 15 minutes | Category: Breakfast

This tasty barbecue dish is the best thing that ever happened to the entire Chicago! I assume you know why. The sauce is thick, flavorful, l and well garnished. It pairs well with citrus drinks. It is made with ketchup and a combination of spices like garlic, kosher salt, black pepper, celery seed etc.

Ingredients

- 1/3 cup ketchup
- 1/3 cup pineapple juice
- 1/4 cup packed brown sugar
- 2 tbs granulated sugar
- 2 tbs apple cider vinegar
- 1 tsp hot sauce
- 1 tsp hot sauce
- 1 tsp mustard powder
- 1 tbs Worcestershire sauce
- 1 tsp kosher salt
- 1 tsp black pepper
- 1 tsp garlic powder
- 1 tsp onion powder
- 1/2 tsp ground celery seed

Steps to Cook

1. Add all ingredients to a large saucepan and mix well.
2. Simmer over medium heat for 30 minutes.
3. Let the sauce cool to room temperature.
4. Recipe may be doubled.

Note:

Each serving contains 194.7 calories. Feed your delights with the sheer awesomeness of Illinois from the millennium park. Music lovers will absolutely enjoy it!

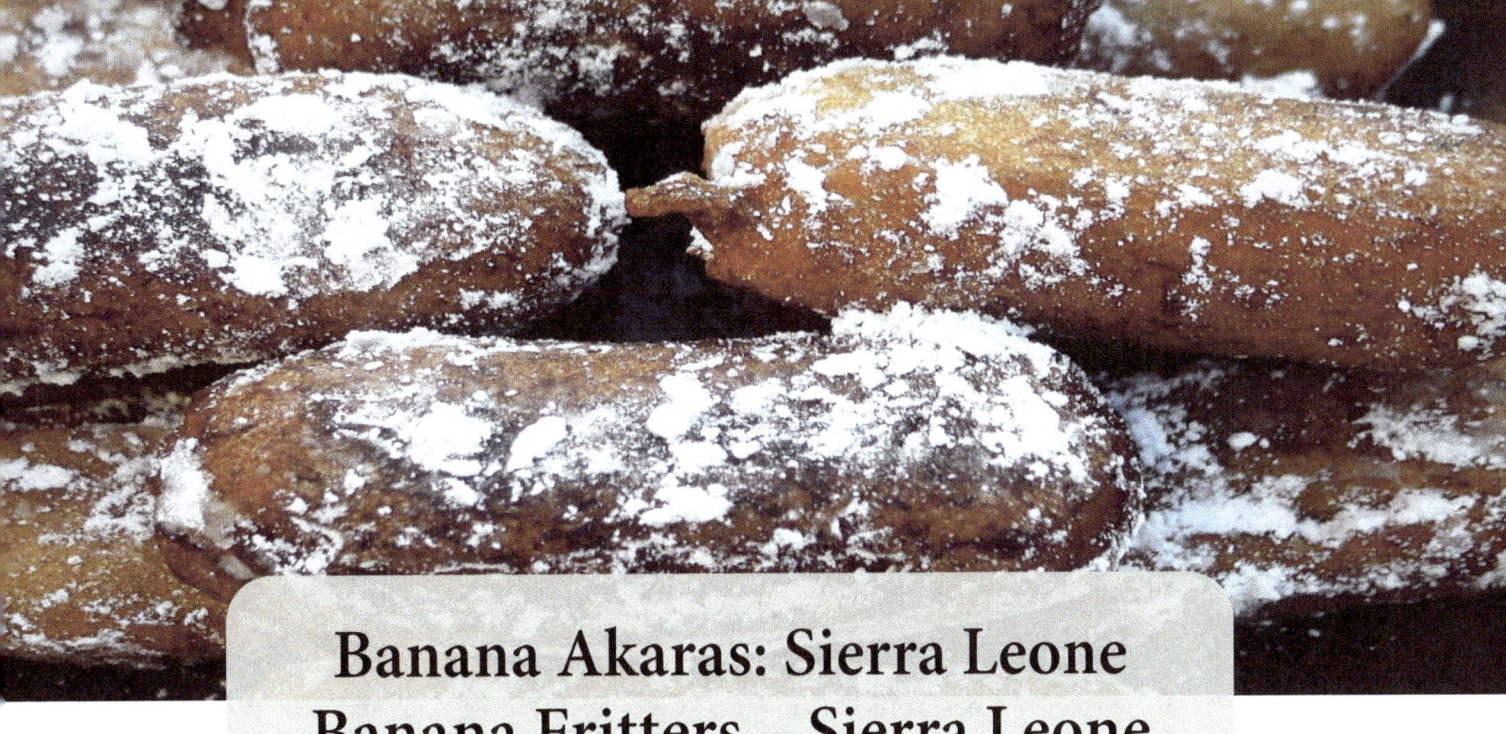

Banana Akaras: Sierra Leone
Banana Fritters – Sierra Leone

Cooking time: 15 minutes | Category: Breakfast

Akaras appear in a multitude of recipes throughout the world, both sweet and savory.

These banana akaras are a favorite breakfast in Sierra Leone. Light and fluffy, but also gluten-free, the taste and texture of these fritters are like banana pancakes combined with doughnuts.

They're also ready in just 20 minutes, from start to finish, so they're the perfect breakfast for your days off when you want to cook yourself breakfast, but don't want to spend your entire morning in the kitchen.

Ingredients

- 4 bananas, ripe
- 1 cup rice flour
- 1/2 cup sugar
- 1 vanilla bean, split and scraped, or 1 teaspoon vanilla extract
- 1/2 cup hot water
- Oil, for deep-frying
- Powdered sugar, to garnish

Steps to Cook

1. In a mixing bowl, mash the bananas, vanilla, and sugar until reaching a smooth consistency.
2. Gradually add the rice flour and then hot water while mixing in the food processor bowl. The mixture should be moist but not liquid.
3. Let cool for 20 minutes.
4. Heat oil in a non-stick pan.
5. Drop a spoonful of the batter into the oil. Pay attention to leaving enough space between each fritter and fry on both sides until browned.
6. Sprinkle with powdered sugar.

Note:

Groundnut stew, Sierra Leone's national dish is a bundle of deliciousness. To immerse yourself in the beauty of Sierra Leone's culture, you need a glass of polo. Poyo is palm wine, a favorite native adult beverage. it is meant to be drunk straight out of the tree, it is mildly alcoholic, maybe 1% alcohol. An undiscovered jewel in West Africa, Sierra Leone tucks a wealth of spectacular beaches and wildlife sanctuaries. An adventurous spirit cannot resist its hidden charms like the busy port city of Freetown, Tacugama Chimpanzee Sanctuary, Banana Island, and Kambui Hills Forest Reserve. Eager to take a souvenir home? Just go to Bo's Big Market to shop for West African fabrics and local treats like coconut cake and groundnut shortbread.

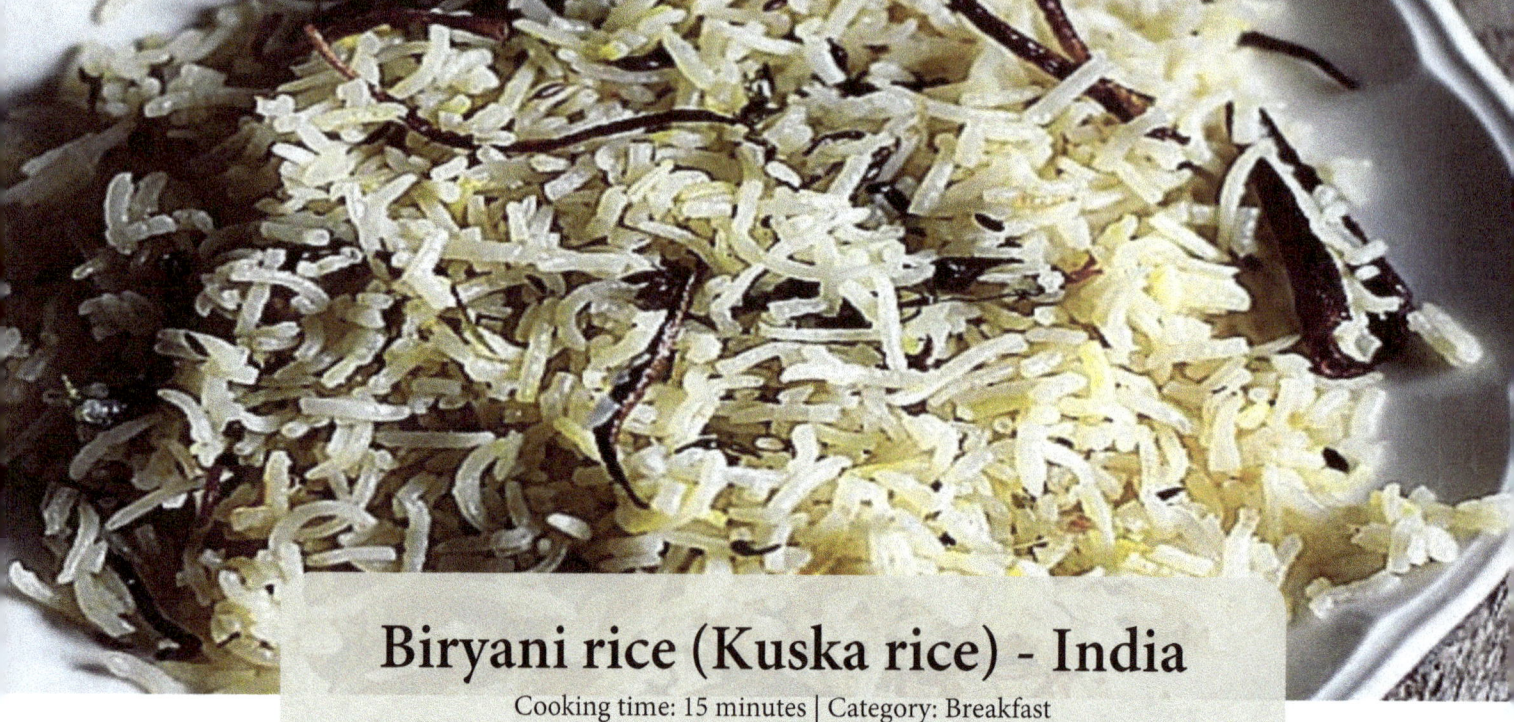

Biryani rice (Kuska rice) - India

Cooking time: 15 minutes | Category: Breakfast

A unique way of preparing the popular biryani recipe without any vegetables or meat with just basmati rice and spices. it is a popular south Indian biryani recipe, particularly from the Hyderabadi cuisine, and is typically served with kurma or salan recipe.

Ingredients

Kuska main Ingredients
- 1 cup Basmati Rice & 2 cups Water
- 1 cup Sliced Onions 2 Medium Sized Onions
- ½ cup Finely Chopped Tomatoes 2 Small Tomatoes
- 1 Green Chili
- 2 tablespoons of Oil
- 1 Cinnamon Piece & 2 Cloves
- 1 Green Cardamom
- 1 Small Piece Kalpasi & 1 Dried Bay Leaf
- 2 tablespoons Curd
- 1 teaspoon Kashmiri Red Chili Powder
- ¼ teaspoon Turmeric Powder
- ¼ cup Finely Chopped Coriander Leaves
- ¼ cup Finely Chopped Mint Leaves
- Salt as needed

Kuska Masala Paste
- 8-10 Garlic Pods
- 2 Ginger Piece
- 2 Green Chilies
- ½ teaspoon Fennel Seeds
- 2 Cinnamon Piece
- 2 Cloves
- 2 Green Cardamoms

Steps to Cook

1. Wash and soak the basmati rice in 2 cups of water for 15-20 mins.
2. Make a paste of all the ingredients under kuska masala paste by adding little water and set aside.
3. In a heavy bottomed pan, heat oil. Add dried bay leaf, cloves, cardamom, and cinnamon. Fry for a few seconds.
4. Add slit green chili along with chopped onions. Fry until translucent.
5. Next add the prepared paste and fry for a few minutes until the raw smell goes off.
6. Add chopped tomatoes and cook until mushy.
7. Next add turmeric powder, red chili powder, and salt as needed. Fry off for 2-3 mins.
8. Add thick curd and mix well, cook for a couple of minutes.
9. Now add finely chopped mint and coriander leaves.
10. Next pour the water from the soaked basmati rice and add salt if needed.
11. As the water begins to boil, add soaked basmati rice – mix well.
12. Close the pan with a lid and cook on low flame for 12-15 minutes.
13. Switch off the heat and let it rest for 5-10 mins before opening it. Fluff up the rice.
14. Serve hot with onion raita.

Note:

The number of calories per serving of Rice Biryani is 145.5calories. Nightlife buzz is a common weekend delight in several cities such as Delhi, Mumbai, and Bangalore are buzzing with activity. Chai is goodness in Indian drinks you would miss upon leaving India! A country with rich history and culture, India is a popular destination for budget travelers due to its amazing views, iconic landmarks, ancient temples, dynamic cuisine, and colorful cities that will leave you enthralled. It is the home of the world-famous Taj Mahal and the world's coldest desert.

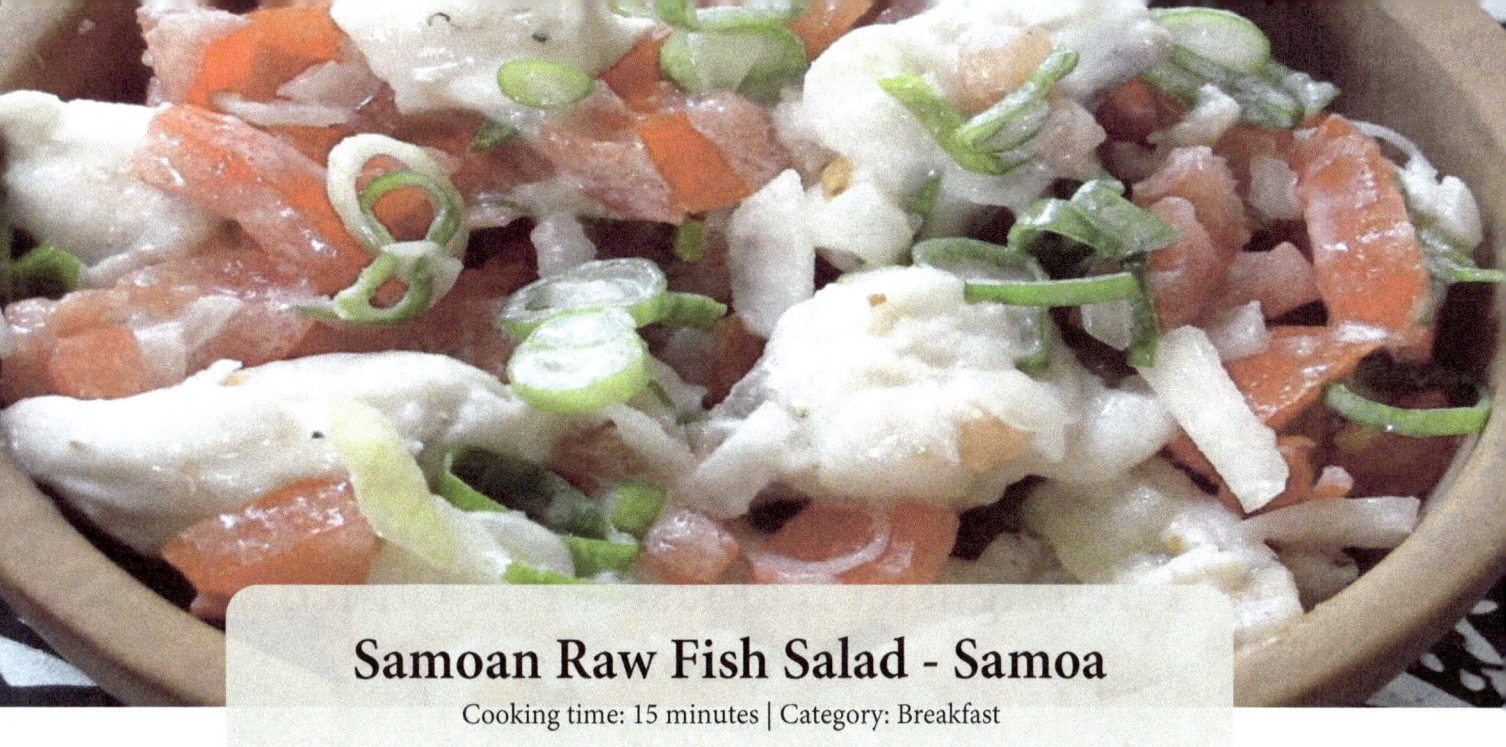

Samoan Raw Fish Salad - Samoa

Cooking time: 15 minutes | Category: Breakfast

This delicious Samoan fish salad is everything healthy. Recipes can be tweaked to suit your choice ingredients; but fresh fish, coconut, and citrus are not optional

One bite of this fish salad leaves you wanting more

Ingredients

- 1 lb. snapper or tuna (any fresh one)
- 1/2 cup Lemon or lime juice fresh squeezed
- 1/4 onion diced
- 2 green onions
- 2 small tomatoes diced
- 1 cucumber Peeled, seeded, and diced
- 1 cup Coconut milk
- 1 serrano minced (optional)
- salt to taste

Steps to Cook

1. Cut up your fish into bite-size pieces
2. Add to a bowl with citrus juice
3. Marinate for 12-15 mins. The fresh citrus cooks the fish
4. Cut the vegetables to bite size pieces
5. Drain the fresh citrus from the fish and add the vegetables
6. Add in the coconut milk
7. Add salt to taste
8. Refrigerate for about an hour to let all the flavors meld together and serve

Note:

The Calories content per serving is 238kcal.

It might interest you to know that Apia is the only city in Samoa boasting a population of about 37,000.

Kava is a famous Samoan beverage known for its sedative properties.

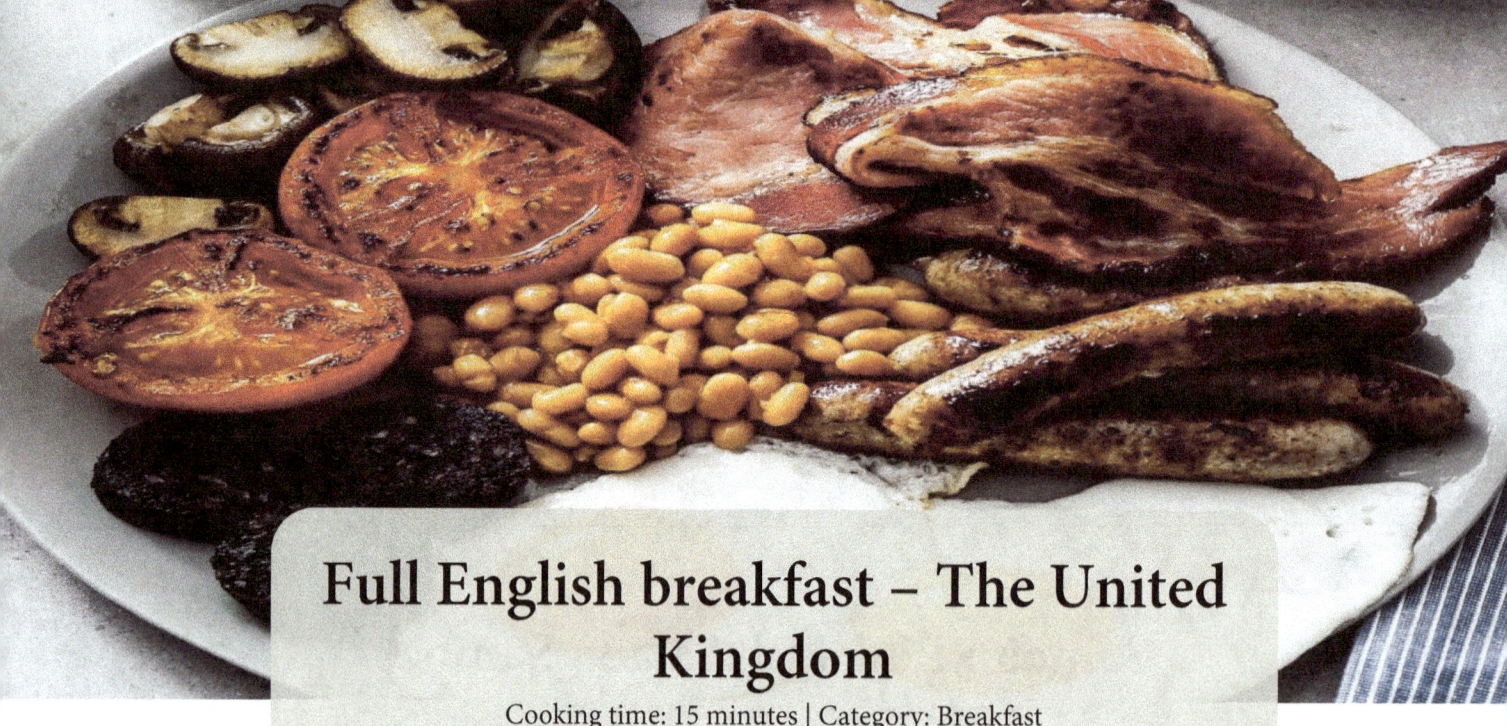

Full English breakfast – The United Kingdom

Cooking time: 15 minutes | Category: Breakfast

Sometimes called a fry-up, a full English is a hearty, hefty breakfast plate served in the UK and Ireland. Full English breakfasts are so popular that they're pretty much offered throughout the day as all-day breakfast.

Full English breakfasts contain sausages, back bacon, eggs, tomatoes, mushrooms, fried bread, and beans.

Ingredients

- 1 can beans Heinz preferred
- 4 links sausages breakfast sausage preferred
- 4 slices back bacon or Irish bacon
- 4 slices of black pudding optional... some say
- 1 cup mushrooms halved or sliced
- 2 small tomatoes halved
- 4 slices of bread
- 4 eggs
-

Steps to Cook

1. Heat the beans over low in a small pot. Keep warm on low.
2. Cook the sausages over medium to medium-low heat, turning occasionally, until brown and cooked through. In the same pan, cook the bacon, flipping as needed. Fry the blood pudding slices over medium heat for 3-4 minutes per side.
3. In another pan, heat a bit of oil and cook the mushrooms, without moving, until brown and caramelized.
4. Remove from the pan, then sear the cut side of the tomato briefly. Remove from the pan, and season everything with salt and pepper
5. Wipe the pan down and heat a bit of oil or butter over medium heat. Fry the bread until golden, flipping and adding more oil or butter as needed.
6. Remove and set aside.
7. Finally, fry the eggs to your liking. Plate everything up: sausages, bacon, black pudding, mushrooms, tomato, bread, and eggs. Enjoy immediately!

Note:

The number of calories per serving is 1684 calories. Fordwich is the smallest town in the U.K, which has around 400 residents.

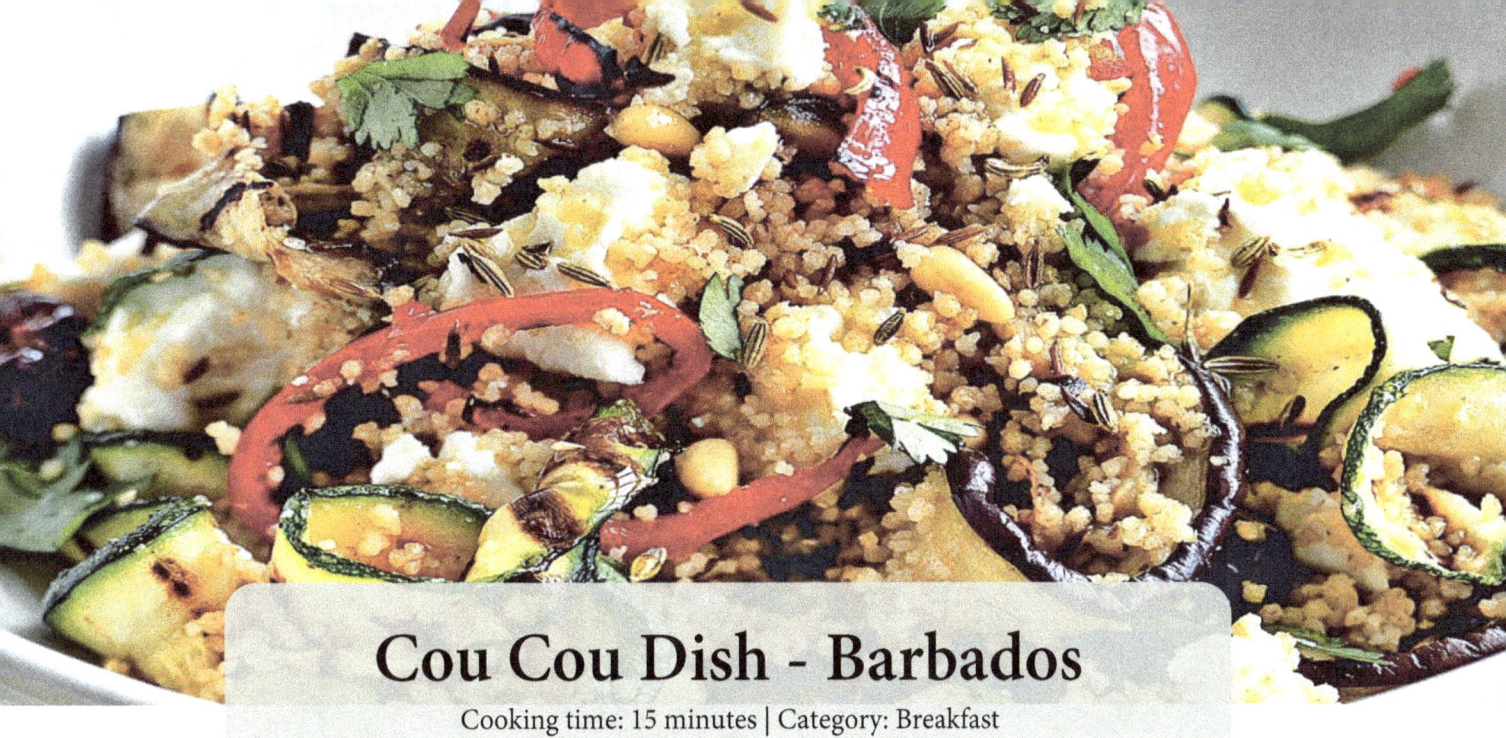

Cou Cou Dish - Barbados

Cooking time: 15 minutes | Category: Breakfast

Cou Cou is a Barbadian dish most often served with the Barbadian national food, flying fish.

It slightly resembles grits or polenta and consists of cornmeal, water, butter, spices, and okra. It is a great side dish to accompany fish and vegetables!

Ingredients

- 1 cup water, plus more for boiling
- 1 cup coarse ground cornmeal
- 4 okra pods
- 1/2 tsp thyme
- 1/2 tsp marjoram
- 3 tbsp butter, plus more for serving
- 1 tsp salt, plus more to taste

Steps to Cook

1. Cut the ends off of the okra pods.
2. Boil about 6 cups of water. Once boiling add the mixture to the two cups of boiling water. Add seasoning and mix to combine.
3. After four minutes, add 3 tbsp of butter.
4. Mix until the mixture becomes stiff (about twenty or so minutes). You will know when the Cou Cou is complete when you remove it from the sides of the pan, and it sticks in place. You can also do the spoon test. If you stick a wooden spoon into the middle of the Cou Cou and it does not fall over (and is fairly easy to remove), the Cou Cou is ready.
5. To serve, take a single serving dish and rub it with melted butter. Form the Cou Cou into the dish, then turn the dish over onto the dinner plate, leaving a mound of Cou Cou! Enjoy!

Note:

You might want to Bask in the essence of Orchid World & Tropical Flower Garden.

The Rum Island is a drink you sure will not miss in Barbados.

The number of calories is 296.4 calories.

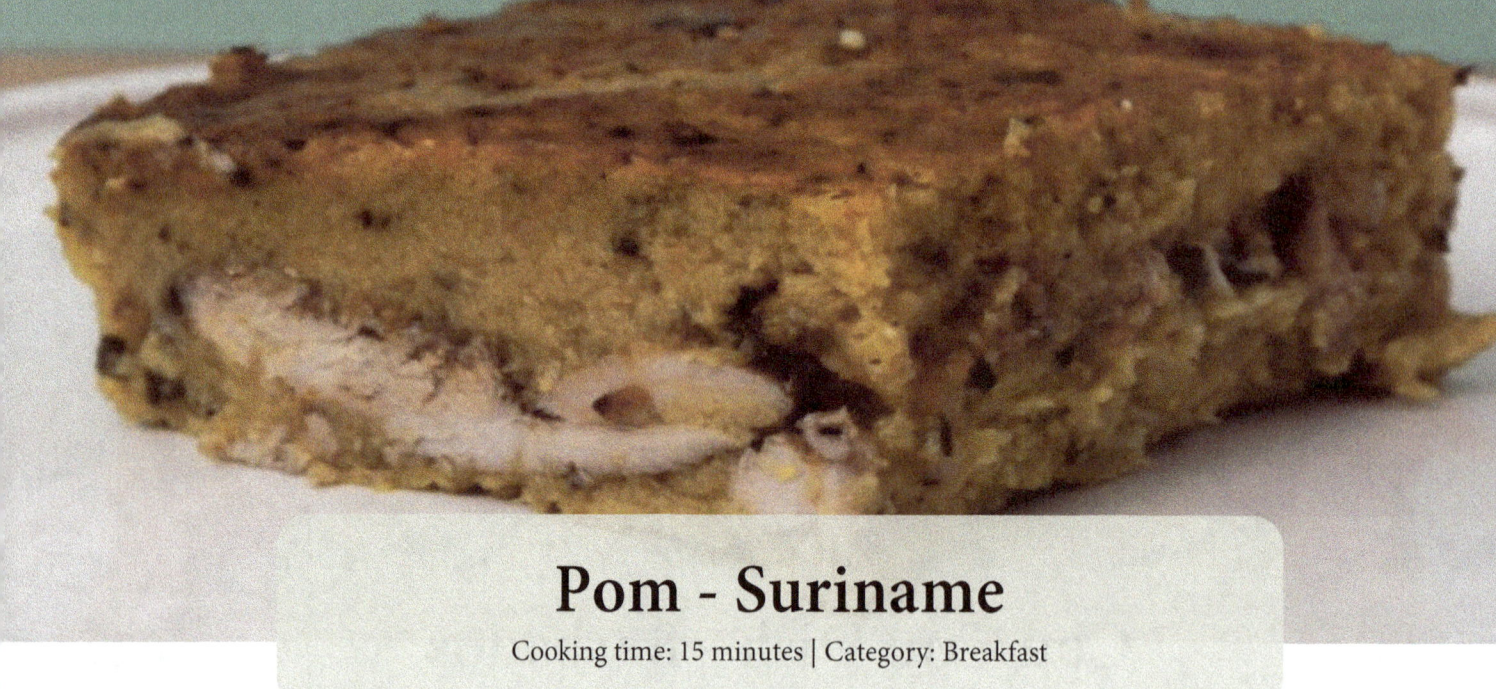

Pom - Suriname

Cooking time: 15 minutes | Category: Breakfast

The pom dish includes chicken and shredded tayer root. It is often served at celebrations, along with roti, an Indonesian grilled flatbread, and this is stuffed with chicken masala, potato, and vegetables. Pom has also become popular in the Netherlands.

Ingredients

Chicken Filling

- 6 tablespoons olive oil divided
- 2 small onions diced
- 1 lb. skinless boneless chicken breasts cut into 2-inch chunks
- 2 teaspoons salt
- 1 teaspoon white pepper ground
- 2 cups tomatoes chopped
- 2 cups chicken stock
- 1 tablespoon tomato puree
- 1/2 cup coconut milk
- 2 oranges juice and zest of
- 1 tablespoon coconut sugar
- 1 teaspoon allspice ground
- 1 teaspoon nutmeg ground
- 1/4 cup piccalilli or spicy relish
- 2 tablespoons sambal oelek or to taste
- 1 cup flat-leaf parsley chopped
- Grated Potato or Pomtajer Topping
- 1 pound russet potatoes peeled and grated
- 1 white onion peeled and grated
- 3 eggs
- 1 teaspoon paprika powder
- 1 teaspoon ground black pepper
- 1 teaspoon salt

Steps to Cook

Cook Onions and Chicken

1. Take the juice of one orange, a dash of salt, and your chicken pieces into a mixing bowl. Massage the salt and citrus juice into the chicken, then let sit for several minutes while you tend to your onions
2. Heat 2 tablespoons of olive oil in a large wok or saucepan over medium-high heat.
3. Add in your onions and stir.
4. Cook the onions for 5-6 minutes as they turn translucent, then take a slotted spatula to remove them. Set aside
5. Drain the orange juice from the mixing bowl of chicken, then add your chicken into the same wok/saucepan with two more tablespoons of olive oil, salt, and pepper
6. Sear your chicken for 2-3 minutes on each side as the outside starts to brown.

Prepare Your Pom Filling

1. As the chicken browns, add back in the onions as well as the chopped tomatoes, chicken stock, and tomato purée. Stir well.
2. Next, add the coconut milk, orange juice, piccalilli (or relish), sambal, sugar, allspice, and nutmeg into the pan. Stir well.
3. Add in some freshly chopped parsley and take the pan off of direct heat. Stir, then transfer the entire mixture into a non-stick (or oiled) casserole dish.

Make and Layer Pom Crust

1. Start by preheating your oven to 375 degrees Fahrenheit.
2. Next, begin grating the peeled potatoes and onion into a large mixing bowl. Stir to combine.
3. Add in eggs, paprika powder, salt, and pepper. Mix thoroughly. Feel free to use your hands.
4. Once the potatoes are well mixed and coated in eggs and spices, carefully spread the grated mixture over top of your casserole dish. You want to cover every possible square inch of surface area so that the chicken is encapsulated in the casserole dish.
5. Place your pom in the oven and bake for 45 minutes or until your potato crust is golden brown and has a nice crunch to it.
6. Serve pom with some stir-fried green beans or just enjoy it on its own.

Note:

Each serving contains 322kcal. Dawat, of Indonesian origin, is a popular summer drink in Suriname. The Suriname style of the traditional vegan Indonesian drink is cool and refreshing

Week - 6

Reflections

- How was your practice of prayer, meditation & gratitude this week?

_____
_____
_____
_____
_____

- What new supermarket did you visit this week?

_____
_____
_____
_____
_____

- What are you observing about yourself?

_____
_____
_____
_____
_____

- Describe how is your body feeling?

_____
_____
_____
_____
_____

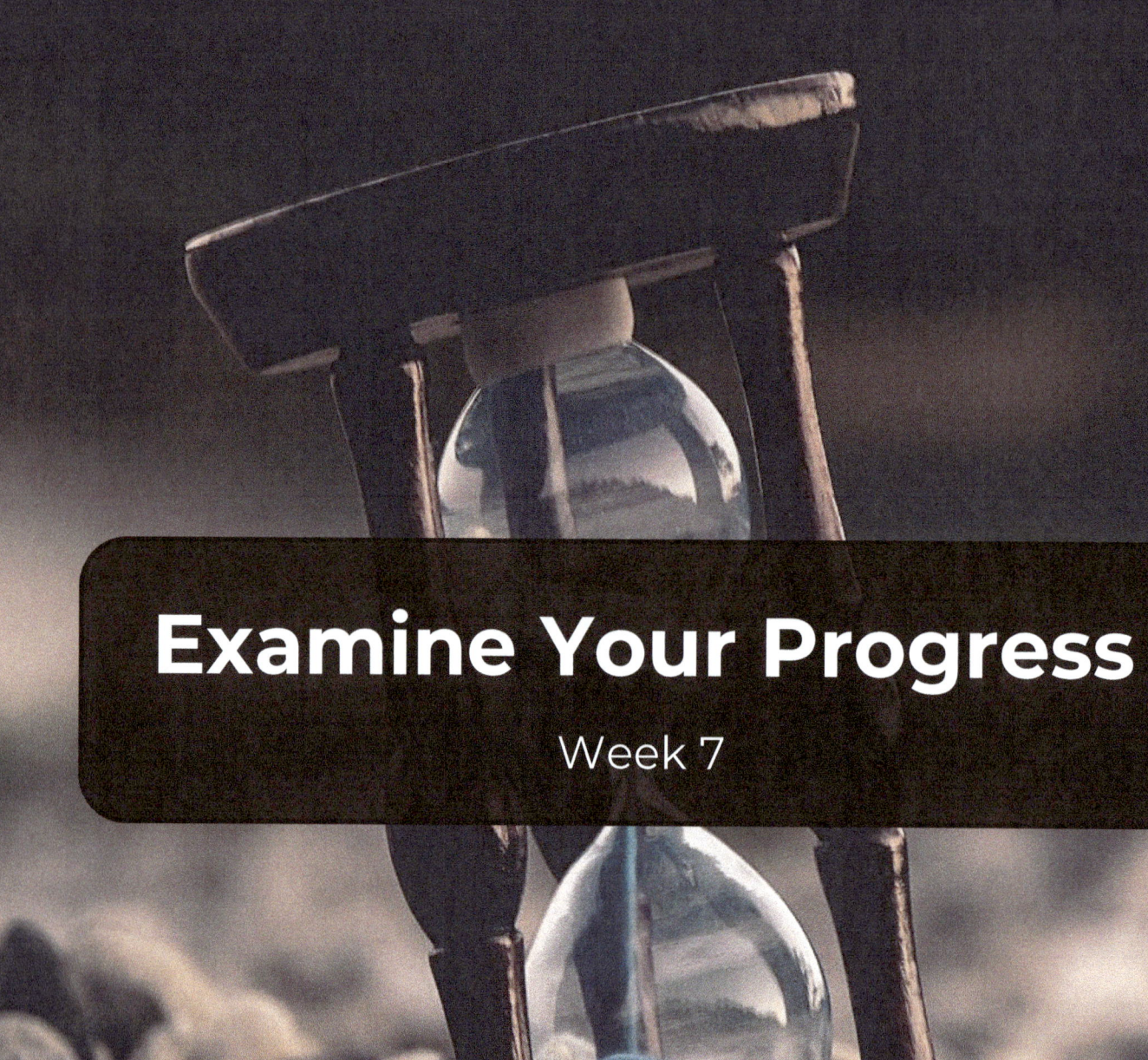

Week - 7

Take Obedient Action

- Spend 20 minutes practicing prayer, meditation & writing in your gratitude journal

---

- Select 2 Dinner recipes from week 7 & prepare them.

- Connect with 4 people from 4 different countries digitally or in person

---

- Connect with old friends from the last 6 weeks

- Try a new leaner protein this week

- Increase your cardio to 2.5 miles of walking or running add 10 minutes of stretching 5 strength training exercises

---

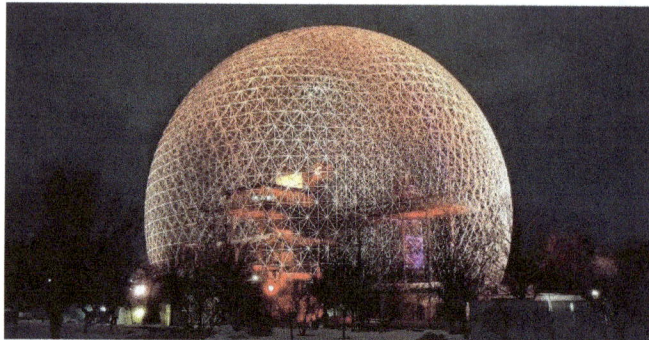

Montreal-Breakfast

Montréal is the largest city in Canada's Québec province.

It's set on an island in the Saint Lawrence River and named after Mt. Royal, the triple-peaked hill at its heart.

Montreal is the second-most-populous city in Canada and the principal metropolis of the province of Quebec.

The city of Montreal occupies about three-fourths of Montreal Island.

It happens to be the second largest French-speaking country after Paris.

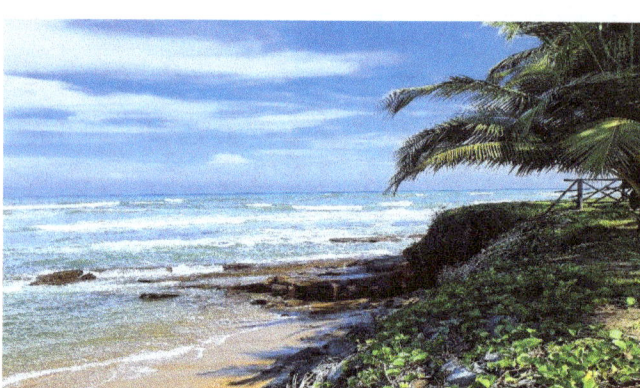

Ghana-Lunch

Ghana is a country of western Africa situated on the coast of the Gulf of Guinea. Although relatively small in area and population. Current population amounts to 31,978,740 .

The West African country is the 2nd largest producer of cocoa. The capital city of Ghana is Accra. Traditional Ghanaian food is typified by the distribution of food crops. With the prominence of tropical produce like corn, beans, millet, plantains, and cassava, most ethnic groups creatively employ these foodstuffs to make mouth-watering dishes for their nourishment.

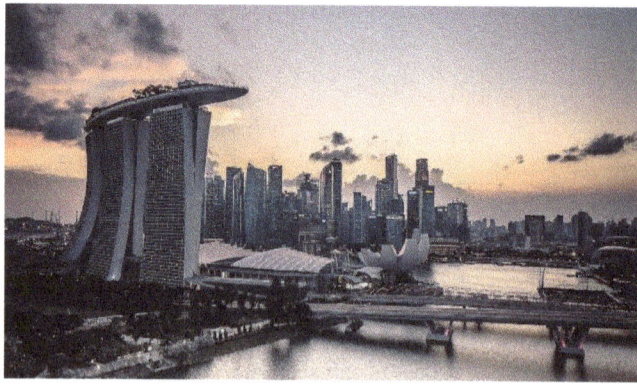

Singapore-Dinner

Singapore is not a single island, but 63 in all, comprising other offshore islands.

The tallest indoor waterfall in the world is in Singapore at the Gardens by the Bay, and it stands at a height of 35 meters.

About 5.8 million people live in Singapore (2021).

Singapore is an island country on the Asian continent.

The country is in Southeast Asia. The country's islands are located between Malaysia and Indonesia.

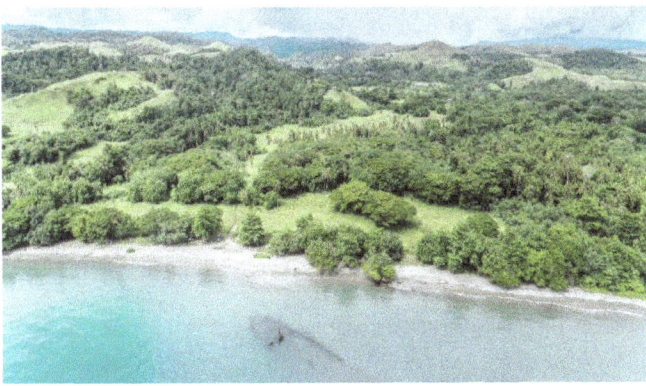

Solomon Islands-Breakfast

The Solomon Islands is a sovereign country in Oceania.

With an average Population of 685,097.

Its Capital city is Honiara.

Only 347 of the islands are populated.

The six major islands are Choiseul, Guadalcanal, Malaita, Makira, New Georgia and Santa Isabel.

Finally, dense rainforest covers around 90% of the islands.

The beauty of bio-varieties in plant and animal life, as well as the marine vegetation.

This informs why fish is considered the staple meat in this country.

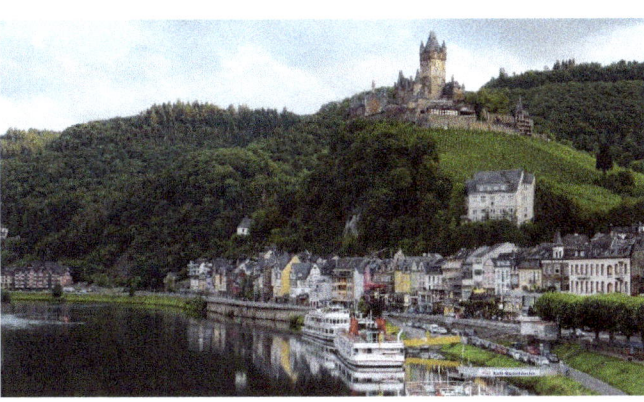

Germany-Lunch

This West European Country has a population of over 82 million people.

Germany is Europe's most industrialized and populous country.

Famed for its technological achievements. Germany has blazed many trails in terms of music, philosophy, and poetry.

Berlin is the capital city of Germany.

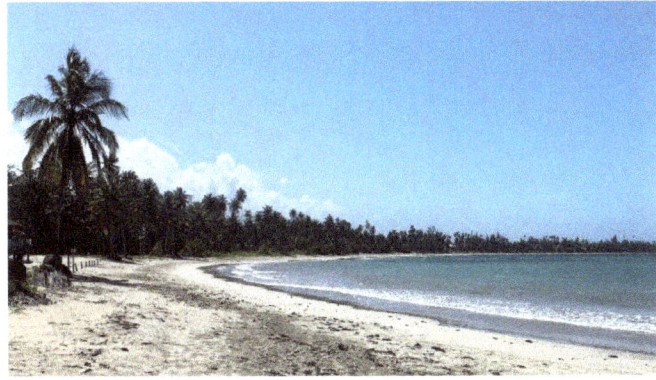

Puerto Rico-Dinner

Puerto Rico is a Caribbean Island and unincorporated U.S. territory with a landscape of mountains, waterfalls, and the historic El Yunque tropical rainforest.

San Juan, the capital and largest city, the Isla Verde area is known for its hotel strip, beach bars and casinos.

Diversity in history and culture, uniqueness in recipes, majestic mountains, relaxation, adventure — all in this Caribbean Island. A feeling of La Isla del Encanto is a feeling of hospitality.

Medieval history, poly-diverse culture, architecture, clement weather, fun attractions, exquisite cuisine, and hospitable people make this Caribbean Island a choice Island for many.

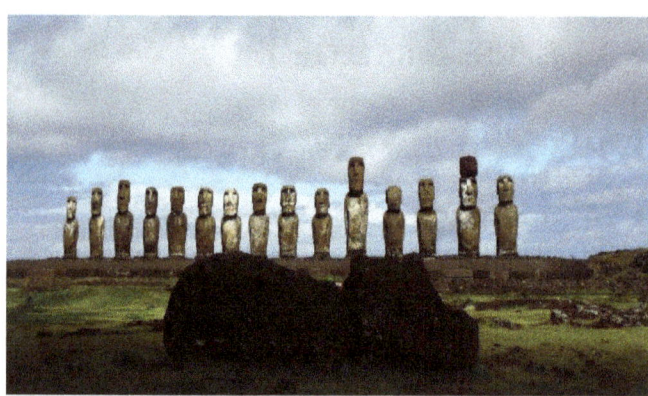

Chile-Lunch

A feel of Chile is a feel of these five major cities Santiago, Puente Alto, Antofagasta, and Vina del Mar.

The capital of Chile is Santiago.

The South American country has the driest place (Atacama Desert) on earth and the largest swimming pool.

How interesting!

Chile boasts of historic mountains, composite volcanoes, and robust wine producing structures.

The current population of Chile is 19,345,681.

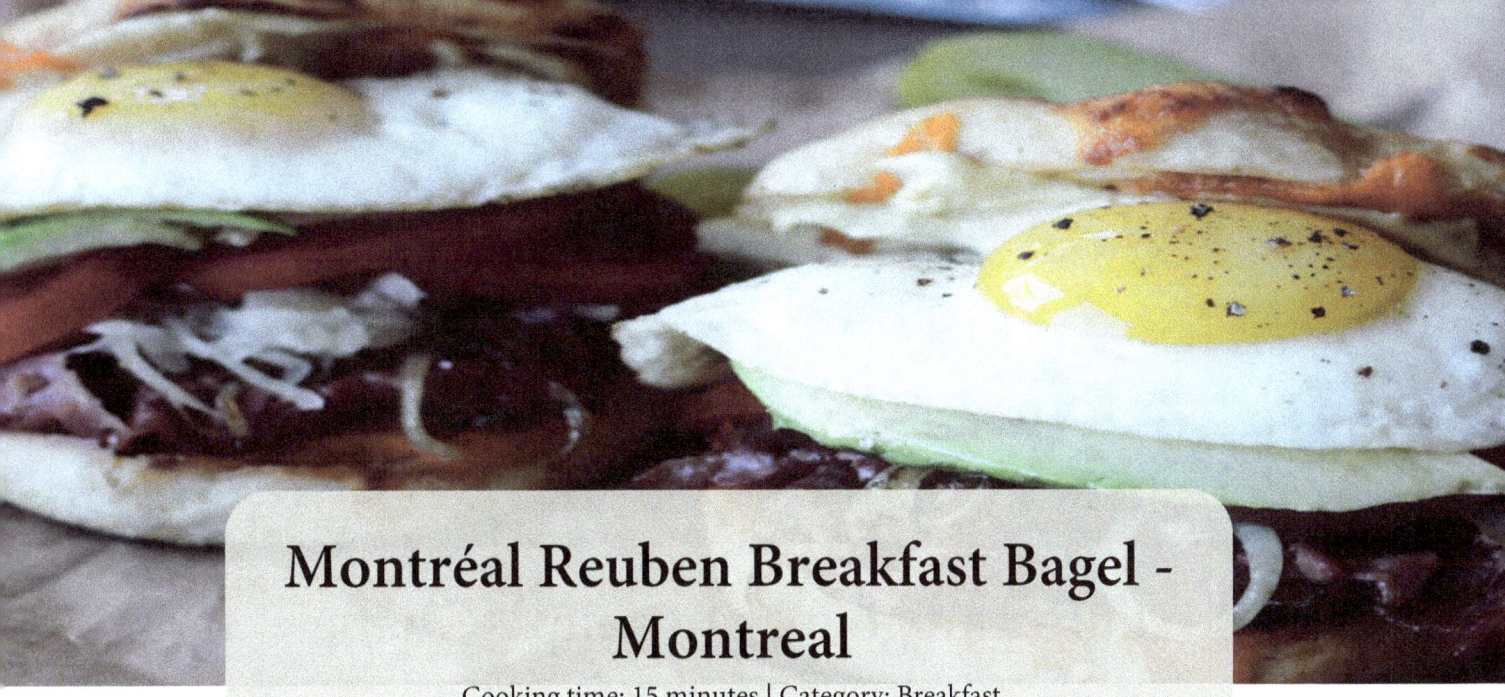

Montréal Reuben Breakfast Bagel - Montreal

Cooking time: 15 minutes | Category: Breakfast

A sandwich full of deliciousness with loads of protein-rich stuff, fried and stacked together beautifully. It's a favorite breakfast for many residents to munch on, in readiness for the day's activities.

Ingredients

- 1 ½ cups water, room temperature
- 2 packages of dry quick-rising yeast (or 1 1/2 ounces fresh yeast)
- 1 teaspoon sugar
- 2 ½ teaspoons salt
- 1 whole egg
- 1 egg yolk
- ¼ cup oil
- ½ cup honey
- 5 cups or more flour (preferably bread flour)
- 3 quarts of water for boiling
- ⅓ cup honey or malt syrup
- Sesame or poppy seeds for sprinkling on top
-

Steps to Cook

1. In a large mixing bowl or in the bowl of an electric mixer that has a dough hook, blend the water, yeast, sugar, and salt. Stir in the whole egg, the yolk, oil and 1/2 cup honey, and mix well.
2. Add the 5 cups flour and mix until the dough is too stiff to mix by hand. Transfer to a lightly floured work surface (if using an electric mixer, attach a dough hook), and knead to form a soft, supple dough. Add a bit more flour as needed to prevent the dough from getting too sticky.
3. When the dough is smooth and elastic, place it in a lightly oiled bowl, and cover it with a sheet of plastic wrap or with a plastic bag. (See note.)
4. Let the dough rest for about 20 minutes. Punch it down and divide it into 18 equal portions. Pour the water into a Dutch oven, along with the remaining 1/3 cup honey or malt syrup, and heat to boiling. Cover, reduce the heat, and allow to simmer while preparing the bagels.
5. Shape the dough portions into bagels or doughnut-like rings by elongating each portion into an 8- to 10-inch coil that is 3/4 inch thick. Fold the ends over each other, pressing with the palm of one hand and rolling back and forth gently to seal. This locks the ends together and must be done properly or the bagels will open while being boiled. Let the bagels rest for 15 minutes on a towel-lined baking sheet.
6. Preheat the oven to 450 degrees. Bring the water back to a boil and remove the lid. Have bowls of poppy seeds and sesame seeds nearby.
7. When the water is boiling, use a slotted spoon, and add three bagels to the water. As they rise to the surface, turn them over, and let them boil for an additional minute before removing them and quickly dipping them in either bowl of the seeds. Continue boiling the bagels in batches of three until all have been boiled and seeded.
8. Arrange the boiled bagels on a baking sheet and bake on the lowest rack of oven until they are medium brown, approximately 25 minutes. Remove from the oven. Once cooled, the bagels can be placed in a plastic bag, sealed, and frozen.

Note:

Montreal Food Tour, the heavenly trip for foodies, a feast on to a variety of cuisines, wines, and soothing music. Montreal Food Tour takes you to a foodie's paradise, letting you indulge in exquisite dishes and drinks, completely satisfying both your palette and soul. Things to do in Montreal list is never complete without a food tour A bustling cosmopolitan located on St. Lawrence, Montreal is the home of major museums, shopping centers, and arts venues such as the Centre-Ville and Vieux-Montreal. The latter is a district of remarkable buildings that date back to the 17th century, resembling a mini-Paris. If you want to take bask in the sunset and see the city in panorama, head to Mont-Royal which also boasts a gorgeous park and monuments of French historical figures. Here you can also find the oldest museum in Canada.

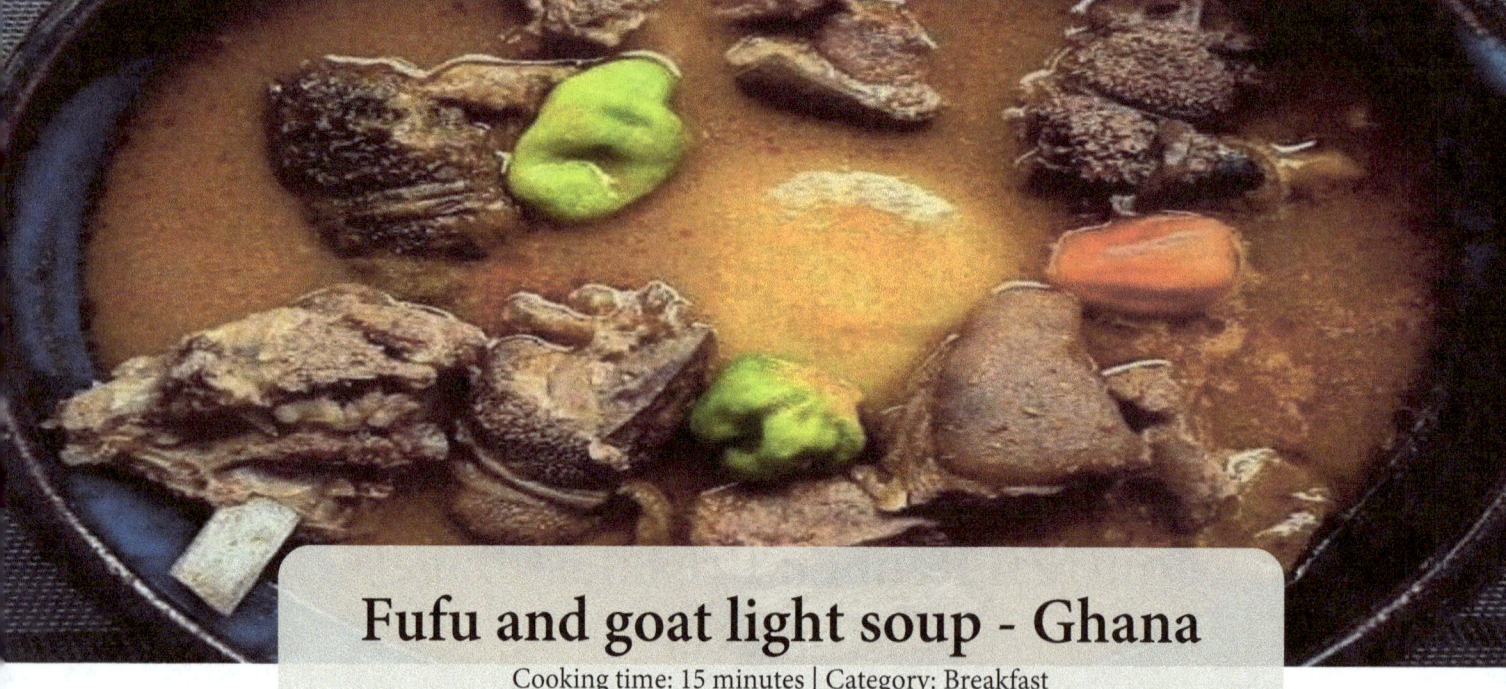

Fufu and goat light soup - Ghana

Cooking time: 15 minutes | Category: Breakfast

In the Eastern and Ashanti regions of Ghana, one meal guaranteed to work its wonder is fufu and goat light soup, the proud dish of the Akan. Fufu is a staple food across West Africa but in Ghana, it is made by pounding a mixture of boiled cassava and plantains into a soft sticky paste to go along with aromatic and spicy tomato soup. Fufu can also be found in Northern Ghana, although it is made with yam in this region. This weekend delight is relished across the country, albeit with slight differences made to the core recipe.

Ingredients

- 1 teaspoon of peeled, fresh grated ginger (about an inch to 1 1/2 inch)
- 2–3 cloves of garlic, crushed
- 1/2 teaspoon of ground aniseed (second) or another seasoning of your choice
- 1 heaping teaspoon of no-salt seasoning of your choice (I'm using Mrs. Dash garlic and herb; many Ghanaians would likely use a couple of seasoning cubes)
- 1/2 to 1 teaspoon of ground dried red chili pepper
- 1 teaspoon salt (or to taste, or substitute seasoning salt) & 2 small bay leaves & 1/2 cup onion, chopped
- 3 whole kpakposhito, whole, if available and (if not, substitute your choice of pepper(s), top(s) sliced off (about a tablespoon), or omit altogether
-

Steps to Cook

1. Put the goat meat in a soup pot and season it with the above ingredients. Stir the goat meat well and add 1/2 cup of water to the pot. Cover, bring the water to a boil, and lower the heat to simmer while you prepare a second pot with:
2. 4 oz of washed tomatoes, whole (1 large or 2 small-to-medium. I used 4 small Campari)
3. ~4 oz of peeled onion (about 1 medium)
4. Fresh whole red chili peppers to taste (probably 1 to 3, depending on type and heat), tops cut off, and seeded if you like
5. 4 cups of water
6.
7. Bring that water to a boil and simmer for 10 or 15 minutes until the vegetables are soft, then remove grind them together (in a blender) and return them to the water in the second pot, along with 4 more cups of water.
8. Stir in 1 tablespoon of tomato paste, let it simmer for a few minutes, and add the broth to the meat. Let the soup simmer until the goat meat is tender, then remove the goat meat and, for a nice clear soup, strain the broth through a sieve, using a spoon if necessary to help force some of the ground vegetables through the sieve (scrape the underside of the strainer with a spoon).
9. 3. Return the meat to the pot and adjust the seasonings (salt, onion, tomato, pepper, etc.) to taste. This may need to simmer for a couple of hours: goat meat tends to be tougher than beef. Add a little more water if necessary

<u>Note:</u>

Hint: To simplify this recipe, grind the vegetables (tomatoes, onion, pepper) at the beginning and add them to the meat pot, along with 8 cups of water. Sorrel Drink in Ghana is called Sobolo. It is a tangy, refreshing, and satisfying drink that tastes amazing and is highly nutritious. It is to be enjoyed on a hot summer day or as a relaxing evening drink! It is made from the petals of a species of Hibiscus, known as Hibiscus sabdariffa (Roselle). Enjoy this natural deliciousness on your tour to the Kakum National Park. Ghana is dubbed West Africa's golden child and for its many gifts, it deserves the title. It is home to many wonderful beaches, vibrant cities with an easy transportation system, and a wildlife. The energy in Ghana is unmatched. It is a mix of indigenous flavors, European and Indian influences.

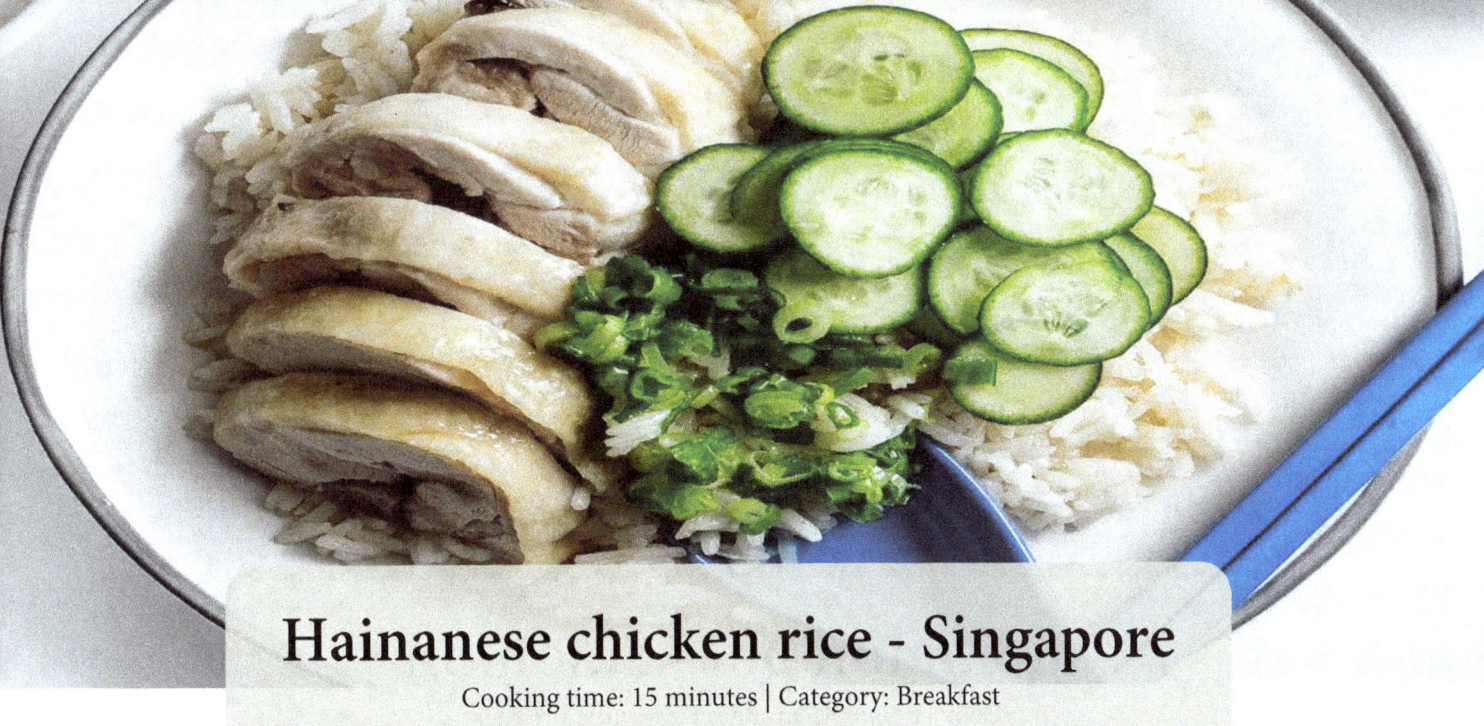

Hainanese chicken rice - Singapore

Cooking time: 15 minutes | Category: Breakfast

Hainanese chicken rice is the national dish of Singapore. The chicken is poached whole and then quickly stopped from cooking by placing it in an ice bath. The rice is seasoned with a chicken made from the chicken and cooked in the poaching liquid.

Ingredients

- 1 large whole chicken at room temperature
- 2 inches fresh unpeeled ginger
- 2 tsp salt
- 1/2 tsp monosodium glutamate or 1 tsp chicken stock powder (optional)
- 1 Tbsp sesame oil
- coriander to serve
- sliced cucumber to serve
- sliced tomato to serve
- Ginger and spring onion oil
- 2 Tbsp fresh grated ginger
- ½ tsp fleur de sol
- 4 spring onions thinly sliced; green tops reserved for chicken poaching.
- ¼ cup peanut oil
- Chicken Rice
- 3 1/3 cups jasmine rice
- 1/4 cup vegetable oil
- 4 garlic cloves
- 2 shallots roughly sliced
- 2-3 pandan leaves optional
- Dressing
- 1 tbsp sesame oil
- 2 tbsp light soy sauce
- 1 cup of chicken stock from poaching chicken
- Chili Sauce for Chicken
- 4-6 red birds-eye chilies
- 6 thick slices of peeled fresh ginger
- 6 garlic cloves
- 2 tsp sugar
- 1/2 tsp salt
- 1/2-1 Cup chicken stock from poaching chicken
- 2 Tbsp lime juice
- 2 Tbsp rendered chicken fat

Steps to Cook

1. Remove the fat deposits from inside the cavity of the chicken, near the tail. Roughly chop the fat and place in a small frying pan over very low heat to render.
2. Render the chicken fat, stirring occasionally for about an hour until all the fat is rendered and the solids are crisp.
3. Remove the solids and use them for another purpose. Reserve the chicken oil. You will use this for both the chili sauce and the chicken rice.
4. For the ginger and spring onion oil.
5. Pound the ginger and salt to a rough paste with a heatproof mortar and pestle.
6. Add the spring onion and pound lightly to combine.
7. Heat the peanut oil in a small frying pan until it is smoking then pour the hot oil over the ginger mixture. Stir, then set aside until ready to serve.

For the chili sauce:

1. Pound the chili, ginger, garlic, sugar, and salt together in a mortar and pestle until very smooth. Pounding chili can take some time so to speed up the process you can start it in a blender or food processor and pound to finish or grate the ingredients into the mortar using a rasp grater.
2. Add the boiling stock to the pounded mixture.
3. Stir in the juice, and adjust the seasoning if necessary, so that the balance of sweet, sour and salty is perfect.
4. Heat the chicken oil in a small saucepan until hot, then pour over the chili mixture and stir to combine.

Note:

Hainanese chicken rice contains 618 calories per serving. Singaporeans love to eat rice and rice noodle dishes. The Singaporean staple diet does not include dairy-based dishes, but you will find many dishes including coconut or rice milk products. Sentosa Island in Singapore has many resorts and family entertainment centers such as Universal Studios, and Water world. There are several lovely beaches for a fun day out or a relaxing couple of days after the hustle and bustle of the city Lovers of gardening should experience Hort Park in Singapore, which has now become a major lifestyle hub in Asia. Perhaps, a trip to Marina Bay sands will not be out of place. The modern face of Southeast Asia, this small city-state is the epitome of wealth, grandeur, and sophistication. Its airport, Changi, deserves a travel piece because it is considered a tourist attraction on its right. Singapore boasts iconic landmarks like the Marina Bay Sands, the towering Super tree Groves at the Gardens by the Bay and the Singapore Flyer. You will also fall in love with its food, diverse and affordable, and you can easily find the best treats from its hawker-style stalls

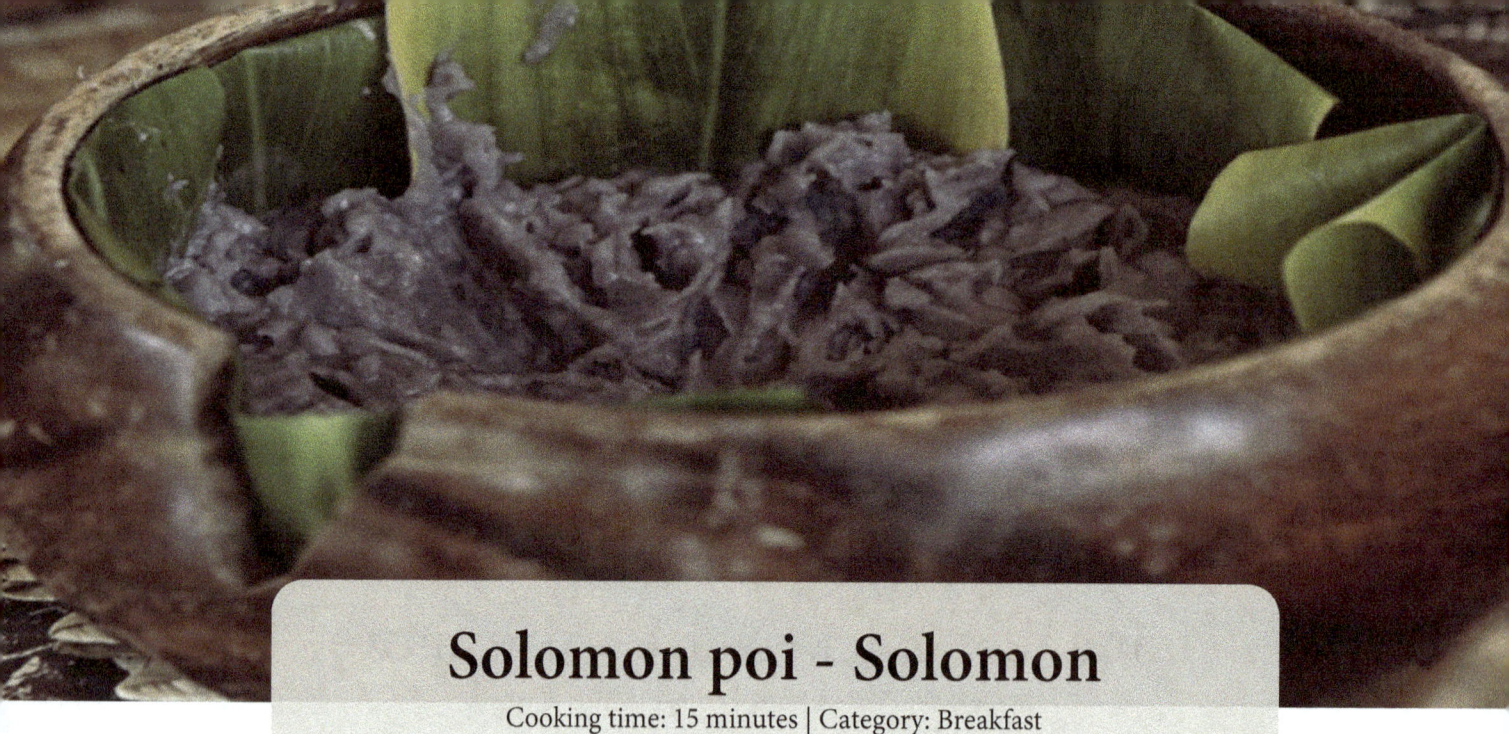

Solomon poi - Solomon

Cooking time: 15 minutes | Category: Breakfast

This lovely dish from the Solomon Islands is a great side for many meals. Poi is the national dish of the Solomon Islands. Taro is an important food crop grown on the islands and it is the main ingredient in Poi. It is prepared by pounding cooked taro roots into a paste. Purple Poi has a distinct flavor. It's okay to be eaten as soon as it is baked. When left to naturally ferment for a few days, it is called sour poi.

Ingredients

- 2 kumara, peeled and grated
- ¼ pumpkin, peeled and grated
- 6 large silver beet leaves, stalks removed and shredded
- 1/2 cup chopped roasted cashew nuts (optional)
- 2/3 cup diluted coconut cream
- Pepper to taste
-

Steps to Cook

1. Set the temperature of the oven to 180°C, to pre-heat.
2. mix thoroughly all the ingredients at once after combining.
3. Using foil, cover the baking pan entirely, allowing for overlaps.
4. Pour the mixed contents into the baking pan.
5. Leave to bake for 70 minutes.
6. Serve Pull out the baked mixture and serve with a choice of veggies or protein.

Note:

Florists will love it at Solomon's Island Memorial Garden to sample the delights of the countryside

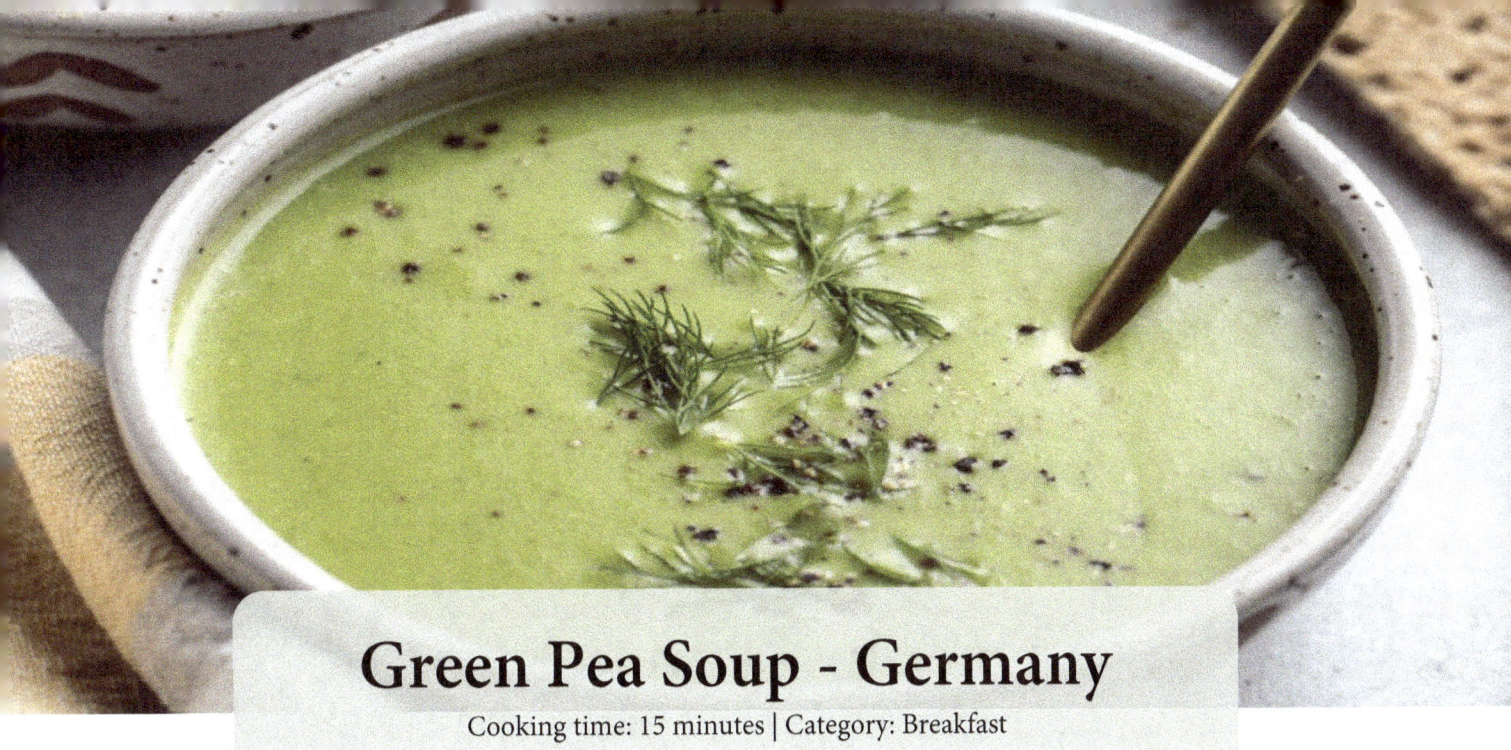

Green Pea Soup - Germany

Cooking time: 15 minutes | Category: Breakfast

Use frozen vegetables to make a hearty stew quickly--no washing, peeling, or slicing required.

It forms a perfect dinner choice for an average German.

Ingredients

- 1.3kg frozen peas
- 110g unsalted butter
- 3 leeks, light green and white parts only, chopped (see tip)
- 1-literer fresh chicken stock, hot
- 500ml fresh chicken stock, chilled
- 300ml double cream
- 400g cooked frankfurter sausages, thinly sliced
- Croutons fried in butter to serve
-

Steps to Cook

1. Put the peas in a colander and run under cool water until almost defrosted. Melt the butter in a very large pan over medium heat until foaming, then add the leeks and cook gently for 10-15 minutes until completely softened.
2. Add the peas to the leeks and cover with the hot chicken stock. Bring to the boil and boil rapidly for 3 minutes, then immediately pour over the cold chicken stock to stop the cooking. This helps to keep the bright green color of the peas.
3. Whizz the soup in a blender, in batches, until very smooth (or use a stick blender). Return to the pan, stir in the cream, and warm gently. Season well to taste.
4. Serve in hot bowls, scattered with frankfurter slices and croutons.

Note:

There are 597 calories per serving of green pea soup.

Lovers of natural fruit extracts will fall in love with engelapfel-school a delicious apple drink with no added sugar, 50 % natural apple juice.

For an experience of Germany, you might want to visit Hamburger, and stop by Zuckermonarchie's coffee shop in Germany.

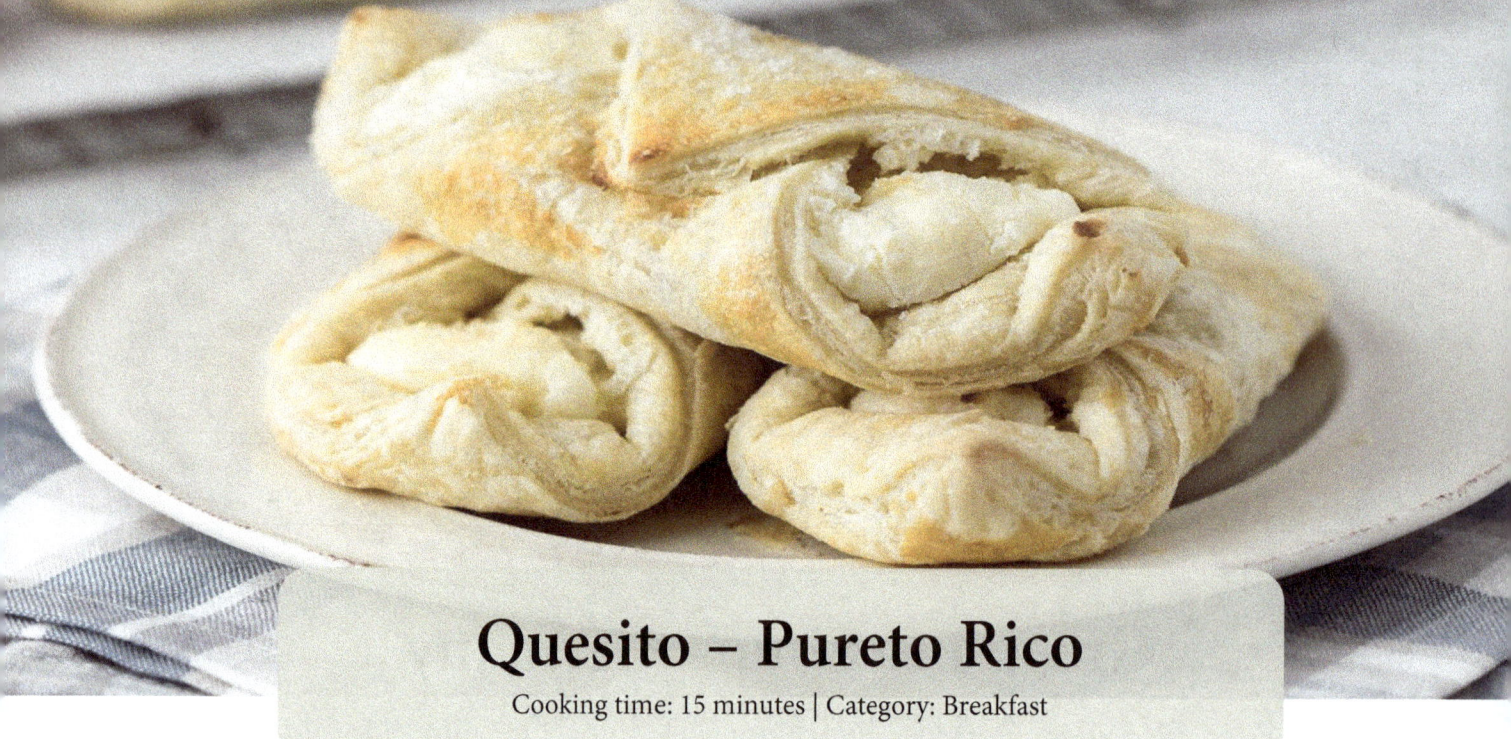

Quesito – Pureto Rico

Cooking time: 15 minutes | Category: Breakfast

Question means "little cheese". This is a good description of this pastry as it is a simple pastry filled with cream cheese. You can choose just to add the cream cheese with a little sugar on top or pick from a few other fillings for this treatment such as guava, pineapple and Nutella. This is another great little pastry to choose to add to your breakfast. It tastes amazing with coffee in the morning, and it is easy to make whether you choose to make the dough on your own or use store-bought They are popular in Puerto Rico for a snack or breakfast and taste amazing with some strong island coffee or café con Leche is just Spanish for coffee with milk (scalded milk).

Ingredients

- 1 Puff pastry sheet
- ½ cup cream cheese
- 1 tbsp vanilla extract
- ¼ cup powdered sugar a bit more to sprinkle on top
- 1 egg
- 1 tbsp granulated sugar

Steps to Cook

1. Preheat the oven to 180ºC (350ºF).
2. Cut the puff pastry sheet into 4×4 inches squares.
3. In a bowl, mix the cream cheese, vanilla extract, and powdered sugar. Mix until the cheese is soft and creamy.
4. Put 1 tsp of filling in the center of each puff pastry sheet. Fold one of the tips over the filling, then fold the diagonal tip to close the quesito.
5. Mix the egg with the granulated sugar.
6. Brush the quesitos with the egg mixture and take them to the oven for 12 – 15 minutes.
7. Sprinkle with some powdered sugar and serve.

Note:

The amount per serving contains 83.7 Calories How to fold quesitos puertorriqueños? Quesitos are easy to fold because the filling is dense and can hold its shape easily. I start cutting the dough pastry sheet into squares of about 4 inches per side (you can make bigger or smaller quesitos, this is just the standard size). I managed to get 9 squares from my puff pastry sheet. Then I add 2 tsp of filling to the center of my puff pastry squares and I fold one of the tips over the filling. Then I grab the diagonal tip and fold it over. This time I stretch a bit the tip to try to get almost to the back of the quesito. That's it! A folded quesito. If you are having a hard time getting your tips folded, you can wet the tip to make it extra sticky. Juan dates to many centuries ago. It tells a beautiful story of the ancient Puerto Rican culture. Wander the cobblestone streets to soak up the unique architecture and colorful local shops, restaurants, and bars scattered throughout the old cityPiñones is a must-go to spot to get a taste of Puerto Rican's culinary palette. A hot cup of café con Leche is a great way to get your day started in Puerto Rico.Puerto Rico is an exciting Caribbean destination that packs a punch – from its splendid, untarnished beaches, lush tropical forests, bioluminescent bay, and historic sites. You will also feel at home by how friendly and warm Puerto Ricans, are known to be the happiest people in the world with their love for life. This is an all-time favorite holiday destination, whether you have your friends or family with you, or even when you're alone. Puerto Rico will offer lots

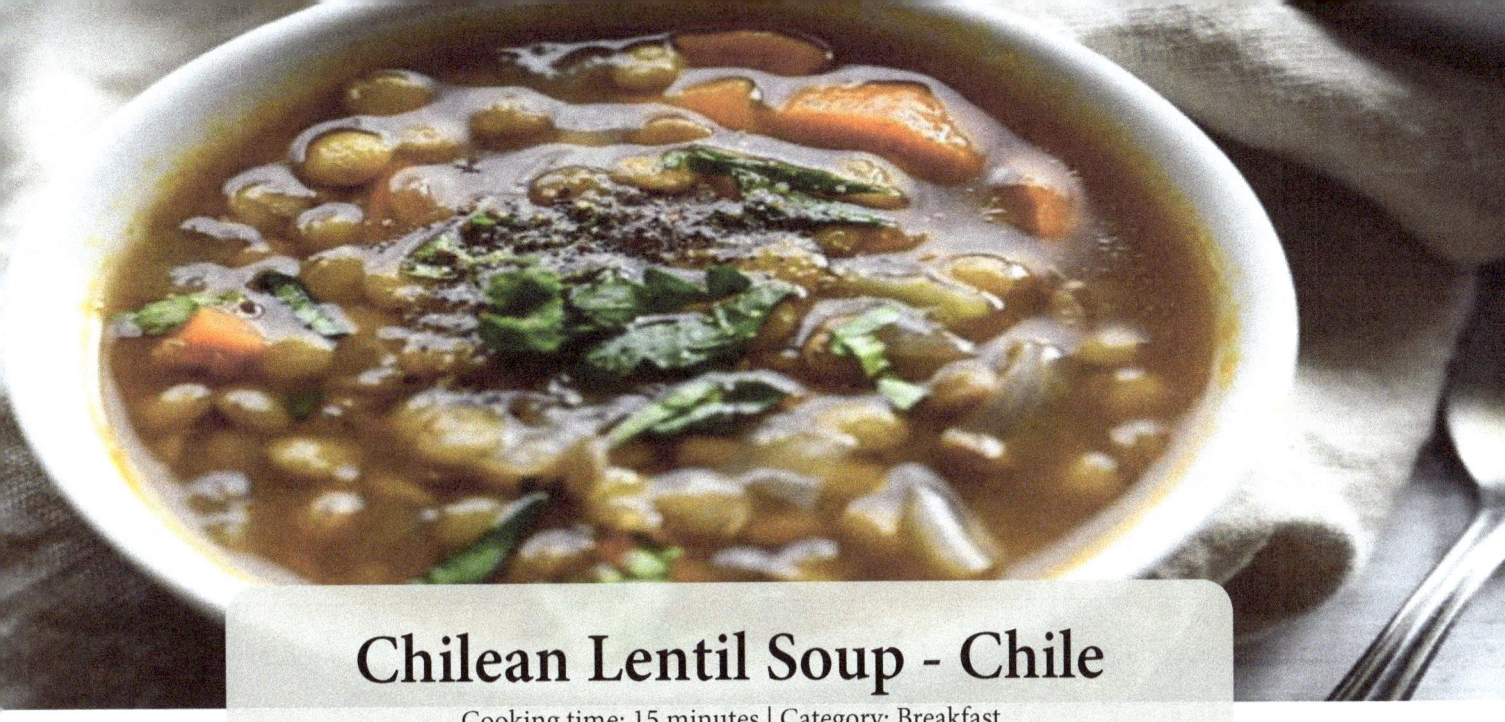

Chilean Lentil Soup - Chile

Cooking time: 15 minutes | Category: Breakfast

Lunch is one of the larger meals of the day in Chile. Traditional lunch foods include cazuela, a clear broth made with rice, potato, corn, and meat. Pastel de choclo, a corn casserole made with meat, olives, and vegetables, is a popular lunch summer dish.

Ingredients

- 1 tablespoon Chilean color or vegetable oil
- 1 medium yellow onion, finely chopped
- 1 clove of garlic, finely chopped
- 1/2 teaspoon ground cumin
- 2 celery sticks finely chopped
- 1 carrot, chopped into small cubes
- 1/2 bell pepper, any color, chopped into small cubes
- 2 sausages cut into 1 cm slices.
- 1/2 cup raw rice, ideally short grain
- 1 large or 2 medium potatoes, peeled, cubed
- 1 cup raw green or brown lentils
- 1/2 bundle of chard with about 8 leaves cut stems and leaves or a bundle of spinach without stems, optional
- salt and pepper

Steps to Cook

1. Soak the lentils in plenty of cold water the night before, and discard stones or damaged lentils. Strain.
2. Heat the oil, in a medium pot, over medium-high heat. Add the onion and cook for 5 minutes.
3. Add the carrot, celery, bell pepper, and garlic, and brown for 1 minute. Season with salt and pepper.
4. Add the sausages and rice and stir for 1 minute.
5. Add the lentils and potatoes and stir well. Add 2-3 cups of cold water, and season with salt and pepper.
6. Cook over low heat, simmering for 20 minutes. Test that the lentils and rice are cooked.
7. Add the chopped chard or spinach and cook for 5 more minutes.
8. Add more water as many times as necessary. You want it always to be covered by a thin layer of water on top, like 1 cm.
9. Taste and adjust the seasoning.
10. Serve hot.

Note:

Calories per serving: 483 Lovers of volcano climbing. white water rafting; kayaking; canoeing; horseback riding; and, come winter, skiing can freely indulge in their favorite sport(s) in the Chilean Lake District. Immerse yourself in fun, while enjoying a Taste of Pisco, a Chilean spirited drink.

Week - 7

Reflections

- How was your practice of prayer, meditation & gratitude this week?
_____
_____
_____
_____

- What new recipes did you try?
_____
_____
_____
_____
_____

- What are you observing about your abilities to connect with others?
_____
_____
_____
_____
_____

- What new learner protein did you try this week?
_____
_____
_____
_____

- How is your body feeling?
_____
_____
_____
_____

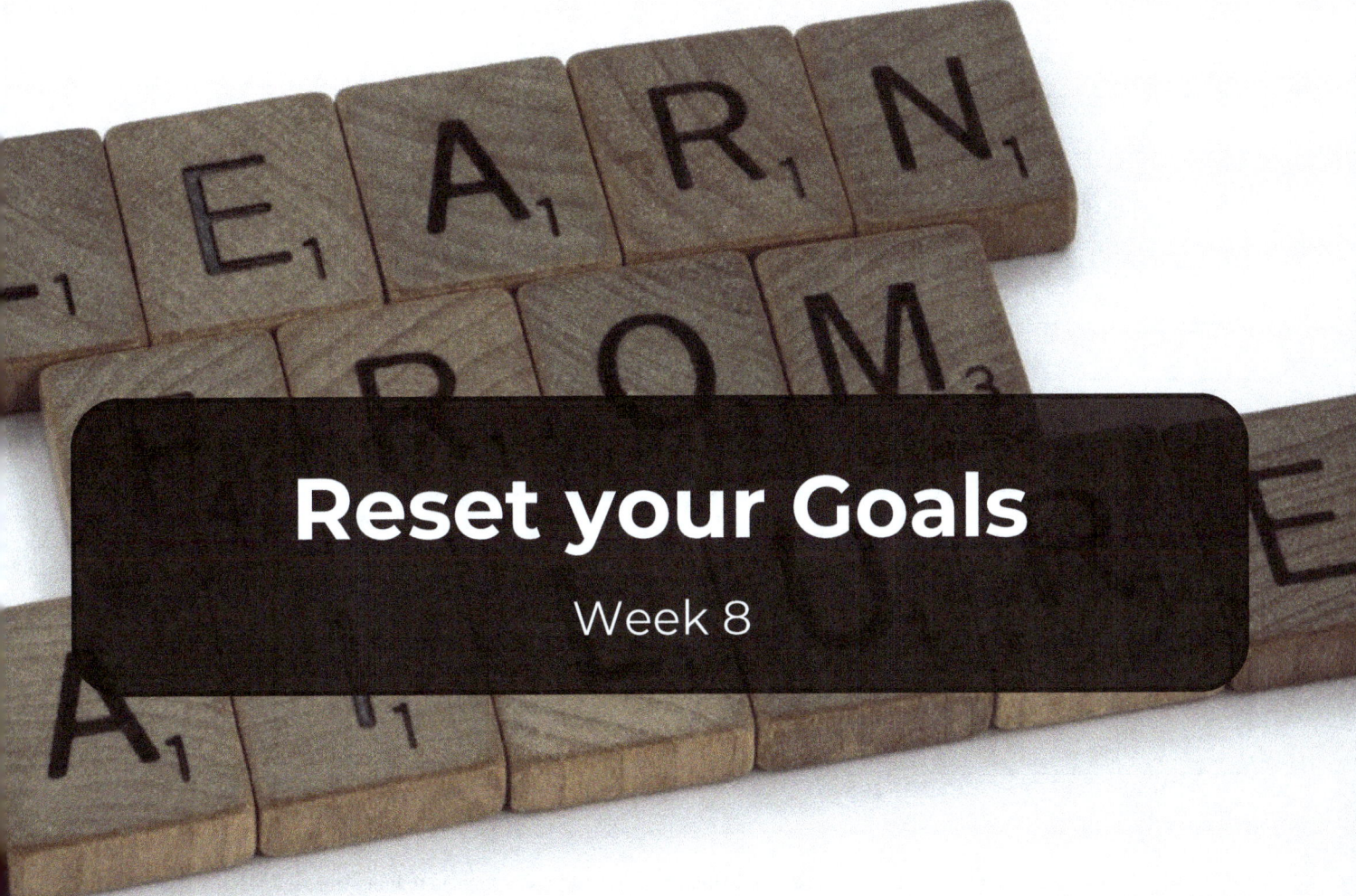

Reset your Goals

Week 8

Week - 8

Take Obedient Action

- Spend 25 minutes practicing prayer, meditation & writing in your gratitude journal

_____
_____
_____
_____
_____

- Select 2 lunch,1 Breakfast recipes from week 8 & prepare them this week.

_____
_____
_____
_____
_____

- Share a meal with old friends & someone from a different country

_____
_____
_____
_____
_____

- Maintain your cardio 2.5miles walking or running adding 10 minutes of stretching & 5 strength training exercises

_____
_____
_____
_____
_____

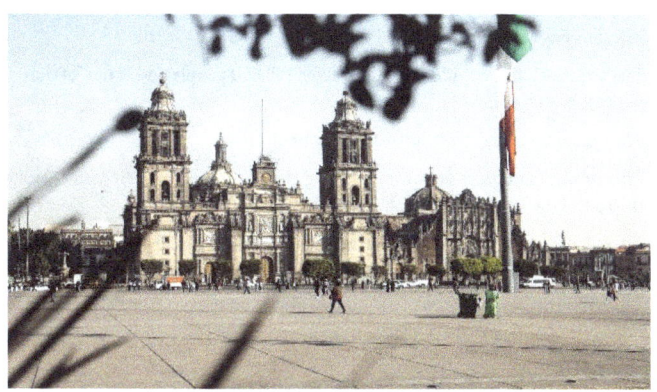

Mexico City-Dinner

Mexico City is the state capital of Mexico. This North American country has the second largest economy in Latin America. Magical towns, beaches, archaeological sites, and eye-popping beaches are commonplace.

México is one of the most bio-diverse countries in the world. Mexico City has an estimated population of over 9,209,944 residents.

Mexico City has a long, rich history and is known for being one of the largest financial centers in the continent and the largest Spanish-speaking city in the world.

The largest city, Mexico City, contributes over 12 million people to the country's total population. Other cities include Iztapalapa, Ecatepec de Morelos, and Guadalajara

There are popular traditional dishes unique to sub-urban outskirts in the Mexico City environs.

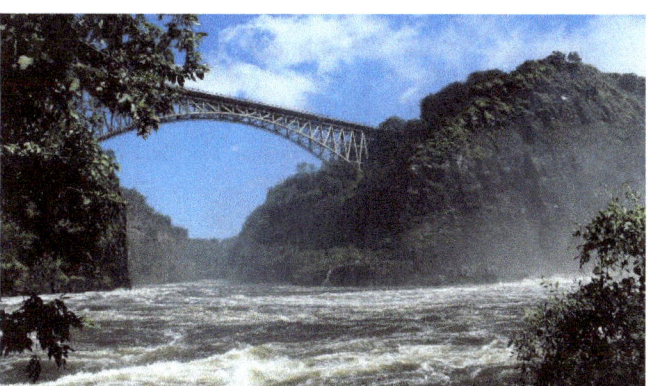

Zimbabwe-Breakfast

Zimbabwe is not complete without a trip to Victoria Falls, National Park, the scenic views of Nottingham Estates.

The prevailing biodiversity of Malilangwe Game Reserve, the rich resources of Sondelani Safaris, and many more characterize the glory of Zimbabwe.

Harare is the capital and most populous city of Zimbabwe. Other cities include Bulawayo, Mutare, Kwekwe. Kadoma. This African country is one of the top 10 producers and exporters of tobacco in the world. However, only 20% of the population consumes cigarettes.

Zimbabwe is home to Lake Kariba, the world's largest man-made lake and reservoir by volume. The main staple of Zimbabwean cuisine is maize/ corn which is used in a variety of dishes. Food in Zimbabwe has remained traditionally African. Whawha is a traditional maize beer, however Zambezi is Zimbabwe's national beer. Mazoe orange drink is a favorite drink and is unique because it is all fruit and chemical-free.

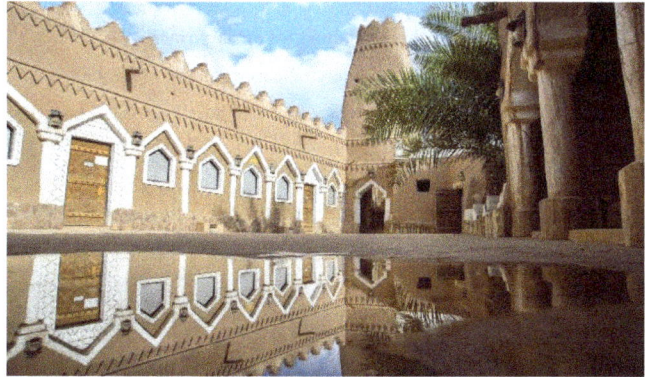

Saudi Arabia-Lunch

Saudi Arabia, officially the Kingdom of Saudi Arabia, is a country in Western Asia. It is the largest country in the Middle East and the second-largest country in the Arab world. However, if you like to spend your winter, Saudi has an exciting experience waiting for you. Discover an exciting range of activities and Saudi destinations that are perfect for the cooler months of the year. Experience the thrill of Riyadh Seasons, the world's largest lifestyle festival, with a huge variety of entertainment and events for the whole family.

The current population of Saudi Arabia is 35,573,004.

Riyadh which lies in the Central Region, is the capital city of Saudi Arabia and the center of its architecture.

Other cities in the country include the holy cities of Makkah and Madinah, Jeddah and Dhahran.

Lunch is traditionally the main meal of the day, and it almost always includes a rice dish.

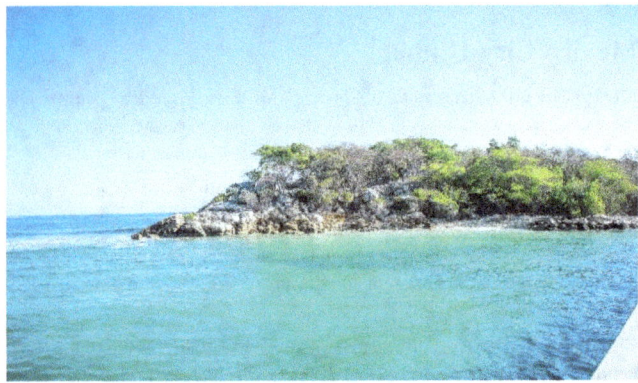

Micronesia-Dinner

Micronesia- is a country located in the western Pacific Ocean.

The country has a population of just over 100,000 people and is one of the poorest in the world.

The economy is based on subsistence agriculture and fishing.

There is little industry or commerce, and the country is not well connected to the rest of the world.

The people of Micronesia are Warmblood horses and are descendants of horses brought to the islands by the Spanish in the 16th century.

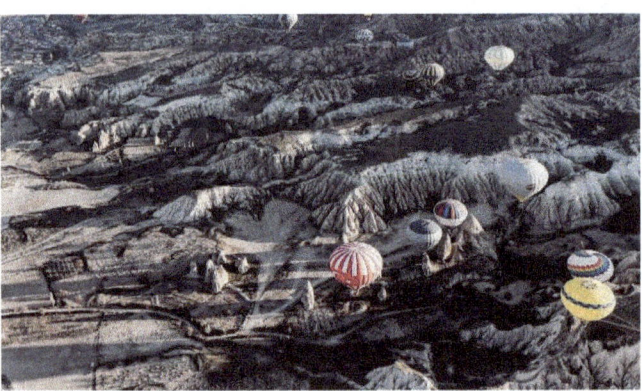

Turkey-Breakfast

Turkey is a country in the Middle East. Turkey has a population of over 83.2 million.

The largest city is Istanbul, while the national capital is Ankara.

Spoken languages are Turkish (official), Kurdish by Kurdish people, and Arabic by Turkish Arabs.

The Economy of Turkey is based on agriculture, industry, and services.

Turkey maintains a mostly free-market economy, which is driven by the industry and the service sector.

The Turks love tea. Turkey is responsible for the production of 75% of the world's hazelnuts.

Nuts are commonly used in many Turkish desserts such as baklava.

One of the oldest (and largest) markets in the world, the Grand Bazaar welcomes up to 400,000 visitors a day.

It's often described as one of the oldest shopping malls in existence.

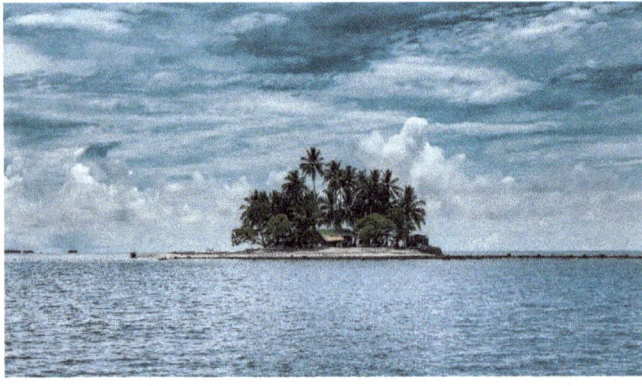

Haiti-Lunch

The capital city of this Caribbean country is Port-au-Prince.

Haitian foods draw influences from ingredients from far-reaching nations.

This most mountainous country in the Caribbean boasts many islands and fun places to discover and indulge oneself. Haitians are music lovers and kompa is a household name in the music industry.

The artistic and colorful country has made a huge advancement in the tourism sector. The national dish of Haitians griots with rice and beans. Joumou (pumpkin soup) is the country's most revered dish.

Modern Recipe Design for Word | 97

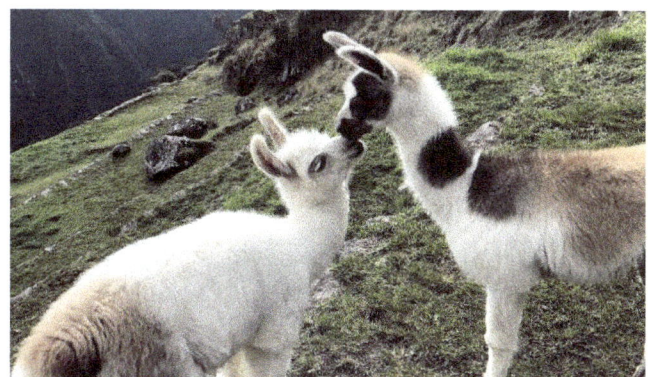

Bolivia-Dinner

A country of extremes, landlocked Bolivia is the highest and most isolated country in South America.

It has the largest proportion of indigenous people.

The country has the second-largest reserves of natural gas in South America, but there have been long-running tensions over the exploitation and export of the resource.

Bolivia is also one of the world's largest producers of coca, the raw material for cocaine.

The official capital of Bolivia is Sucre. Bolivia has an estimated population of 10.8million persons.

The vast country with different and varied climates offers a great variety of natural products, including hundreds of varieties of potatoes and corn, fruits, and spices, which are well used by its people to enrich their cuisine.

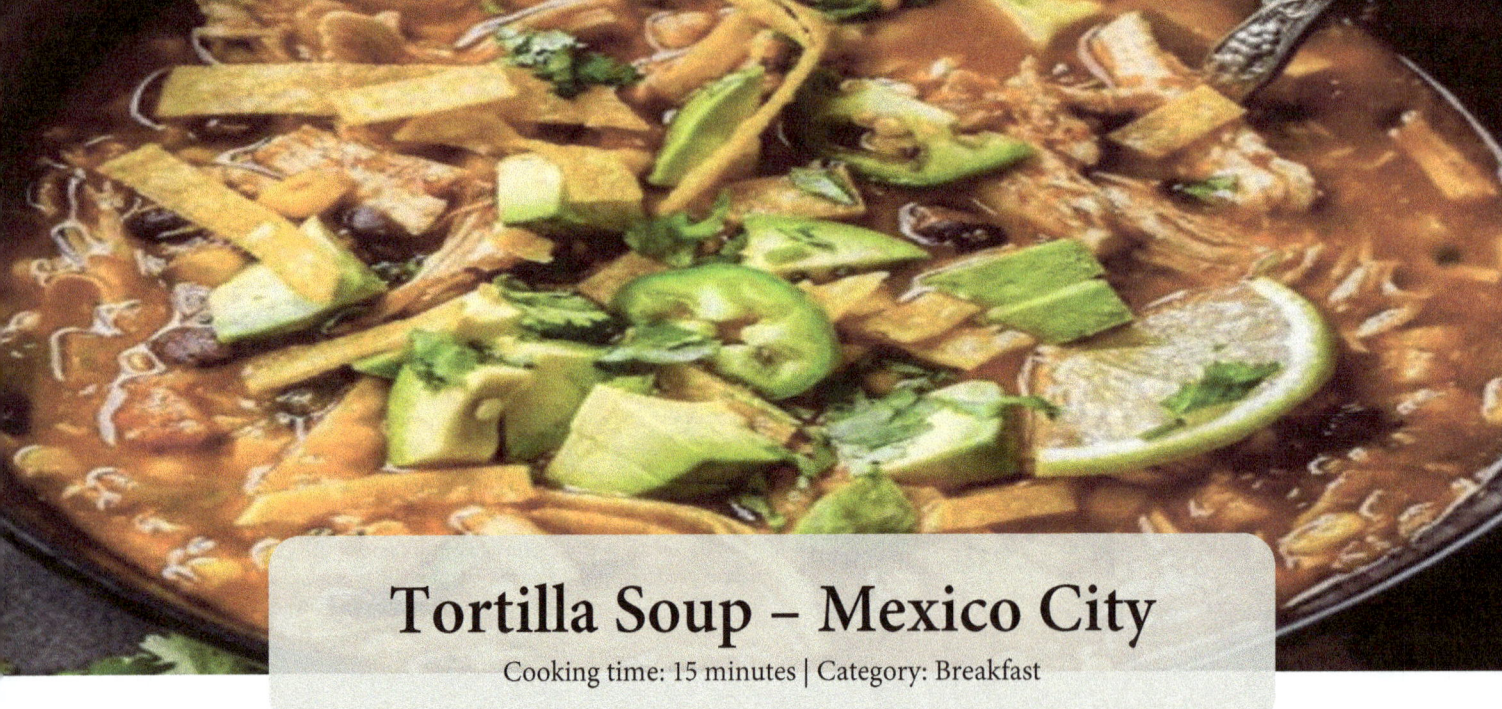

Tortilla Soup – Mexico City

Cooking time: 15 minutes | Category: Breakfast

This vegetarian tortilla soup is so flavourful and easy to make! It's full of zesty flavor, featuring black beans and adobo sauce.

Ingredients

- 6 6-inch corn tortillas
- Olive oil &
- Kosher salt

For the vegetarian tortilla soup

- 1 yellow onion
- 1 green bell pepper
- 4 medium garlic cloves
- 2 15-ounce cans of black beans
- 2 tablespoons extra-virgin olive oil, plus more for brushing
- 2 teaspoons dried oregano
- 1 teaspoon cumin & 1 28-ounce can of crushed tomatoes (fire roasted, if possible)
- 1½ cups frozen corn or a 15-ounce can of corn
- 1 tablespoon adobo sauce (from 1 can of chipotle peppers in adobo sauce)
- 1 quart (4 cups) vegetable broth
- 1 teaspoon kosher salt, plus more for sprinkling
- 4 radishes, for garnish & 1 lime, for garnish
- 1 handful of cilantros, for garnish

Steps to Cook

1. Heat oven to 375°F.
2. Make the tortilla strips: Brush the tortillas lightly with olive oil on each side. Using a pizza cutter, slice them in half, then into thin strips. Place the strips on a baking sheet and sprinkle with kosher salt. Bake for 10 to 12 minutes until crispy and lightly browned.
3. Prep the veggies: Peel and dice the onion. Dice the green pepper. Peel and mince the garlic. Drain and rinse the beans.
4. Make the soup: In a large pot or Dutch oven, heat 2 tablespoons olive oil and sauté the onion until translucent, about 5 minutes. Add the green pepper and the garlic and sauté for 2 minutes. Stir in the oregano and the cumin for 1 minute. Add the tomatoes, beans, corn, adobo sauce, broth, and kosher salt. Bring to a boil, then simmer for 10 minutes. Taste and add additional adobo sauce or kosher salt if desired.
5. Prep the garnishes: Slice the radishes. Slice the lime into wedges.
6. Serve: To serve, ladle the soup into bowls and allow it to cool to warm. Garnish with the tortilla strips, radishes, torn cilantro leaves, hot sauce, and plenty of lime juice.

Note:

The number of calories per serving is 283

A favorite cocktail, the classic margarita, is a Mexican staple. The traditional recipe is either served on the rocks or blended and made from lime juice, tequila, and triple sec, served in a sugar-rimmed glass to soften the bitterness. The Veracruz festival beautifully captures Mexican culture. December is a good time to engage yourself in the wonders of the Cancun International boat show.

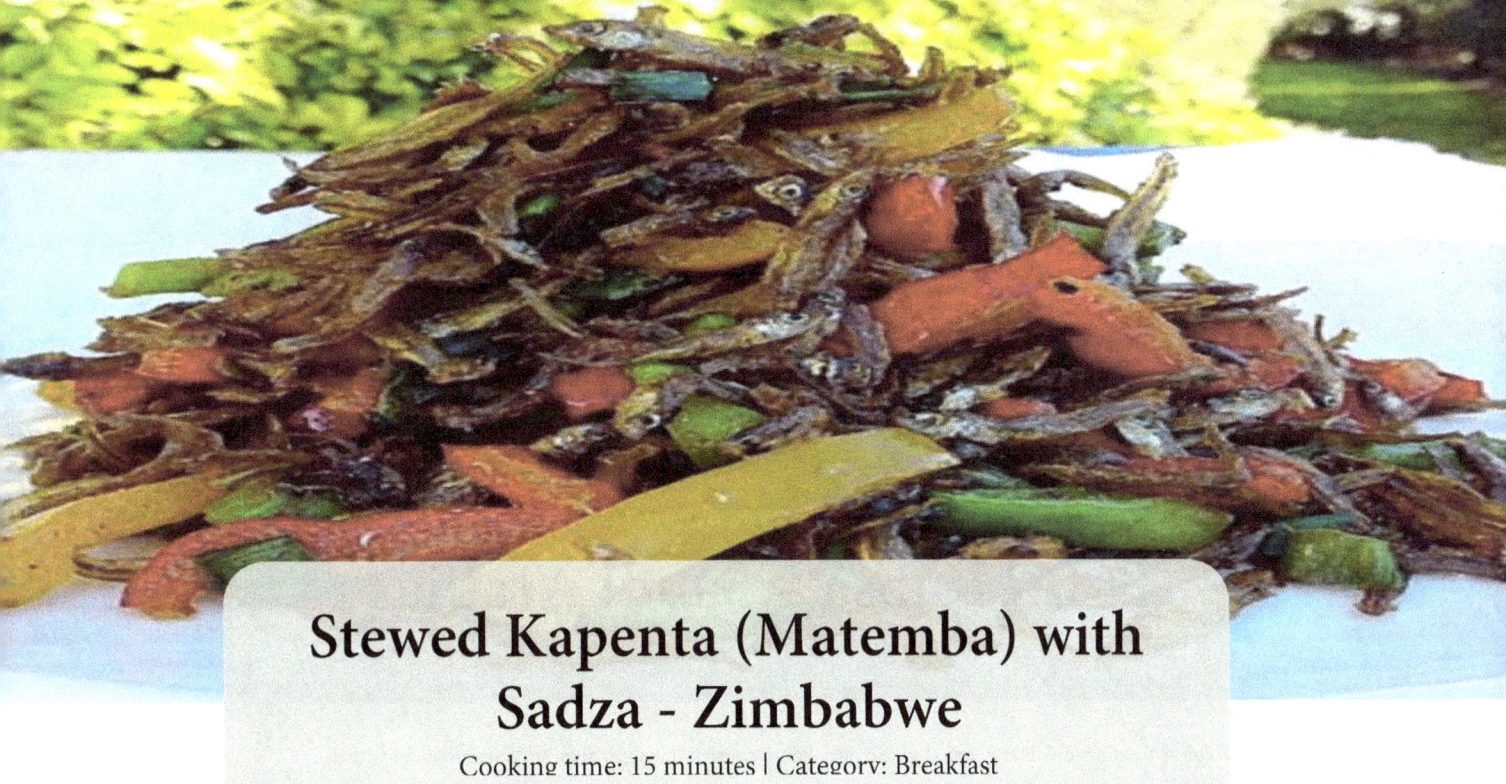

Stewed Kapenta (Matemba) with Sadza - Zimbabwe

Cooking time: 15 minutes | Category: Breakfast

Kapenta (or matemba as it is locally pronounced) is a beautiful fish that is eaten almost exclusively in the African regions of Zimbabwe and Zambia due to the large fisheries. Traditionally, before cooking, the kapenta is dried in the sun on a rack for a day and, because of this, it can go for periods without refrigeration and provides an important source of protein to locals. Kapenta is therefore an epitome of the type of traditional cuisine eaten across the country. This delicacy is often served with sadza which is made of ground maize, but you can also serve kapenta stew with rice.

Ingredients

- 1 lb Dried kapenta fish
- 1 Large onion
- 1 Large tomato
- 4 cloves of Garlic
- 1 tbsp Olive oil
- Salt & pepper to taste

Steps to Cook

1. Prepare a large pot of boiling water and place it in your kapenta, boil for 15 minutes.
2. After 15 minutes, remove your kapenta, pat it dry and then chop it into thin chunks ready for frying.
3. Finely chop your onion and garlic and add to a hot frying pan of olive oil and cook until browned.
4. Finely chop the tomato and add to the pan along with salt, pepper, groundnut powder, and a 1/2 cup of water.
5. Add your kapenta to the pan, making sure to immerse it in the sauce. Cover the pan and leave to simmer for 10 minutes on low heat, stirring halfway through.
6. Take your fish stew off the heat and leave it to rest for 2 minutes to allow the sauce to thicken.
7. Your stewed kapenta is now ready to eat, serve with sadza or boiled rice.

Note:

Amount per serving: calories: 202

Enjoy fishing? A fishing spree at Lake Kariba, sipping mazoe alongside will not be a bad idea at all!

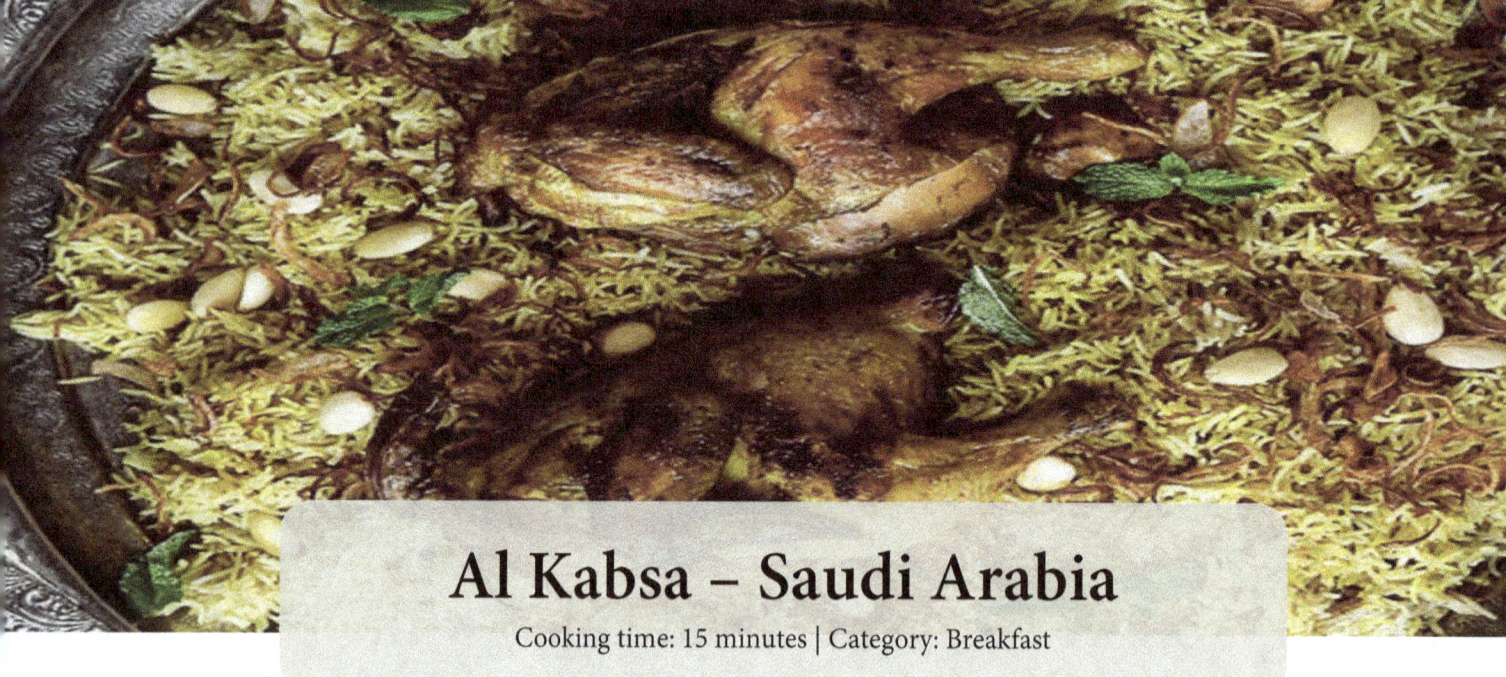

Al Kabsa – Saudi Arabia

Cooking time: 15 minutes | Category: Breakfast

A beautifully spiced chicken and rice dish that is perfect for a crowd. Be sure to make the super spicy shattah sauce to go with it.

Ingredients

- 1/4 cup butter
- 3 lbs chicken cut into 8-10 pieces
- 1 large onion finely chopped
- 6 garlic cloves minced
- 1/4 cup tomato puree
- 14 ounces canned chopped tomatoes with liquid (or fresh)
- 3 carrots grated
- 2 whole cloves
- 1/4 teaspoon grated nutmeg
- 1/2 teaspoon ground cumin
- 1/2 teaspoon ground coriander
- salt & freshly ground black pepper to taste
- 4 cups of hot water
- 1 chicken stock cube
- 2 1/4 cups basmati rice don't rinse or soak this
- 1/4 cup raisins
- 1/4 cup slivered almonds toasted

Kabsa Spice Mix

- 1/2 teaspoon saffron
- 1/4 teaspoon ground green cardamoms
- 1/2 teaspoon ground cinnamon
- 1/2 teaspoon ground allspice
- 1/2 teaspoon ground dried limes

Steps to Cook

1. Melt butter in a large stock pot, or Dutch oven.
2. Add chicken pieces, onion & garlic & sauté until onion is tender and chicken is browned.
3. Stir in tomato puree & simmer over low heat for a couple of minutes.
4. Add tomatoes, carrots, cloves, and all the spices including the kabsa spice mixtures & salt and pepper.
5. Cook for a couple of minutes.
6. Add the water & chicken stock cube.
7. Bring to a boil, then reduce heat and cover.
8. Simmer over low heat for 30 minutes.
9. Add rice to the pot & stir carefully.
10. Re-Cover & simmer for 35 - 40 minutes - add the raisins for the last 10 minutes - cook until rice is tender.
11. Place the rice on a large serving dish, topped with the chicken & garnished with almonds.
12. Serve with a hot sauce called 'shattah'.

Note:

Nutrition

Calories: 538kcal

Enjoy the temperate climate of the Red Sea for winter sun, sand, and marine adventure. Explore Saudi's national parks and ward off the evening chill with a roaring campfire beneath the glorious desert stars, or head for the colder climes of Saudi's mountainous north for a chance to see the desert. Saudi Champagne is one of the most popular non-alcoholic beverages you would not want to

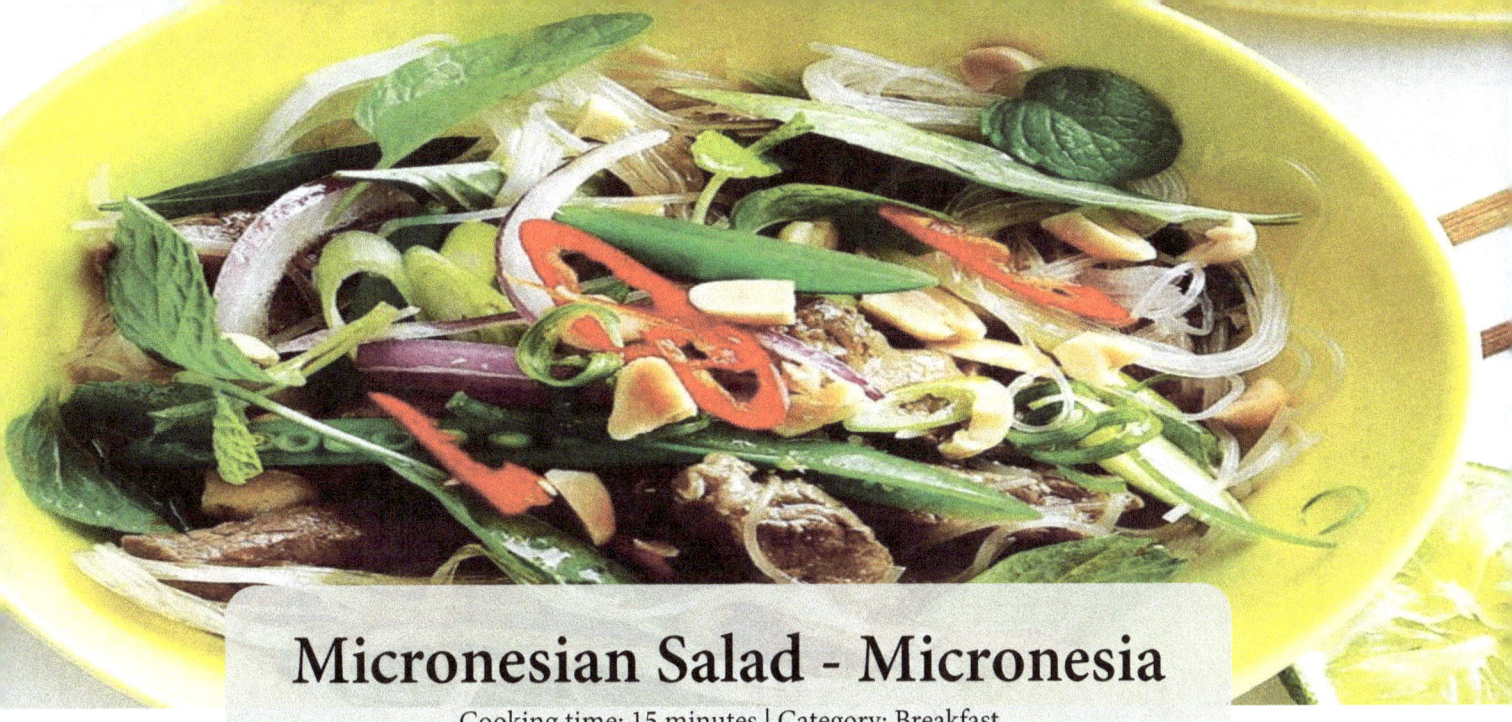

Micronesian Salad - Micronesia

Cooking time: 15 minutes | Category: Breakfast

Ingredients

- Boiled breadfruit 1
- Hard-boiled eggs 2
- Tomatoes 1 chopped
- Beans 1 cup boiled
- Cucumber 2 sliced
- Onions 1 chopped
- Dijon mustard 1/2 teaspoon
- Fried pork or chicken 1 cup
- Mayonnaise 1/4 cup
- Vinegar 2 tablespoon
- Sugar 1 pinch
- Salt 1/4 teaspoon
- Crushed Black Pepper 1/4 teaspoon.

Steps to Cook

1. Mix all veggies and chicken with mayonnaise in a bowl.
2. Mix vinegar, Dijon mustard, salt, black Pepper and mix well
3. Pour onto the salad.
4. Chill for ½ hour and then serve.

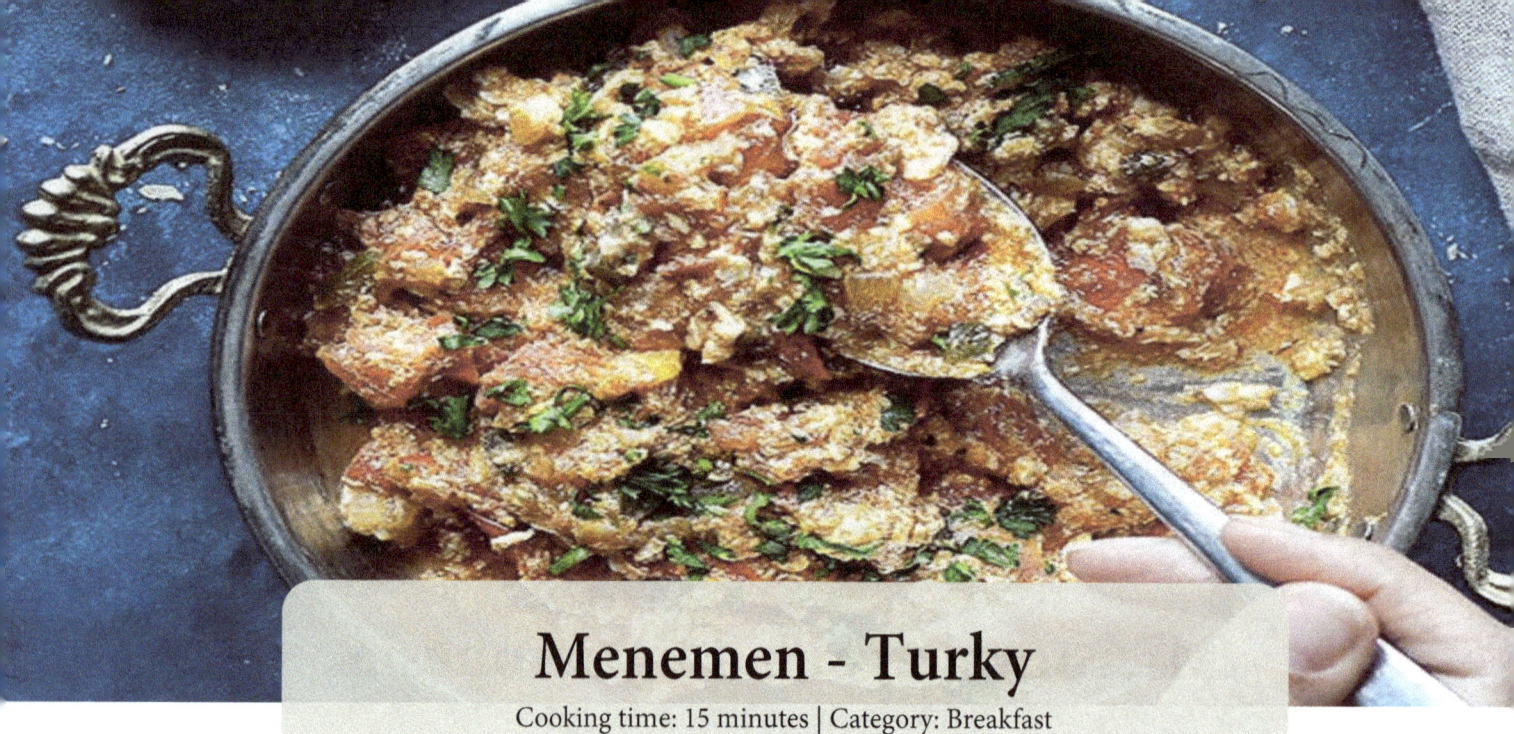

Menemen - Turky

Cooking time: 15 minutes | Category: Breakfast

Menemen is a traditional Turkish dish that is mostly served as a hearty breakfast. It is a simple one-pan dish with eggs, tomatoes, and green peppers. This simple egg dish gets its name from a Turkish town called Menemen, which is located in Izmir. It is said that this egg dish was made first by the Cretan Turks who moved to this town.

Ingredients

- 2 tablespoons olive oil
- 3 green peppers, chopped (Turkish peppers or any sweet green pepper)
- 4 tomatoes (1 cup peeled and diced)
- ½ tsp salt
- ½ tsp paprika
- 4 eggs
- ½ tsp black pepper
- ½ tsp red pepper flakes
- Parsley for garnish

Steps to Cook

1. Heat olive oil in a pan.
2. Cook chopped peppers in it for 2-3 minutes.
3. Add in tomatoes.
4. Season with salt and paprika and cook over medium-low heat until tomatoes are tender, stirring occasionally. Now reduce the heat a bit.
5. There are two options after this step:
6. First option: In a bowl, beat the eggs and pour it all over the tomatoes. Give it a gentle stir so that the beaten eggs can spread everywhere. Cook, it uncovered until the eggs are set. It takes no longer than 3-5 minutes. Don't overcook.
7. Second option: Using a spoon, make rooms for each egg and break eggs into those hollows. Let it simmer uncovered until the eggs are slightly cooked for 8-10 minutes. Help egg whites cook well with a spoon. If you like the yolks hard, cook them longer.
8. Sprinkle black pepper and red pepper flakes over it. Garnish with herbs like parsley or chopped green onions and serve. Serve it with your favorite crusty bread.

Note:

The number of calories per serving is 214.

The Aryan drink is very unique to the Turkish people.

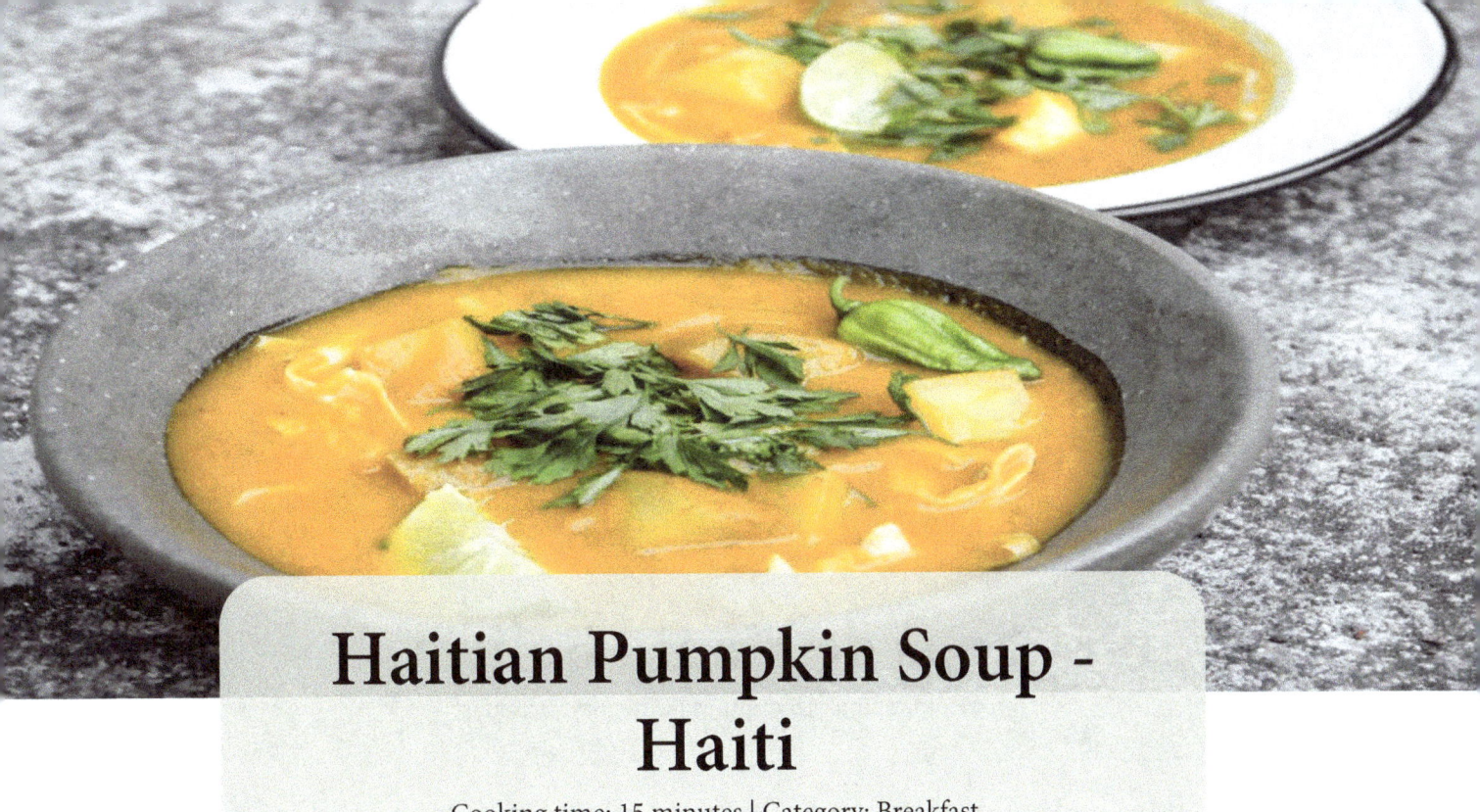

Haitian Pumpkin Soup - Haiti

Cooking time: 15 minutes | Category: Breakfast

Now, who will dislike this yummy and eye-popping soup. This Haitian delicacy, being richly garnished with garlic and onion gives it an inviting taste. You will love the deliciousness of this dinner delight.

Ingredients

- 1 tbsp. extra-virgin olive oil
- 1 large onion, coarsely chopped
- 4 cloves garlic, minced
- 4 lb. pumpkin (any kind but preferably sugar pie)
- 4 c. low-sodium chicken broth
- Kosher salt
- Freshly ground black pepper
- 1/2 c. heavy cream, plus more for garnish

Steps to Cook

1. In a heavy soup pot or Dutch oven over medium heat, heat oil.
2. Add onion and garlic and cook until golden.
3. Meanwhile, halve, peel, and scrape out the seeds of the pumpkin. Cut into chunks.
4. Add pumpkin chunks and broth to the pot. Season with salt and pepper. Bring to a boil, uncovered, and then reduce heat to a simmer. Simmer until pumpkin is fork-tender, about 30 minutes.
5. Remove pot from heat and, using an immersion blender, blend the mixture until smooth. (Alternatively, let the soup cool, and then blend in a blender.) Stir in cream and season to taste.
6. To serve, ladle soup into bowls, add a swirl of cream, and garnish with pepper.

Note:

On a trip to Haiti?

Get ready to smack your lips repeatedly with a taste of the Haitian tropical rum punch and the akasan (a mix of milkshake and a smoothie) You will love the tasty beverages.

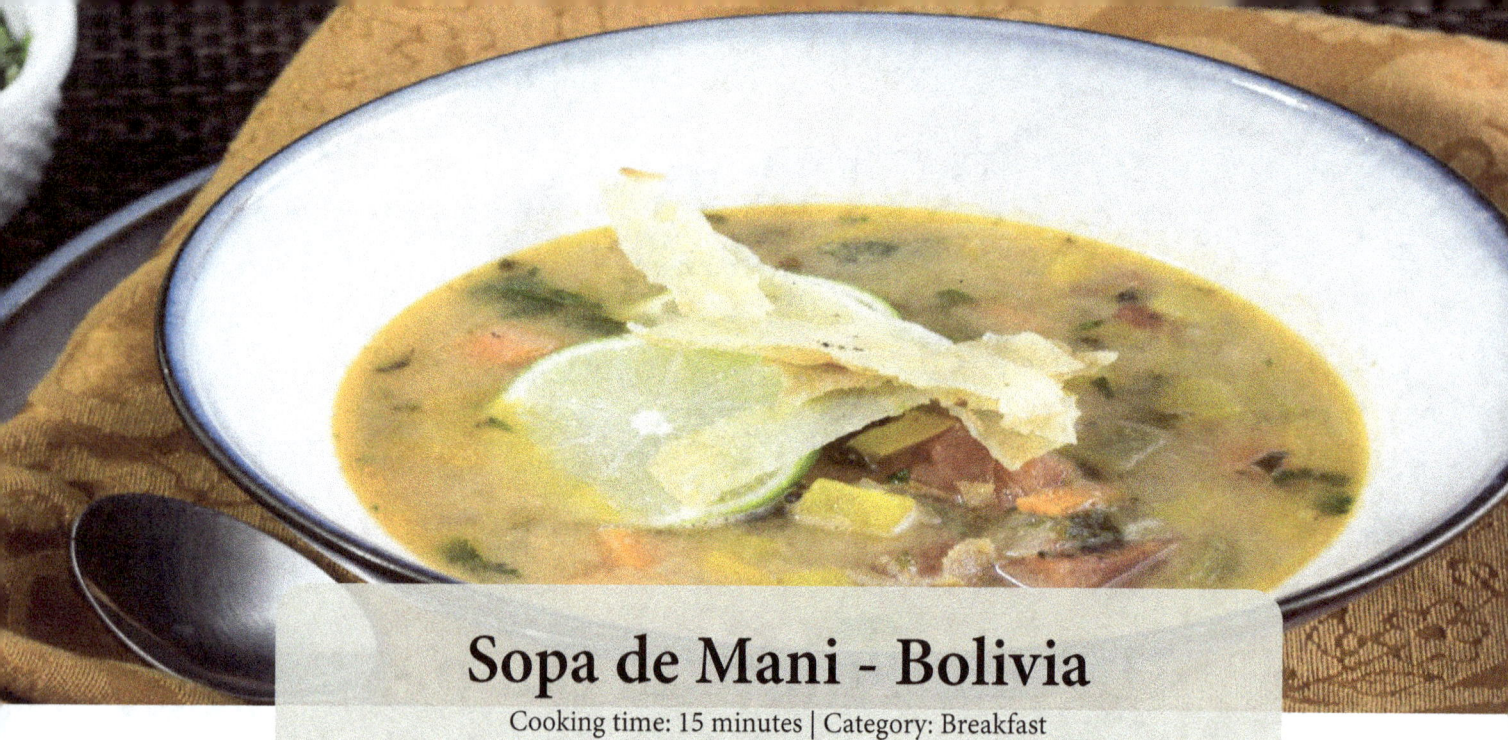

Sopa de Mani - Bolivia

Cooking time: 15 minutes | Category: Breakfast

The people of the Andean zone, with its cold climate, favor very spicy foods full of carbohydrates. Sopa de mani is one of the most delicious and traditional soups in Bolivia. It is made with peanuts, pasta, peas, and potatoes, and is accompanied by pieces of beef or chicken

Ingredients

- 3 lbs. beef with bone (neck or rib), cut into pieces
- 4 oz. raw peanuts
- 1 white onion, peeled and chopped
- 1 carrot, diced
- 3 oz. peas (fresh or frozen)
- 1 stalk celery, finely chopped
- ½ red bell pepper, diced
- ¼ cup vegetable oil
- 3 cloves garlic, chopped
- 6 cups beef broth (or vegetable broth)
- 4 potatoes, cut into large cubes
- 1 teaspoon cumin
- ½ teaspoon oregano
- ½ lb macaroni pasta
- 1 small bunch of flat parsley, chopped
- Salt
- Black pepper

Steps to Cook

1. Toast the macaroni in a dry pan, stirring constantly over medium heat until golden brown (about 8 minutes). Set aside.
2. Soak the peanuts in hot water for 2 minutes so that they can be peeled easily. Drain them.
3. In the bowl of a blender, mix the peanuts and a cup of cold water until you obtain a paste. Set aside.
4. In a large pot, heat the oil over medium heat and sauté the garlic.
5. Add the onion, carrot, peas, and celery.
6. Sauté over high heat for 5 minutes, stirring constantly.
7. Add the meat, red bell pepper and broth, and sauté over medium heat for 5 minutes.
8. Add the blended peanuts and stir well.
9. Add the potatoes. Add salt, black pepper, cumin, and oregano. Mix well.
10. Cover and cook over medium heat for 15 minutes.
11. Add the toasted macaroni.
12. Cover and cook over low heat for 15 minutes, stirring regularly.
13. Sprinkle with chopped parsley at the time of serving.

Note:

The number of calories per serving is 459.

Week - 8

Reflections

- How was your practice of prayer, meditation & gratitude this week?

_____
_____
_____
_____

- What are you observing in your body & mind?

_____
_____
_____
_____

- What new recipes did you try?

_____
_____
_____
_____

- How did you feel connecting with old friends?

_____
_____
_____
_____

- What is your time for 2.5miles of running or walking?

_____
_____
_____
_____

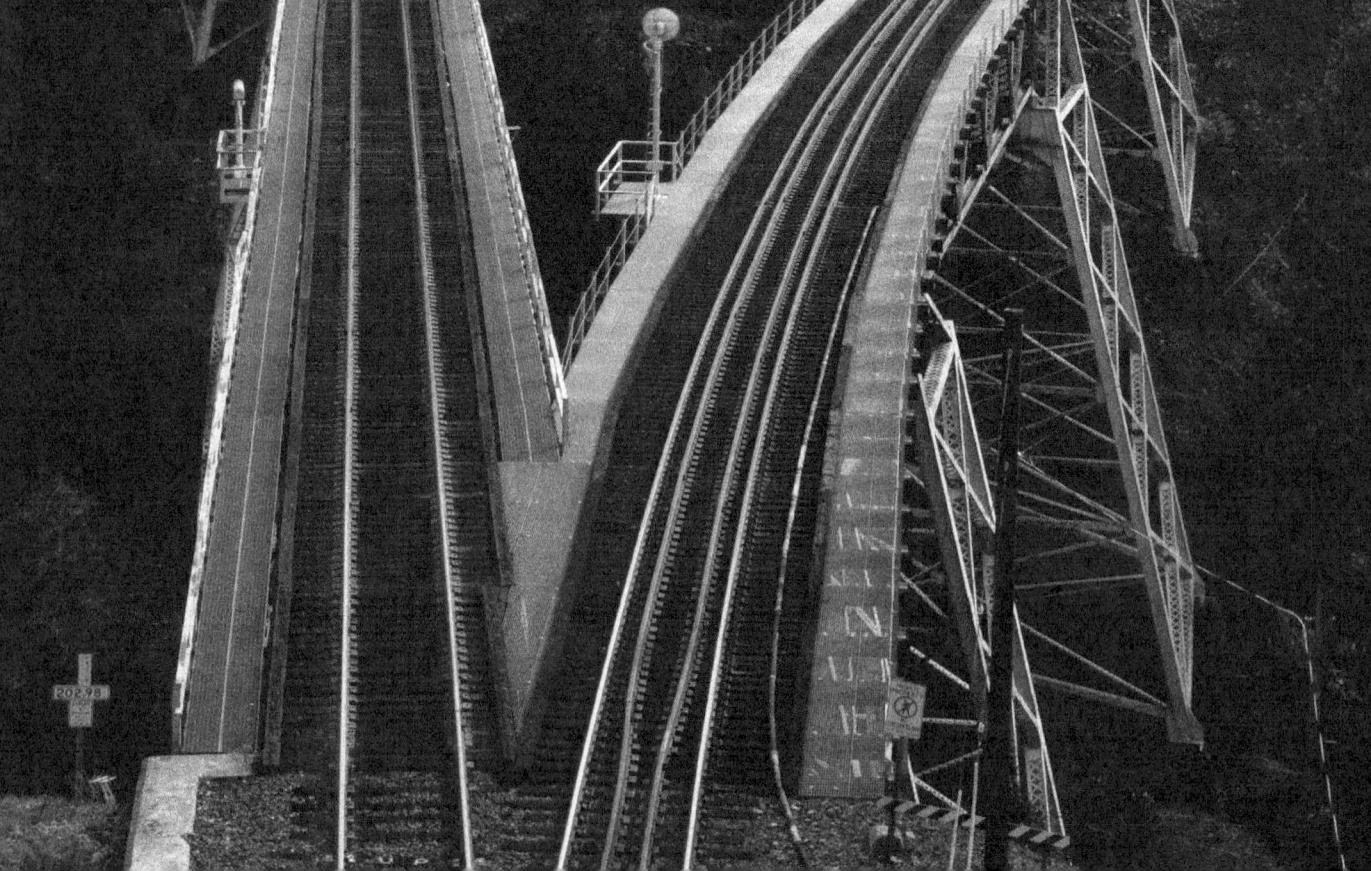

Identify your strongholds
Week 9

Week - 9

Take Obedient Action

- Spend 25 minutes practicing prayer, meditation & writing in your gratitude journal

_____

_____

_____

_____

- Try a new cooking oil this week.

_____

_____

_____

_____

- Select 2 Lunch, 2 Dinner & 2 Breakfast recipes from week 9 & prepare them.

_____

_____

_____

_____

- Connect with new people from different countries digitally or in person

_____

_____

_____

_____

- Increase your cardio to 3 miles walking or running add 10 minutes of stretching & strength training exercises

_____

_____

_____

_____

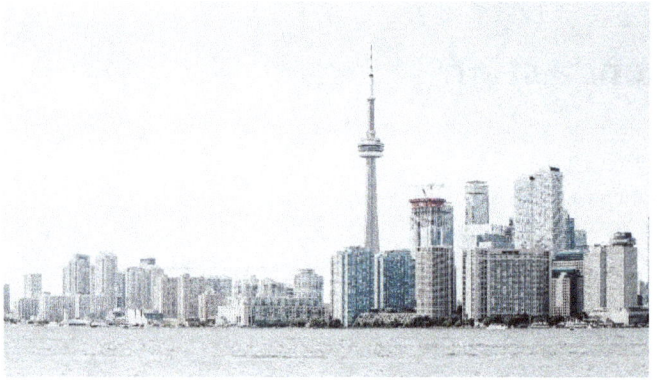

Toronto-Dinner

Toronto is the capital city of the Canadian province of Ontario. With a recorded population of 2,731,571 in 2016. It is the most populous city in Canada. The Toronto Zoo is the largest in Canada, and one of the largest in the world. It is popular in Ontario, but it's also world-renowned.

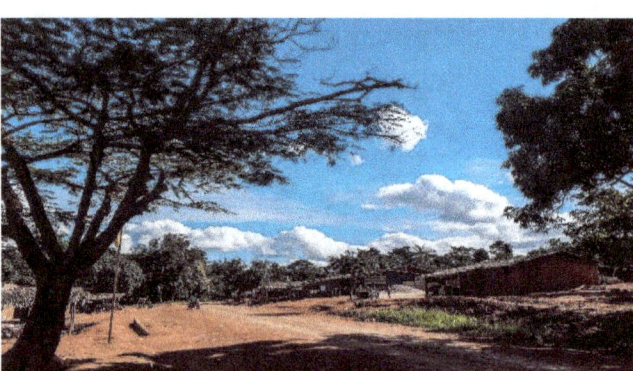

Cameroon-Breakfast

This Central African country has its main capital in Yaoundé.

Its seaport in Douala.

Cameroun is poly-diverse in culture and geography with an average population of about 27615638.

Cash crops for exports are majorly cotton cocoa, coffee, bananas, and oil seeds.

Its quality soil properties make for one of the most fertile grounds for agricultural production.

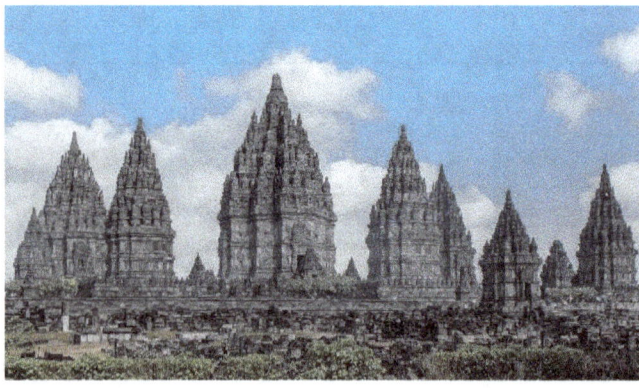

Indonesia-Lunch

The country is famous throughout the world for its islands and beautiful landscapes.

Its capital city is in Jakarta.

Rice, coconuts, soybeans, bananas, coffee, tea, palm, rubber, sand sugar cane.

It's the world's fourth most populous nation.

Indonesians are separated by seas and clustered on islands. The largest cluster is on Java, with some 130 million inhabitants.

On a vacation to Indonesia?

Perhaps a visit to Lorentz National Park will re-orient your mindset for good about this Asian country.

Rice, coconuts, soybeans, bananas, coffee, tea, palm, rubber, and sand sugar cane are very common food products in Indonesia.

It might interest you to also know that this country has the largest gold mine in the world.

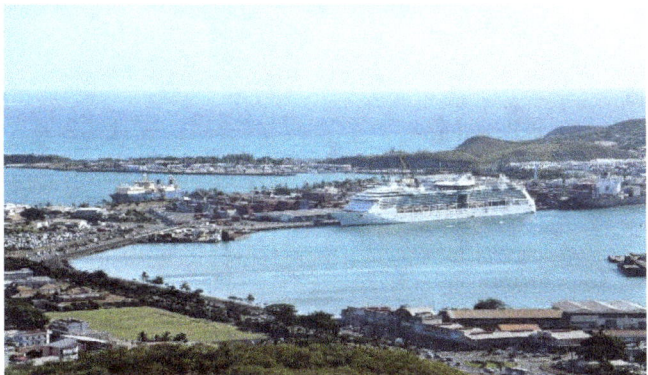

New Caledonia-Dinner

The current capital city of this French country is Nouméa.

It's known for its green vegetation, exotic beaches, and lovely aquatic scenery and is just a bit of New Caledonia.

It boasts a population of 289,875.

The French lifestyle largely rubbed off this South Pacific country in terms of mouth-watery cuisines and clothing lines.

Fine French flavors are not absent in this country's rich marine life dishes.

Prawns, lobsters, and shrimp are abundant.

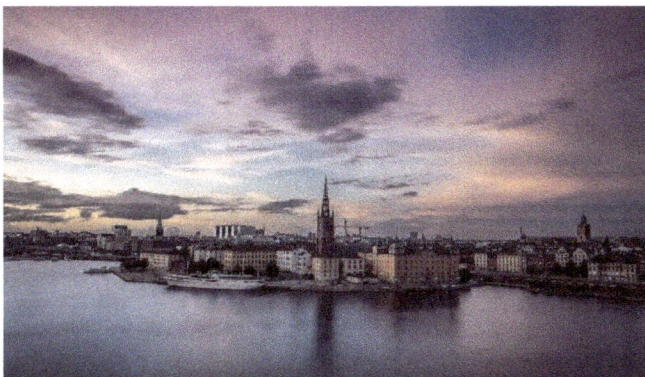

Sweden-Lunch

The Swedish population of 10.3 million people is concentrated in the southern part of the country. The capital and largest city is Stockholm. Approximately 57% of Sweden is forested. Sweden's yuletide drink of choice is a carbonated beverage, or soda, called Julmust.

Julmust is a fermented, though alcohol-free, malt drink like root beer. Fika is a communal and pretty much compulsory thing. It's a recognized break twice daily where workers enjoy coffee, cake, and chat. Swedish cuisine could be described as centered around cultured dairy products, crisp and soft (often sugared) bread, berries and stone fruits, beef, chicken, lamb, pork, eggs, and seafood. Potatoes are often served as a side dish, often boiled.

Swedish meatballs might be the most iconic dish from Sweden. There are several ways you can serve meatballs, but the most common is with mashed potatoes, creme sauce, and lingon. Meatballs and macaroni with ketchup are especially popular among kids.

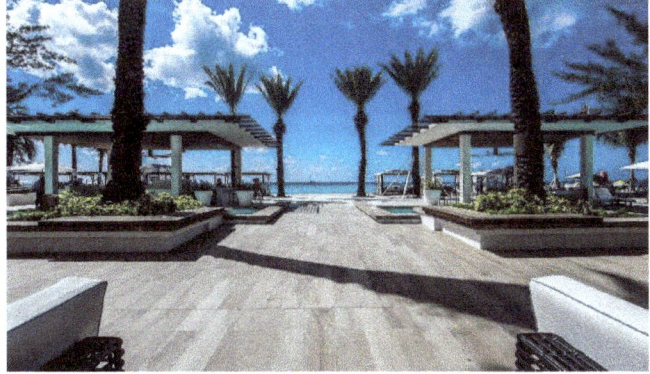

The Cayman Islands-Dinner

This territory has its capital location in George Town. There are 3 major islands.

The Grand Cayman (the largest island, famed for exotic beach resorts and a must-try spot for divers. Cayman Brac is a favorite spot for fishers. This British Overseas territory inhabits about 66,955 currently Popularly revered as the culinary capital of the Caribbean.

This territory gallantly appeals to the finest flavors for sea-food foodies.

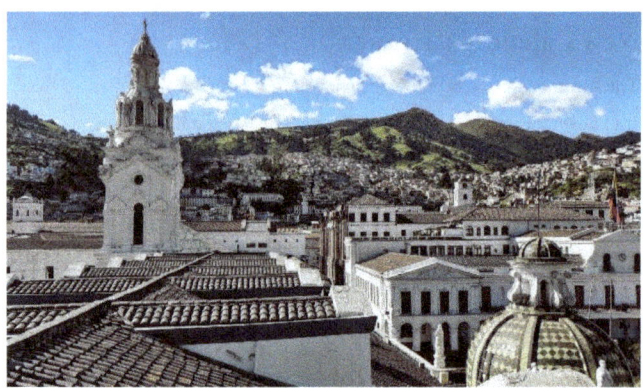

Ecuador-Breakfast

The capital state of this South American country (Quito) is famous for certain sacred buildings. Ecuador boasts of large petroleum reserves, and this accounts for a large portion of her national capital. Ecuador is a big exporter of coffee, wood, and fish. It is also renowned to produce staples like corn, palm, and coffee, shrimp, sugar cane, rice.

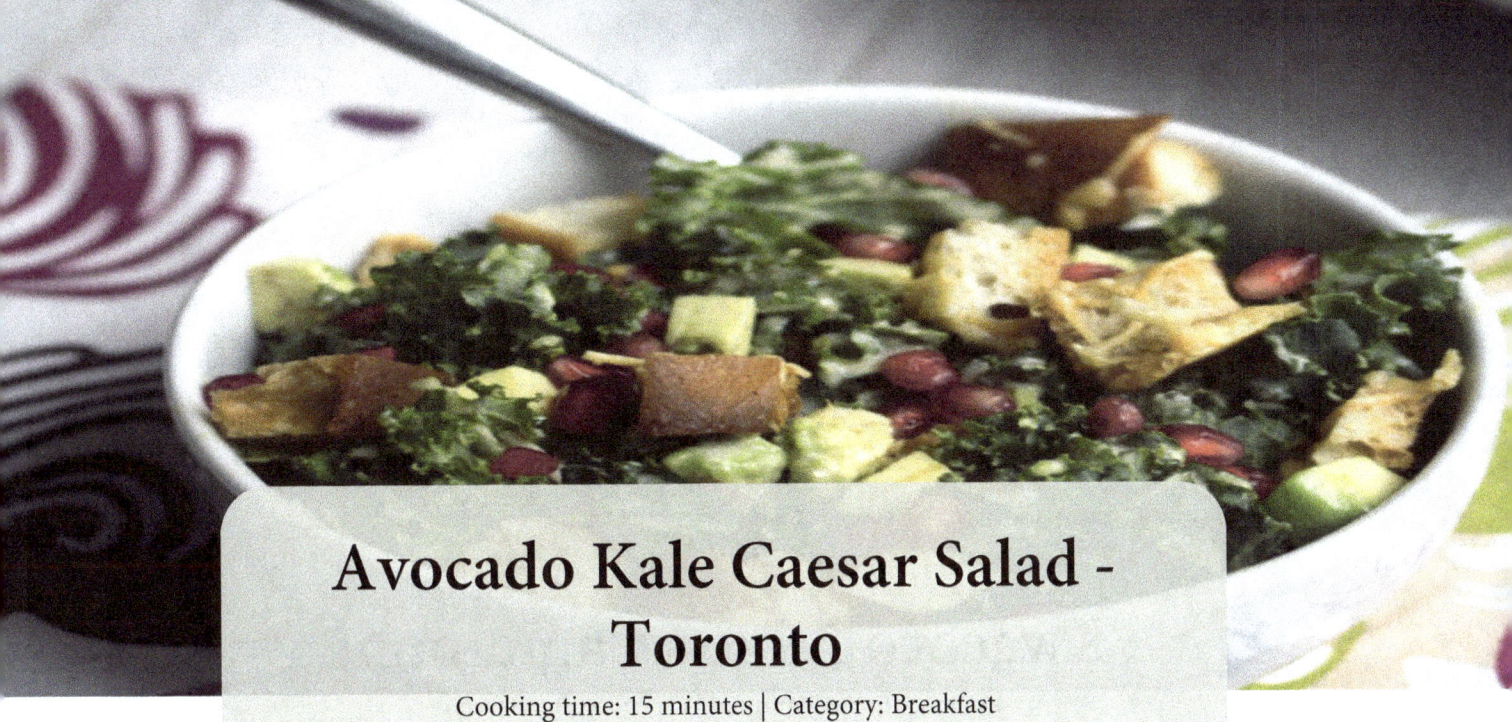

Avocado Kale Caesar Salad - Toronto

Cooking time: 15 minutes | Category: Breakfast

Kale Caesar is quickly becoming a classic and here we have a unique twist that adds Fresh California Avocado to both the dressing and the salad. This creates a creaminess that sticks to the kale leaves, delivering the full flavor of Caesar Salad in every satisfying bite.

Ingredients

Salad

- 6 strips of bacon
- 2 bunches of kale, shredded
- 1 romaine lettuce heart, coarsely chopped
- 4 Tbsp Avocado Dressing
- Salt
- 4 Tbsp grated Parmigiano- Reggiano
- 1 avocado, sliced
- 1 cup croutons
- 1 lemon, cut into wedges (optional)

Avocado dressing

- 2 avocados, peeled and pitted
- Juice of 1 lemon
- 1/4 cup avocado oil
- 1/4 cup cold waterf
- 2 Tbsp grated Parmigiano-

Reggiano

- 1/2 clove garlic, finely chopped
- 1/4 anchovy filet, finely chopped
- 1 Tbsp salt

Steps to Cook

Avocado Dressing

1. Place avocado, lemon juice, avocado oil, and water into a blender and blend for 1 to 2 minutes, until smooth and creamy.
2. Add Parmigiano-Reggiano, garlic, anchovy, and salt and purée for another 30 seconds, until well incorporated.
3. (If the mixture is too thick, add more cold water.)
4. Refrigerate until needed. Makes approximately 1 cup.

Salad

1. Preheat the oven to 400°F. Place bacon on a baking tray and bake for 7 to 8 minutes, or until crispy.
2. Place kale and romaine in a large bowl, add dressing, and mix thoroughly to coat.
3. Add a pinch of salt to taste and add more dressing if desired.
4. Place dressed leaves in a large serving bowl, sprinkle with Parmigiano-Reggiano and top with avocado, bacon, and croutons. Serve with lemon wedges, if using.

Note:

The number of calories per serving of Avocado Kale Caesar Salad is 310 Caribana is one of Toronto's most celebrated traditions. It is a multi-weekend cultural celebration that aims to celebrate Caribbean culture and traditions. Perhaps a motorcycle ride through Yonge Street (the longest street in the world) will not be a bad idea at all. Niagara Falls is a must-go place to have real fun.

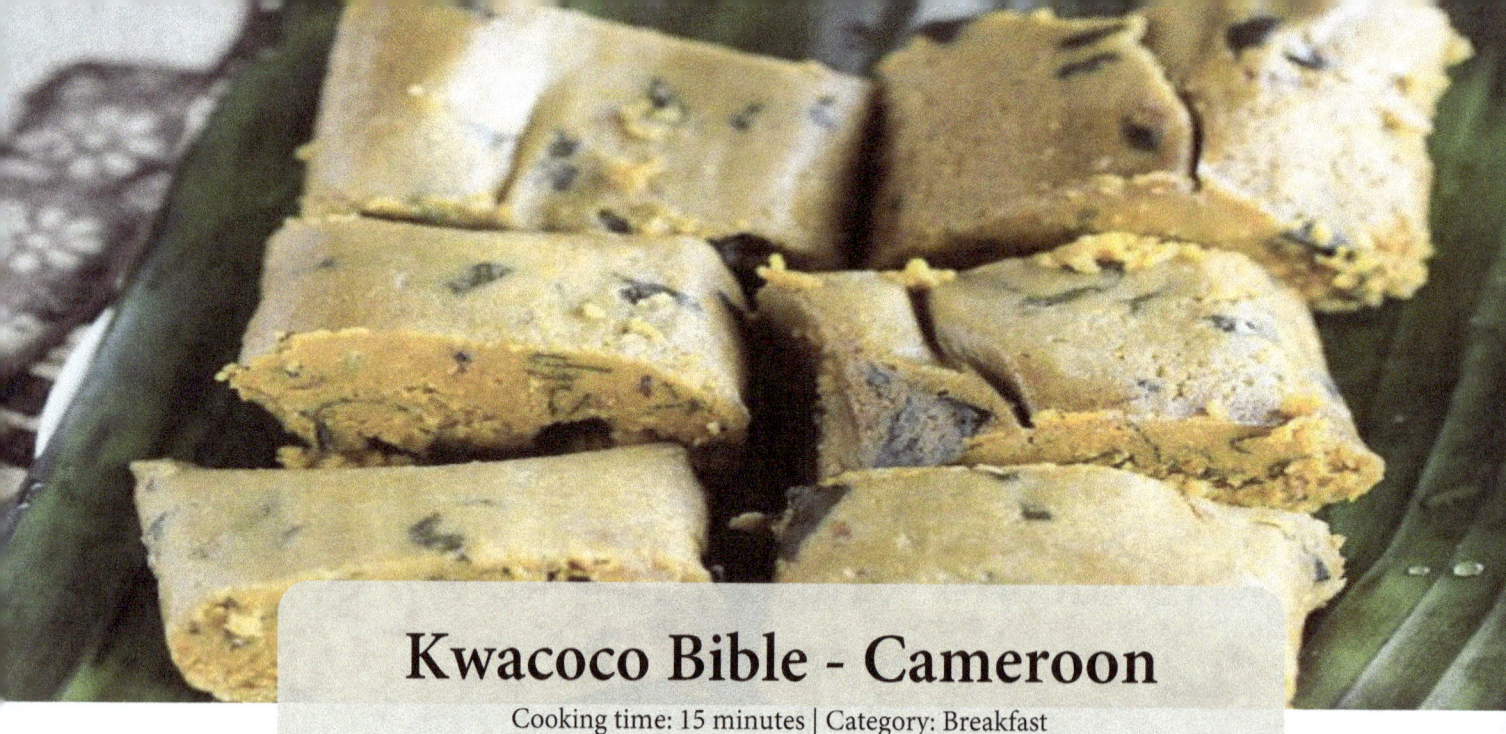

Kwacoco Bible - Cameroon

Cooking time: 15 minutes | Category: Breakfast

This traditional dish is simply cocoyams grated, fortified with fish, crayfish wrapped in plantain leaves, and steamed until cooked through. This will take you to the heart of the Bakweri tribe.

Ingredients

- 3 pounds cocoyam peeled and cleaned
- 4 -5 cups fresh spinach chopped
- 1 cup red oil or more adjust according to preference
- 1– 1 ½ cup smoked turkey cut in bite-size pieces
- 2 teaspoons salt adjust to taste
- 1 scotch bonnet pierced
- 1 teaspoon bouillon powder or Maggie
- ½ teaspoon country onion spice optional
- ½ cup crayfish
- 1 1/2 cup smoked fish

Steps to Cook

1. Add about Lightly boil smoked turkey, smoked fish, crayfish with pepper, and Maggie in a medium pot for about 3-5 minutes.
2. Reserve the stock for later use. If you want more heat press the pepper for a long time. Remove scotch bonnet pepper and set aside.
3. Peel the coco
4. Cut into large chunks and wash immediately to prevent discoloration and leave them in cool water until ready to use.
5. Grate cocoyam using a grater or pulse the cocoyam in a food processor with water until puree (try not to make it too fine).
6. In a large bowl add a mixture of fish, spinach, red oil, crayfish, smoked turkey, stock, salt, and country onion to the grated cocoyam.
7. Cut the banana leaves into rectangles, remove any edges, submerge them in water to clean, and drain. Use aluminum paper

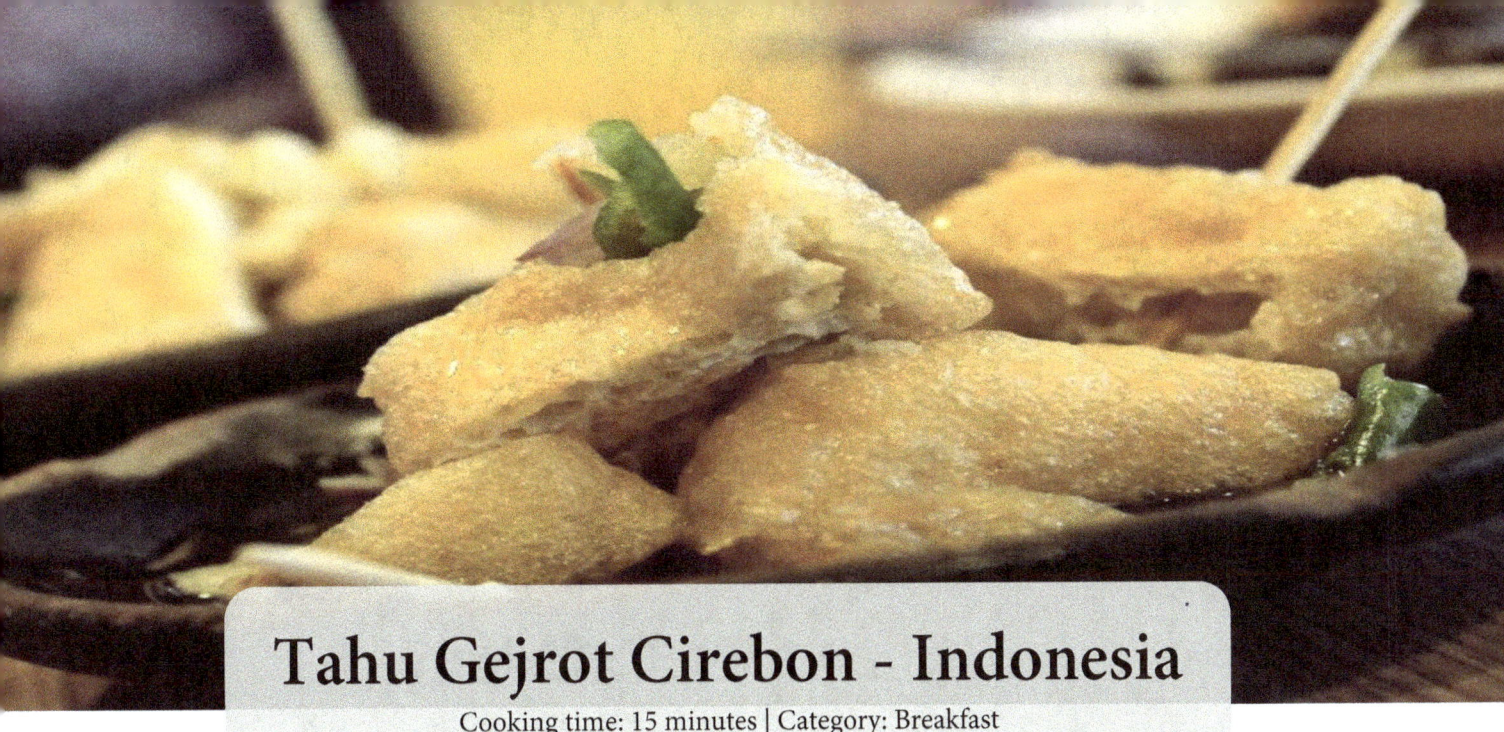

Tahu Gejrot Cirebon - Indonesia

Cooking time: 15 minutes | Category: Breakfast

Street food is a common sight in Indonesian life, and though it may sound unusual to non-Indonesians, we have quite a variety of tofu-based street food snacks or light meals.

Ingredients

- 450 grams of tofu
- 200mls of water
- 50 ml (3 tablespoons + 1 teaspoon) sweet soy sauce
- 25-gram (0.9 oz) coconut palm sugar
- 1/2 teaspoon salt
- 1/2 tablespoon cane sugar vinegar/rice vinegar
- 2-5 bird-eye chilies, or 1-3 cayenne/serrano/jalapeno, thinly sliced
- 50-gram shallot, minced
- 2 cloves garlic, minced

Steps to Cook

1. The tofu is dried with a kitchen towel and cut into many pieces
2. Pour a little oil into a frying pan and it is fried until it is brownish color. Cut into smaller pieces and the parts are arranged in smaller bowls.
3. Pour some water into a saucepan, and add some sweet soy sauce, coconut palm sugar, salt, vinegar, shallot, and garlic.
4. Stir together and allow to boil
5. Reduce heat and simmer for 5 minutes.
6. Dress prepared tofu with toppings from the sauce and serve immediately.
7.

Note:

The number of calories per serving is 323.5.

Feeling cold in Indonesia?

Bandrek is the perfect drink for you. It is made from ginger and brown sugar, while pandan leaves and spices such as cinnamon and cloves can be added to increase the richness of the drink. You will smack your lips in affirmation of its deliciousness.

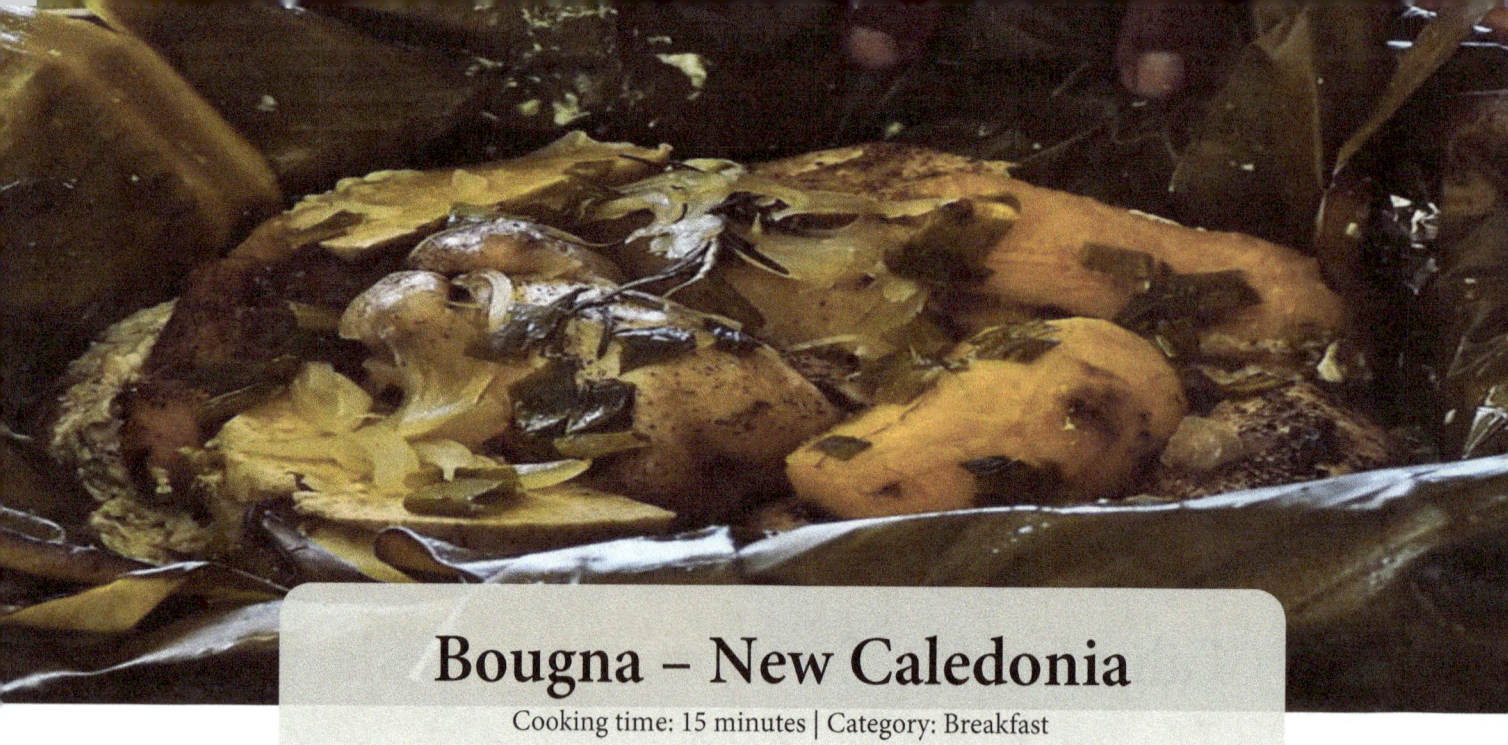

Bougna – New Caledonia

Cooking time: 15 minutes | Category: Breakfast

This New Caledonian dish is peculiar to Kanak cuisine. It is common among the locals.

It is a combination of chicken, lobster, or fish mixed with yams, sweet potatoes, and coconut milk, wrapped in banana leaves. There are variations in the choice of condiments across different regions.

Ingredients

- 4minced garlic
- 3 parsley
- 2 cups of coconut milk
- 2 cups of chicken stock
- Salt and pepper
- 1 carrot
- 1 chicken
- 3 small tomatoes (into 4 chunks)
- 1 sliced onion
- 2 sprigs of thyme
- 1 parsnip

Steps to Cook

1. Peel the root vegetables and cut them into small pieces. Then put them in water to prevent them from turning black. Peel the bananas and cut them in half. Cut the tomato into quarters, slice the onion, the bunch of spring onions, and finally the chicken.

2. Put a tablespoon of oil in the pan and add the chicken pieces. Place the root vegetables, onion, spring onions, tomato, and bananas on top. Add salt and pepper and pour in a liter of coconut milk. Put the lid back on and simmer for 30 minutes.

3. Remove the lid and pour in half a glass of water. Replace the lid for a further 30 minutes.

4. Return to the pan and make sure the root vegetables are cooked through. To do this, pierce them with a sharp knife. If it goes in easily, the bougna is cooked. Bon appétit!

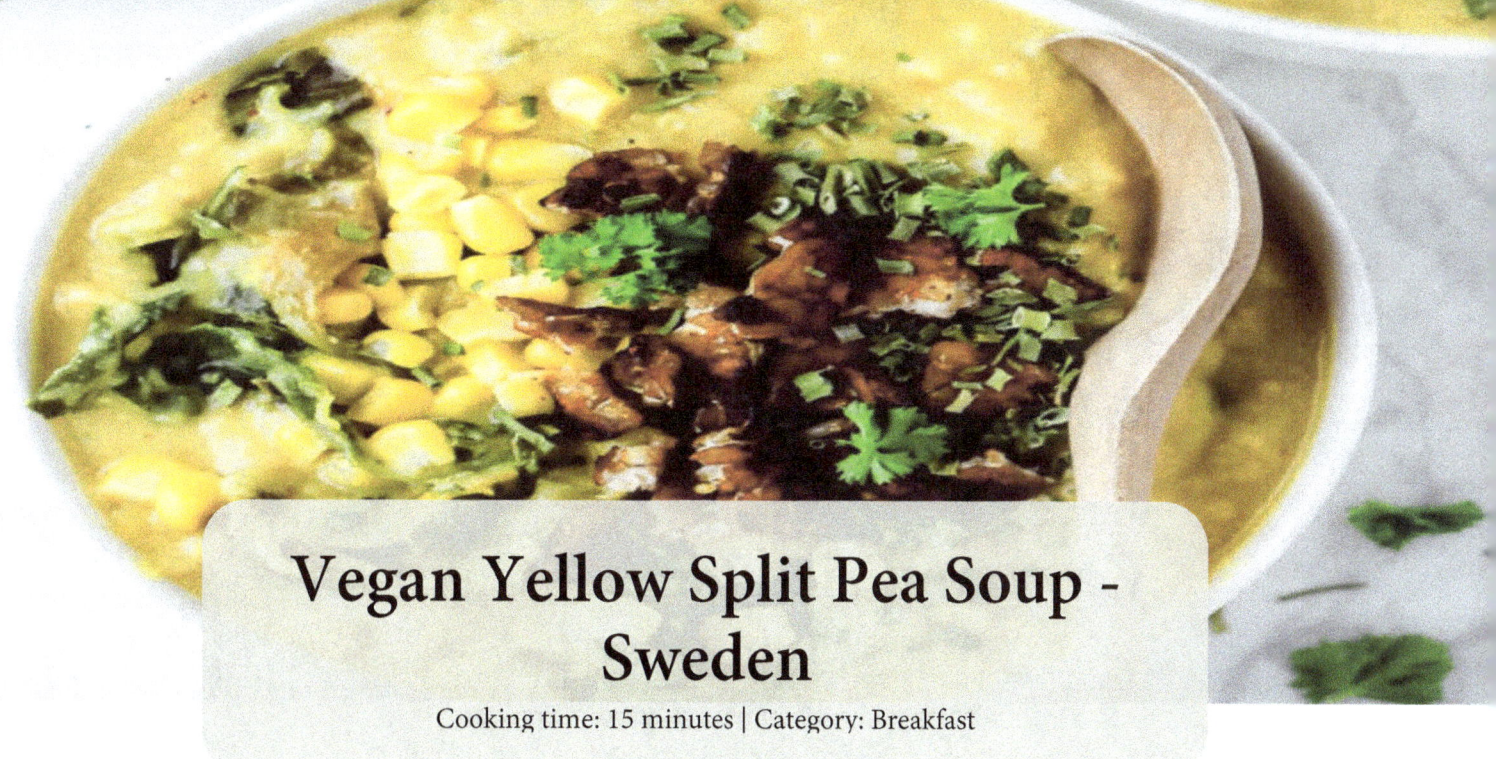

Vegan Yellow Split Pea Soup - Sweden

Cooking time: 15 minutes | Category: Breakfast

Vegan yellow split pea soup is a healthy, protein-packed, and frugal soup that is delicious and satisfying!

It can also be made with green split peas or yellow lentils. Loaded with protein and super affordable, this thick, warm soup is the perfect way to stay warm during those long, cold Swedish winters.

Ingredients

- 1 tablespoon extra-virgin olive oil
- 2 cups chopped onions
- 1 and 1/2 cups chopped carrots
- 1/4 tsp freshly cracked black pepper
- 1 and 1/3 cups dried yellow split peas, rinsed
- 6 and 3/4 cups water, divided
- 1/2 teaspoon fine sea salt (plus more to taste)
- Optional: 1/4 cup chopped fresh flat-leaf (Italian) parsley or dill, divided

Steps to Cook

1. In a large saucepan, heat oil over medium-high heat. Add onions, carrots, and pepper; cook, stirring, for 6 to 8 minutes or until vegetables are softened.
2. Stir in peas, 6 cups water, and salt. Bring to a boil. Reduce heat to medium-low, cover, and simmer, stirring occasionally, for 35 to 40 minutes or until peas are very tender.
3. Transfer 1 cup of the soup solids to a food processor. Add remaining 3/4 cup water and process until smooth.
4. Return purée the pan and stir in half the parsley or dill, if using. Simmer, stirring often, for 5 minutes to blend the flavors, thinning soup with water if too thick. Serve sprinkled with the remaining parsley or dill.
5. Number of calories per serving is 236.
6. A visit to the Gamla Stan in Stockholm city is a must-do fun activity to immerse oneself completely in the Swedish culture.

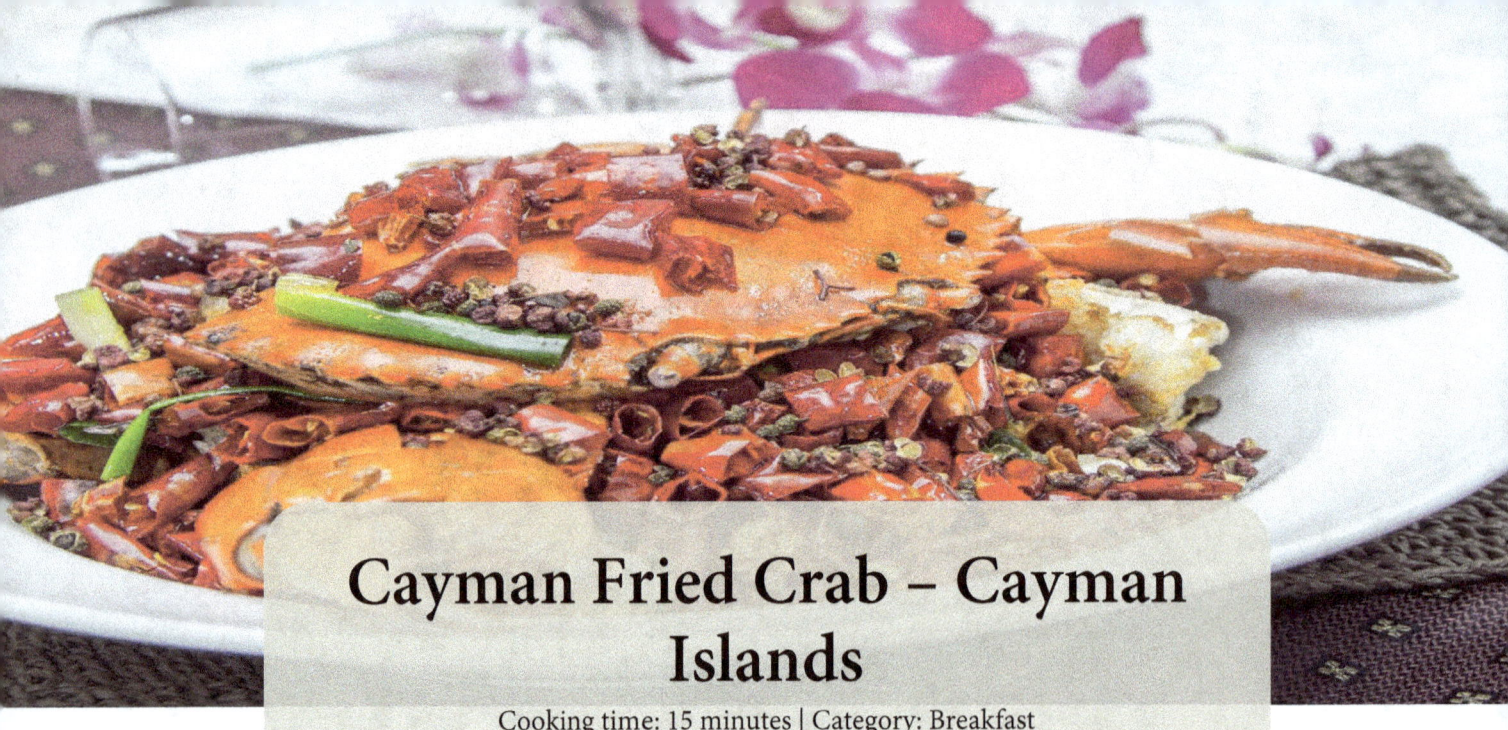

Cayman Fried Crab – Cayman Islands

Cooking time: 15 minutes | Category: Breakfast

This lunch recipe is prepared with fresh crabs; the meat from crab boiling is removed and mixed with the other stuff. It's a healthy protein-rich choice for an average Cayman and even tourists.

Ingredients

- 1 lb. crab meat
- 2 medium onions
- 1 scotch bonnet pepper
- ½ tsp. black pepper
- salt (to taste)
- ¼ cup cooking oil

Steps to Cook

1. Wash crabs and boil in a large pot of water for 15 minutes, remove from boiling water, and cool. Crack legs and open backs to remove all meat and set aside.
2. Remove seeds from scotch bonnet pepper and dice pepper and onions. Sauté onions and scotch bonnet peppers in oil over medium heat until onions begin to get transparent.
3. Add crab meat, black pepper, and salt, stirring occasionally. Cook over medium heat for an additional 5 to 10 minutes.
4. Serve with "bread kind", a local dish that consists of a variety of starchy vegetables including pumpkin, squash, plantain, potato, cassava, and breadfruit.
5. Optional: Seasoned crab meat may also be stuffed in cleaned crab backs and baked. Cover stuffed backs with foil paper and bake at 350 degrees for 30 minutes.

Note:

Cray brew beer is a must-try beverage on your next visit to Cayman Island. It's an infusion of locally sourced ingredients. The Cayman Islands are renowned to possess a plethora of recipes to satisfy your marine-life cravings!

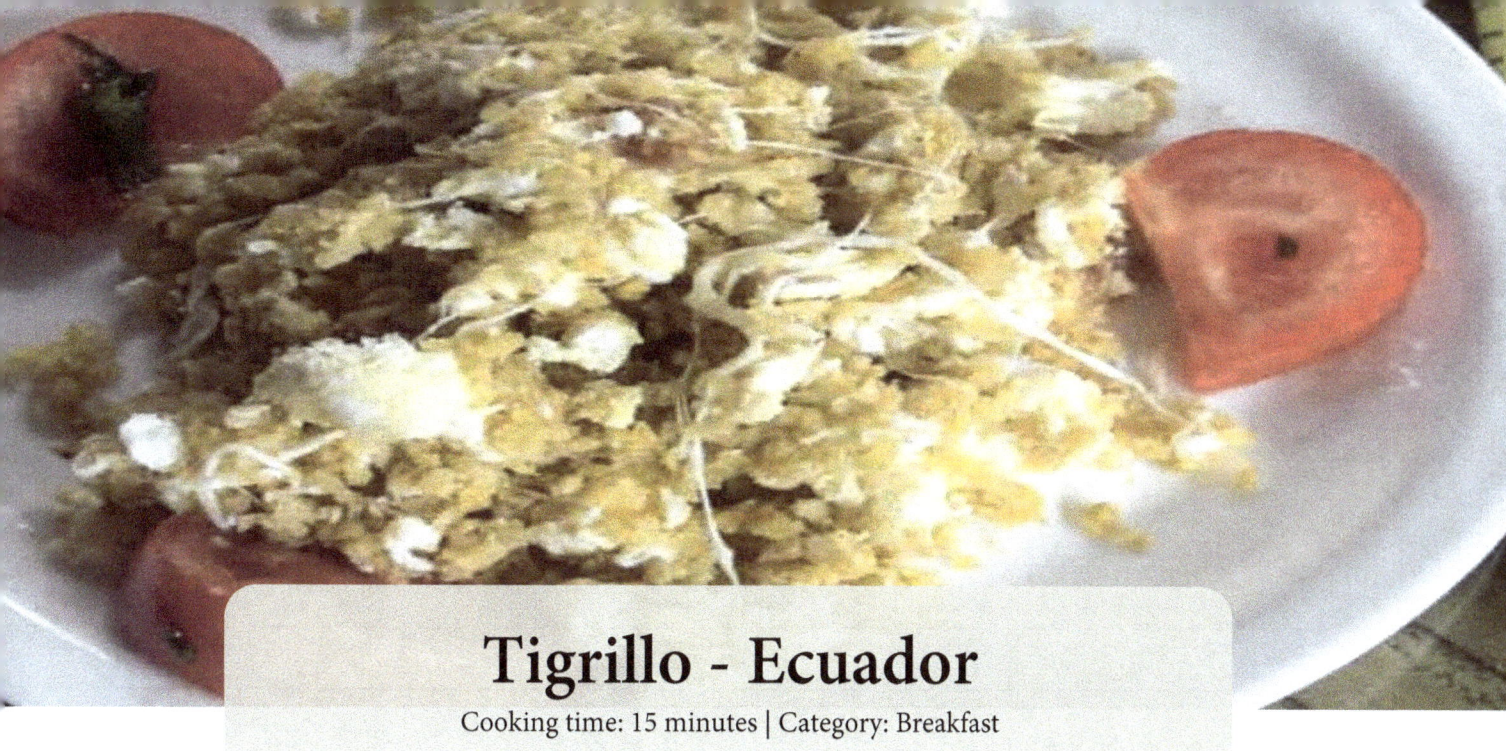

Tigrillo - Ecuador

Cooking time: 15 minutes | Category: Breakfast

This unique breakfast is peculiar to an average Ecuadorian. It consists of a mixture of plantains, scrambled eggs, cheese, and coriander spice. Plantains can be substituted for potatoes if desired.

Ingredients

- 2 plantains
- 2 spoons of butter
- 2 – 3 eggs
- 100 g grated cheese
- 30g coriander
- half an onion, chopped
- Salt and Pepper

For the cream:

- Some broth, milk, or cream
- Fried egg
- Up to your taste
- Chicharron (crispy pork skin)

Steps to Cook

1. Boil some water in a pot, chop the onions and coriander, grate the cheese and prepare the butter.
2. Peel and halve the bananas, cut them in half, and place them in the boiling water.
3. After about 10 minutes, the bananas are soft enough to crush like the potatoes in mashed potatoes.
4. While the bananas are cooking, heat some oil in a pan and prepare a classic scrambled egg.
5. Then melt the butter in another pan. Add the onions, and sauté lightly. Then add the crushed banana mixture and let it heat up.
6. To make your tigrillo creamier, add some broth or cream. Add the scrambled eggs and cheese, let it warm for a short while, and refine with delicious coriander, salt, and pepper.

Note:

Ecuador, (the largest exporter of bananas in the world), boasts of unique biodiversity as displayed by its scenic geographic sites:

The Galapagos Islands and Yasuni are favorite national parks, for wildlife enthusiasts

Week - 9

Reflections

- How was your practice of prayer, meditation & gratitude this week?

_____
_____
_____
_____
_____

- Favorite meal to prepare this week?

_____
_____
_____
_____
_____

- What new oil did you use this week?

_____
_____
_____
_____
_____

- How did you connect with others this week?

_____
_____
_____
_____
_____

Reframing Your Obstacles

Week 10

Week - 10

Take Obedient Action

- Spend 30 minutes practicing prayer, meditation & writing in your gratitude journal

___

- Select 3 Lunch recipes from week 10 & prepare them

___

- Host a luncheon or dinner party to share your new recipes from the last 9 weeks

___

- Maintain cardio of 3 miles of walking or running, add 10 minutes of stretching & 5 strength training exercises

___

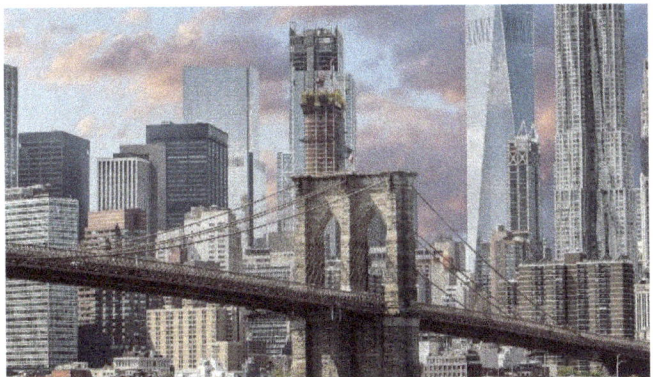

New York City-Breakfast

New York City is the most populous city in the United States. Its capital is called Albany. It is the most influential American Metropolis.

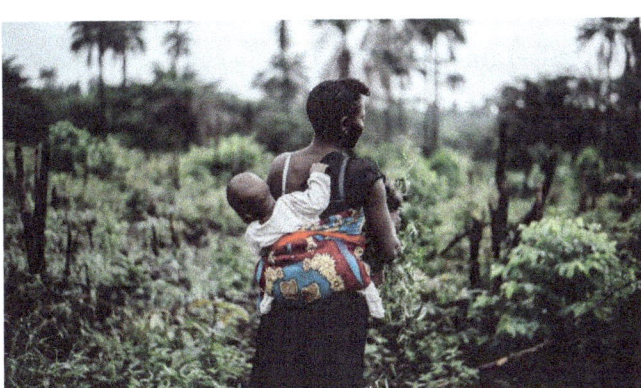

Togo-Lunch

This West African Country has its capital in Lome. Rich phosphate reserves, scenic countryside, and captivating mountaintops are all typical of this country.

Major cash crops are coffee, cocoa, and cotton. The French- speaking country is a proud producer of corn, sorghum, rice, yams, manioc, peanuts, beans, and soy which forms most of its cuisine staples.

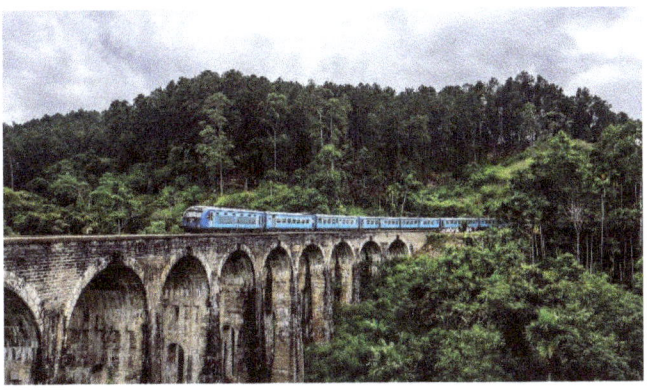

Sri Lanka-Dinner

The current population of the South Asian country is 21,556,478. Uppuveli and Nilaveli are large expanses of sandy beaches to feed your desire to unwind. Wildlife enthusiasts will surely love the spinner dolphins, giant elephants, blue whales and a variety of animal life to make you go wild!

Colombo's Ministry of Crab houses the finest reserves of the Sri Lankan crab. Little wonder, it was nominated as one of Asia's 50 best eateries in 2016.

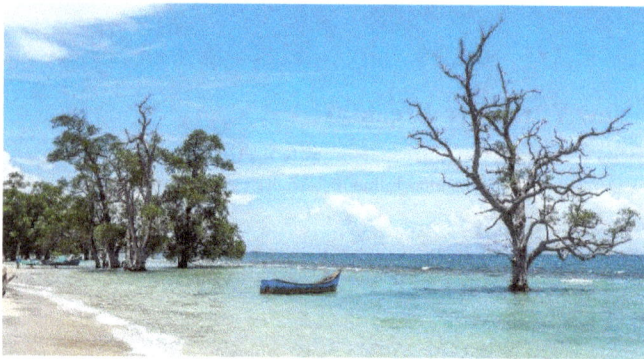

Kiribati-Breakfast

This island country in the central Pacific Ocean houses about 20 habitable Islands. The current population is estimated at 122,371.

The capital city is South Tarawa.

Sparsely dispersed land masses and fine aquatic scenes, phosphate-rich Banaba Island are sites that could leave you thrilled!

A majority of Kiribatian dishes are based on coconuts, fish, and taro. They are abundant!

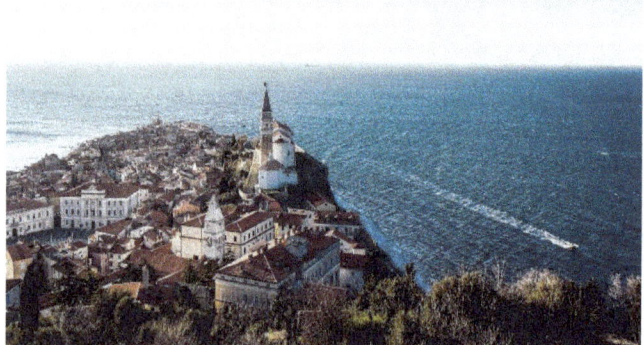

Slovenia-Lunch

The current population is estimated at over 2.1 million people. Ljubljana is Slovenia's capital known for its glacial scenes. The Central European country is famous for its lovely mountain top view, ski resorts, and the tourist-attracting lakes in the entire continent. The jaw-dropping spots will feed your adventure cravings. Lovers of natural greenery and traditional landscapes will love it here!

Slovenian cuisines are healthy and sumptuous with a variety of locally sourced spices!

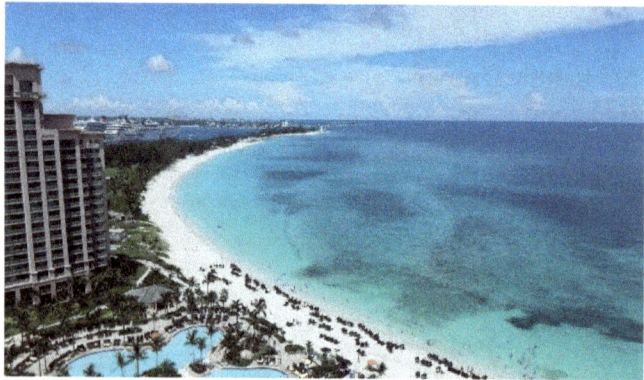

The Bahamas-Dinner

The current population of this Caribbean country skyrocketed to 400,516 in 2022 compared to 2021. Water sports are common within its capital: Nassau.

The Bahamas is the go-to spot to satisfy your pleasure cravings, with San Salvador Island as a great resort center for tourists.

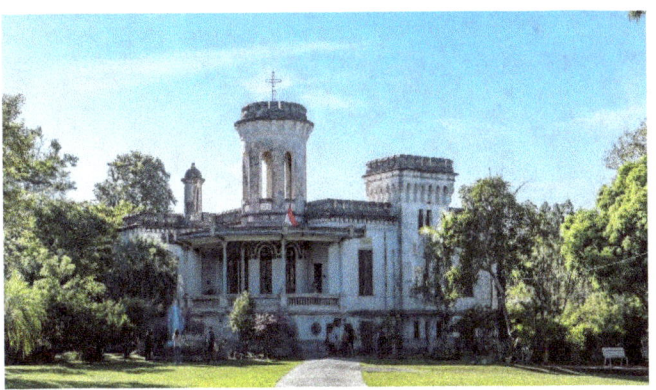

Paraguay-Breakfast

This South American country is heralded by forests, swamps, and savanna bordering. The capital city is Asunción and a population of over 7 million residents.

Paraguay plays home to one of the world's most sophisticated power plants as well as a formidable naval force. Chipa SOPAsopa is common breakfast staples.

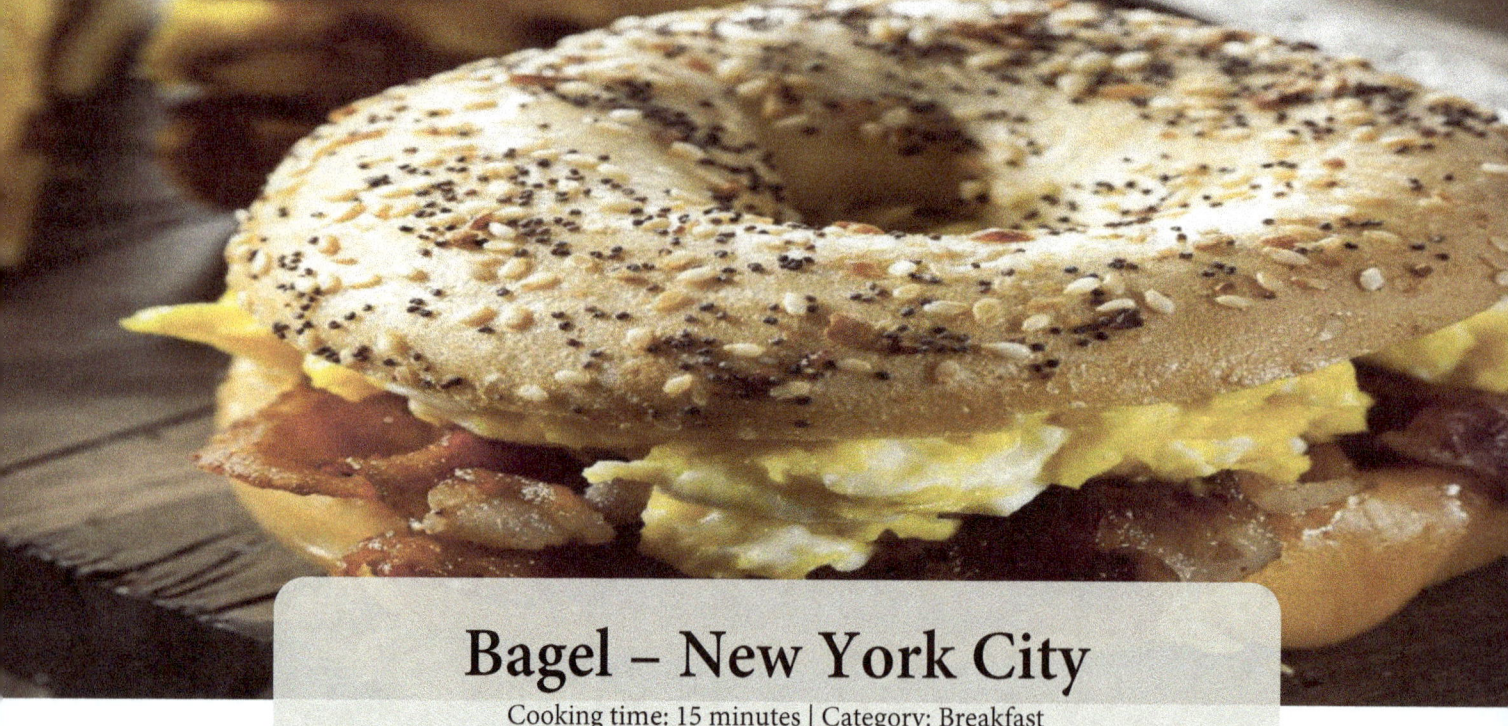

Bagel – New York City

Cooking time: 15 minutes | Category: Breakfast

Fresh bagels can be eaten plain, dressed with butter, or smeared with cream cheese. Like pizza, bagels are a source of pride to New Yorkers. At corner deli, you can find flavors like poppy seed, sesame, and cinnamon raisin are common in most bagel shops, plus a New York favorite called "everything". Topped with poppy seeds, toasted sesame seeds, dried garlic, dried, onion, and salt. Another good news is their thick crust and center.

Ingredients

- 1 cup water, warmed
- 2 large eggs
- 4 cups plain flour
- 1 1/2 tablespoons vegetable oil
- 1 tablespoon sugar (brown or white)
- 1 tablespoon salt
- 2 1/2 teaspoons dried yeast
- 1 egg yolk mixed with 1 tablespoon water, for glaze

Steps to Cook

1. Place all the dry ingredients into your food processor with the dough attachment on. Switch the machine on and then add the wet ingredients and mix until sticky dough is formed.
2. Empty onto a lightly floured board and knead by hand for about 3 minutes. Cover with plastic and leave to rise for about 20 minutes.
3. Divide the dough into equal portions. This mix will make around 12 to 14 decent-sized bagels. Roll each portion into a long snake shape. Wrap each dough snake around your wrist and nip where both ends meet to join them together and place on a baking sheet lined with plastic wrap or a baking mat.
4. At this point you have two options: 1. Leave the bagel rings to rise for around 30 minutes at room temperature before boiling. 2. Place in the fridge for around 48 hours before moving on to the next step. (Leaving them in the fridge allows for a slow rise, which will improve the final texture of the bagel.)
5. Preheat the oven to 375°F. Bring a large pot to a rolling boil and add 2 teaspoons of salt. Carefully add a couple of the bagel rings to the boiling water.

Note:

Use a slotted spatula or carefully drop in with your fingers. The bagel will sink to the bottom and then float within 1-2 minutes. Time 4 minutes from drop; then turn the bagels over and leave for another 3 minutes. Remove the bagels with the slotted spatula and place them back on the baking sheet lined with a baking mat to prevent sticking. Bagels pair comfortably with coffee. Bagels have a calorie content of 250 calories. A feel of a home can be experienced at Aire Ancient Baths. It's a cool way to unwind.

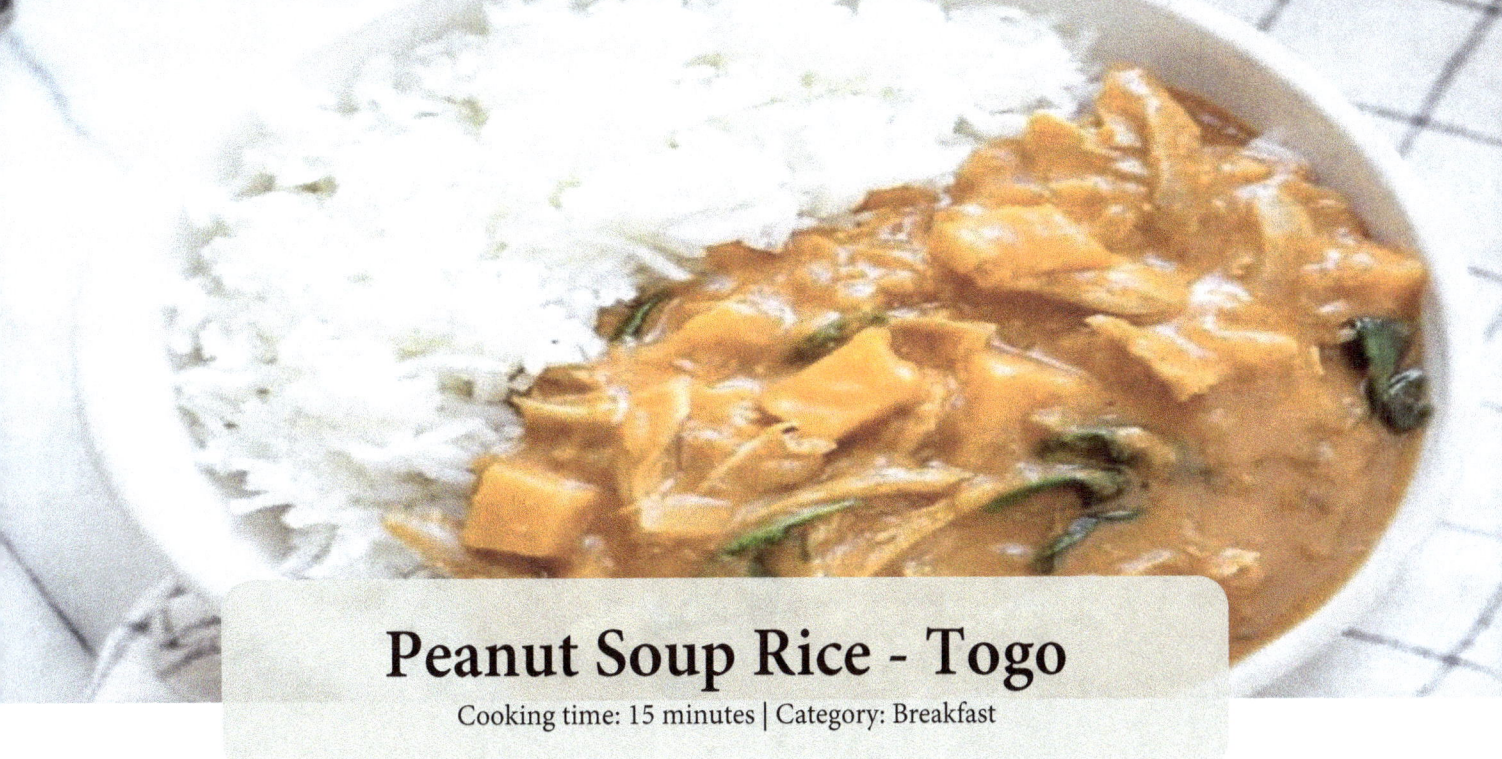

Peanut Soup Rice - Togo

Cooking time: 15 minutes | Category: Breakfast

Peanut soup rice will fill your lunch cravings in Togo. It is made from simply from milk, rice which is boiled white and kept aside. Ground peanuts are used to make a rich oily broth for incorporating upon the rice as a top dressing. Meat or fish is a preferred animal protein.

Ingredients

- 8 chicken thighs or 2 large, sweet potatoes/ 1 squash
- 1 large onion, chopped
- 1-2 cloves garlic, crushed
- 2 fresh medium tomatoes, chopped
- 2 tbs tomato puree
- 1 chicken or vegetable stock cube
- 1 cup of peanut butter
- Salt and pepper to taste
- 2 cups of water

Steps to Cook

1. Season the chicken with salt and pepper.
2. Add 1 tbsp of oil to a large frying pan or casserole dish and brown the chicken on all sides over medium heat. You may need to do this in batches.
3. Add the onions and garlic to the chicken and fry until soft.
4. Meanwhile, in a blender, add the peanut butter, chopped tomatoes, tomato puree, and water. Blend until you have a fine paste.
5. Stir the peanut paste into the chicken and leave on low heat, stirring occasionally. Leave for 30–40 mins to reduce and for the sauce to thicken.
6. Enjoy! Perfect with rice or couscous this stew makes the perfect teatime treat.

Note:

The number of calories per serving is 187.8g

You will be blown by the taste of tchoukoutou (fermented millet) is a healthy choice drink in Northern Togo. Lovers of lager beers are sure to have a field day in Togo.

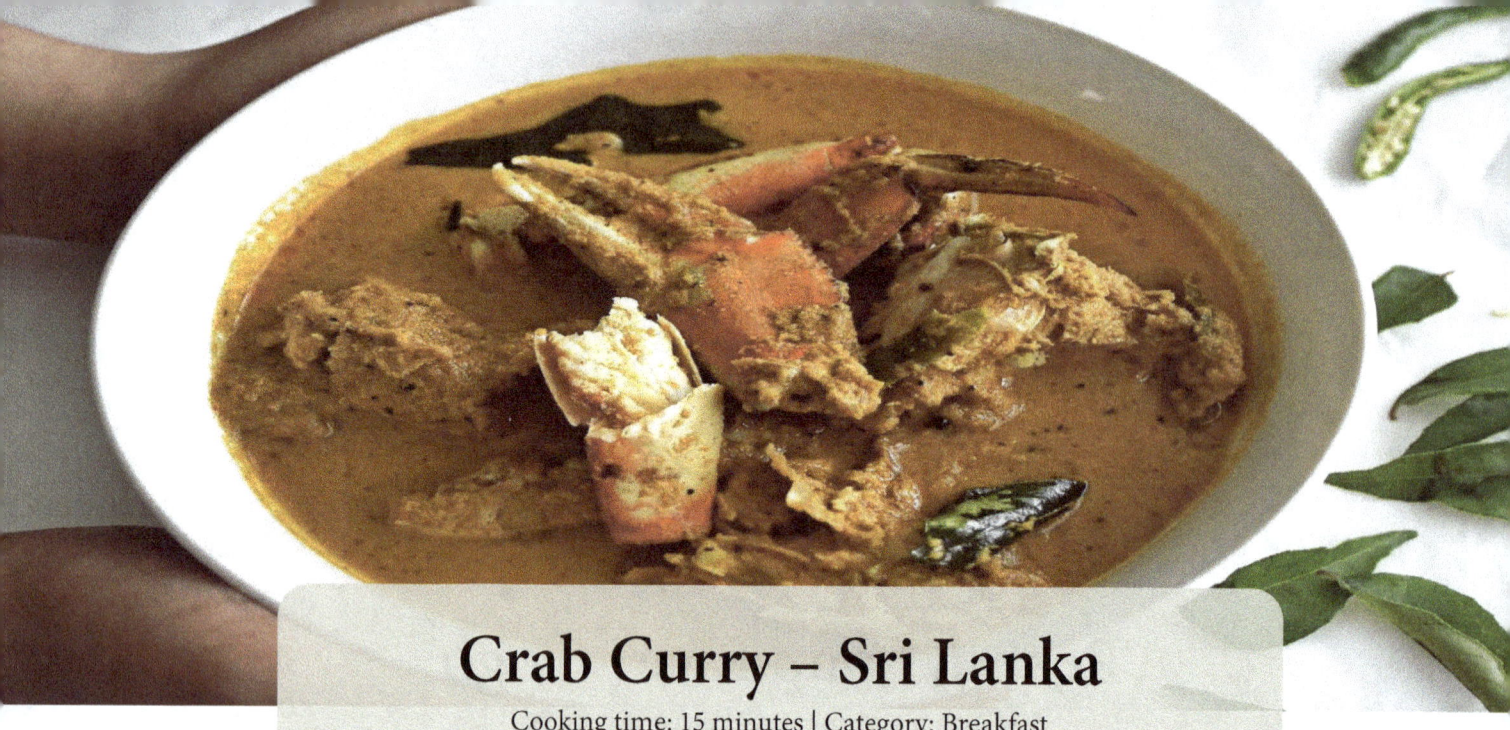

Crab Curry – Sri Lanka

Cooking time: 15 minutes | Category: Breakfast

Seafood lovers are sure to drool over this perfect dinner dish. The spicy bundle of goodness can be tweaked to perfection with a blend of spices.

Ingredients

- 6 Servings
- 800 gm crab meat
- 1 1/2 cup milk
- 1 tablespoon lime juice
- 4 cloves of garlic
- 1/4 teaspoon powdered fenugreek seeds
- 1/2 teaspoon turmeric
- 2 tablespoons grated coconut
- 2 tablespoons sunflower oil
- 1/2 teaspoon salt
- 6 shallots (small onions)
- 1/2-inch ginger
- 1 teaspoon red chili powder
- 1/4-pound powdered cinnamon
- 5 stalks of curry leaves

Steps to Cook

1. Cut the crabs into half down the center into 2 pieces. Discard the lungs, fibrous tissue and shells of the crabs.
2. Separate the claws and lightly crack them.
3. Heat oil in a pan over medium flame. Sauté the ground masala paste for 4 to 5 minutes.
4. Add coconut milk, salt, and lime juice. Cook for 10 minutes.
5. Add the coconut and simmer for 3 to 4 minutes. Now add the crabs and curry leaves.
6. Cook for 5 to 8 minutes until the crabs are cooked and the gravy is thick. Stir occasionally.
7. Serve hot with rice.

Note:

Each serving of baked paper salmon contains 333 calories.

Your tour is incomplete without a feel of Sri Lanka's Ceylon tea or the coc0nut milk-rich hoppers for a quick snack.

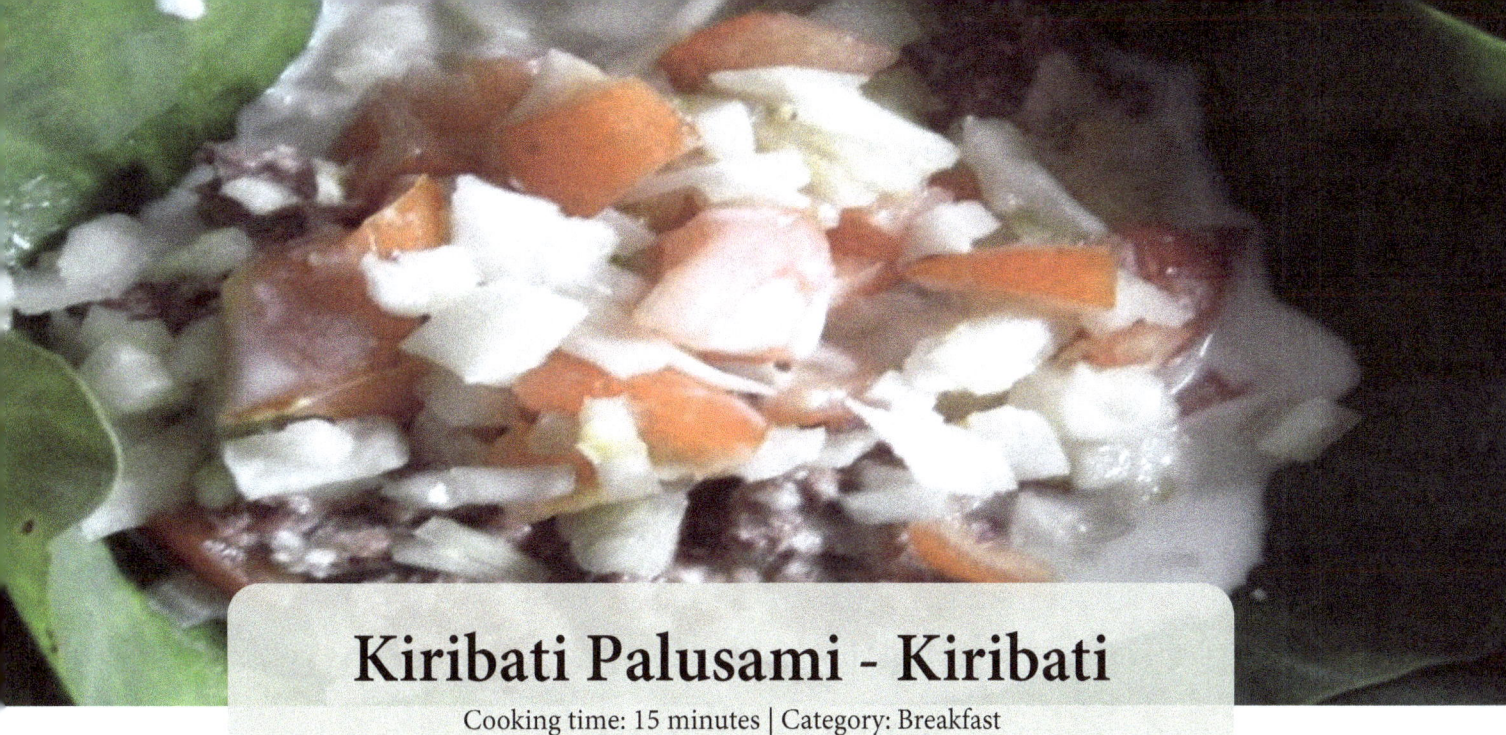

Kiribati Palusami - Kiribati

Cooking time: 15 minutes | Category: Breakfast

This delicious coconut creamed spinach is a local dish of wrapped bundles of taro leaves with a coconut and onion filling. Protein choices can be fish, minced meat, or chicken together with infused coconut cream.

Ingredients

- 13.5-ounce cans of coconut milk, such as Mae Ploy
- 1 1/2 teaspoons salt
- Juice of 3 lemons
- 1 onion, chopped
- 180 taro leaves

Steps to Cook

1. Cut up your fish into bite-size pieces
2. Put in a bowl and cover with the freshly squeezed citrus juice
3. Pour the coconut milk into a large mixing bowl. Stir in the salt, lemon juice and onions.
4. Take 6 taro leaves per palusami and stack them on top of each other, using the largest leaves on the bottom to prevent leaking. Put the taro pile into the open palm of your hand and form a cup with the leaves.
5. Fill the cup with the coconut milk mixture, making sure not to overfill.
6. Close the leaves around the liquid to form a ball, and then wrap the ball in tin foil. Repeat with the remaining taro leaves.
7. Place the palusami balls into a steamer for 3 hours. Remove, let cool and enjoy.

Note:

The number of calories per serving of Kiribati Palusami is 1416 calories.

Kiritimati (ki-ris-mas) is a must-go place for lovers of aviary enthusiasts. It is considered a sacred breeding ground for some seabirds. This Island country is the first country to embrace New Year.

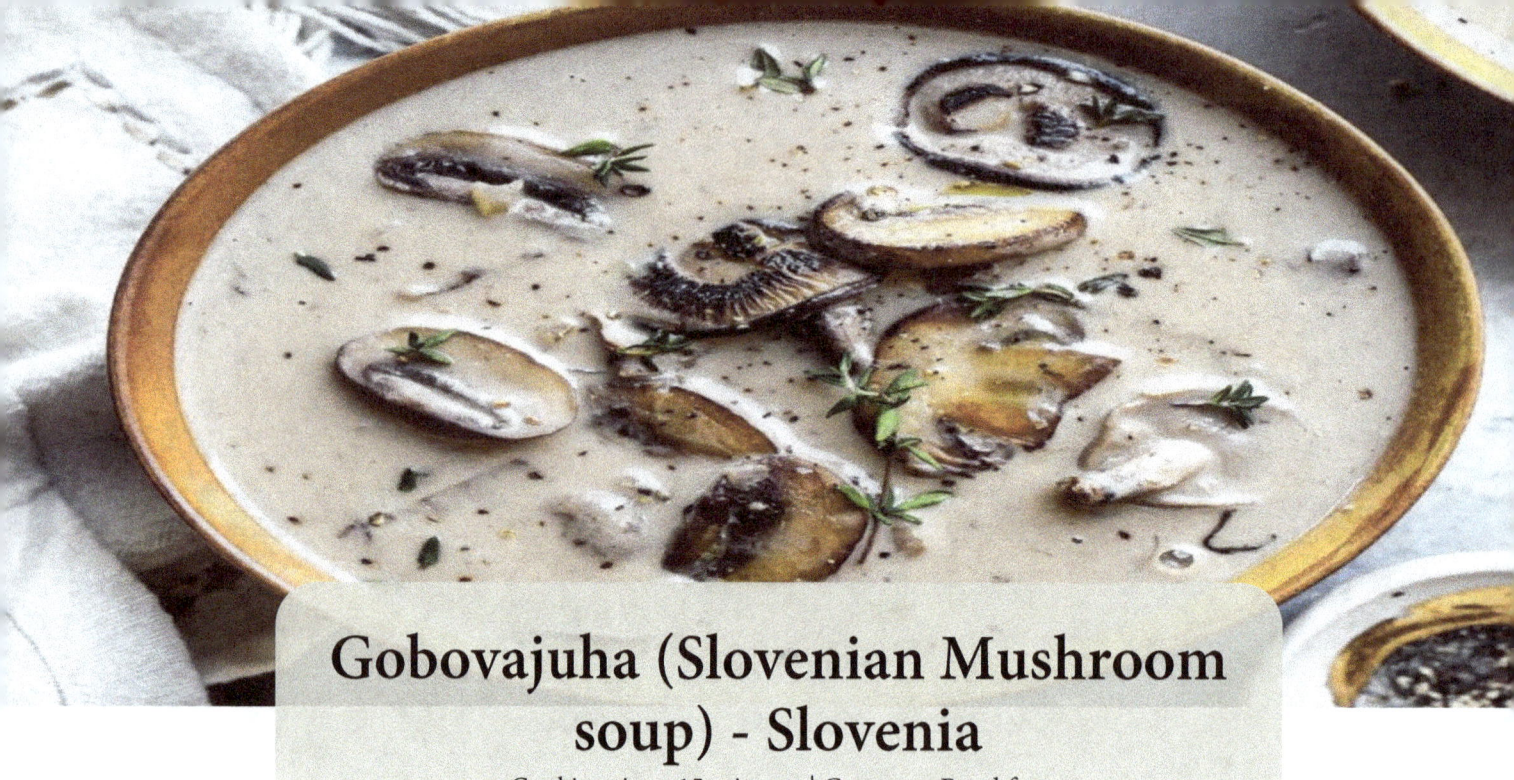

Gobovajuha (Slovenian Mushroom soup) - Slovenia

Cooking time: 15 minutes | Category: Breakfast

Gobovajuha is a traditional Slovenian mushroom soup. The multiple variations in the preparation of this dish make it a popular favorite in most Slovenian homes.

Ingredients

- 1 pound of wild mushrooms
- 1 tablespoon flour
- 1 teaspoon minced garlic
- 3 cups of warm water
- 4 - 5 tablespoons of butter
- 1 medium onion
- 2 medium potatoes- small cubes
- 2 bay leaves
- 1/2 teaspoon black pepper
- Pinch of dried marjoram, crumbled
- 1/2 cup semi-dry white wine or 1 tablespoon of wine vinegar
- Salt to taste
- Garnish:
- 2 tablespoons parsley
- Dollops of sour cream

Steps to Cook

1. Melt butter in a large saucepan and sauté onion. Stir in the flour along with 1/2 teaspoon garlic and cook until frothy, about 30 seconds.
2. Add mushrooms. Add water, bay leaves, pepper, and marjoram.
3. cook on low heat for ten minutes, then add potatoes and reserved 1/2 teaspoon garlic. Continue cooking until potatoes are soft. Add wine or vinegar and adjust seasoning to taste with salt. Pour soup into bowls and sprinkle with parsley. Garnish with sour cream. Serve immediately.

Note:

One serving of Mushroom Soup gives 76 calories. Slovenians are great beekeepers.

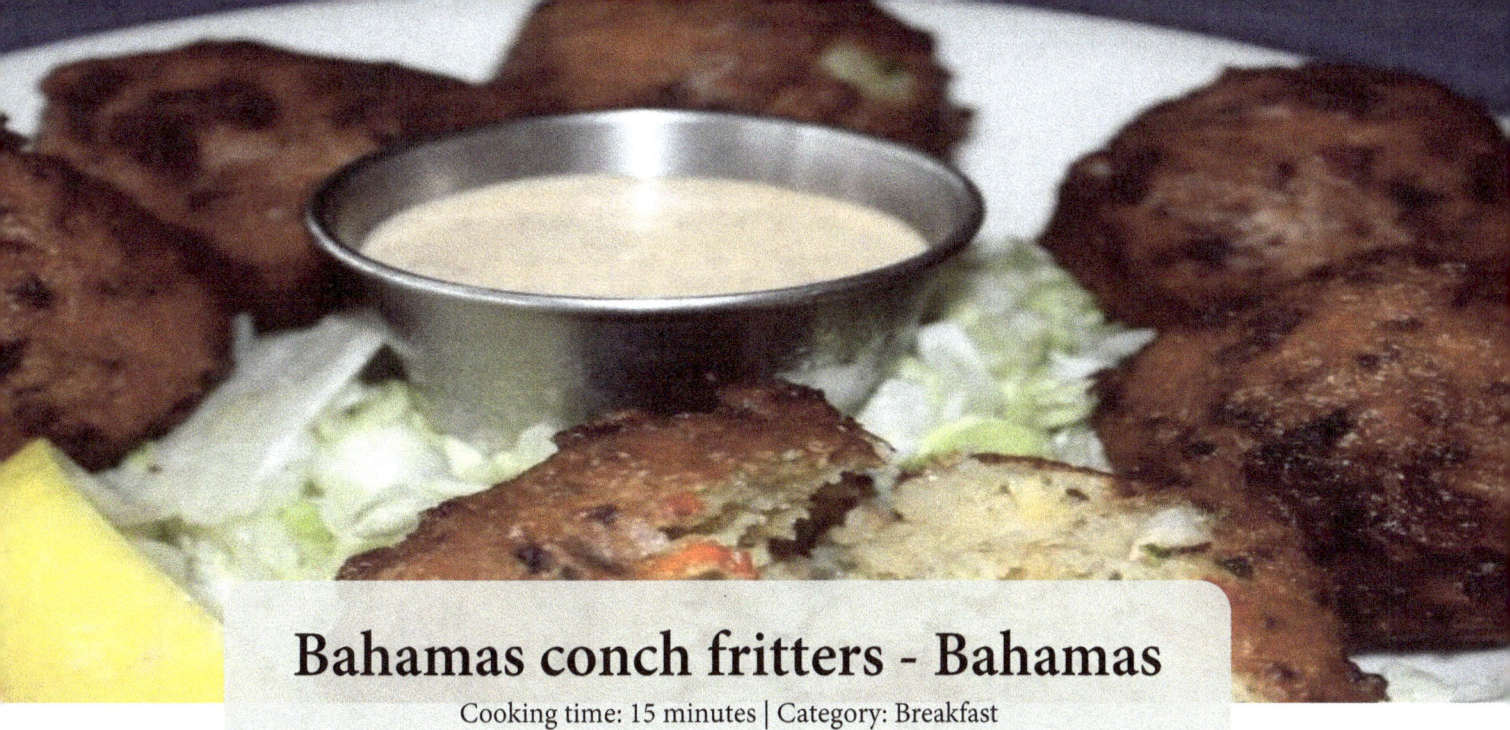

Bahamas conch fritters - Bahamas

Cooking time: 15 minutes | Category: Breakfast

Bahamas conch fritters are the nation's dish. Enjoy Bahamas conch for the first time if you haven't already indulged in this delicacy. Conch fritters are a Caribbean dish to try to have a feel of the Bahamas. It is made with conch meat, onion, peppers, celery, garlic, and spices. Conch fritters pair well with the dipping sauce.

Ingredients

- 1 lb Conch Meat
- 125-gram All-purpose flour
- 1 Tablespoon Baking Power
- 2 Teaspoon Old Bay
- 2 Eggs
- 100 ml whole milk
- 6 ounces Onion - minced
- 1 ounce Garlic- minced
- 2 ounces Celery - minced
- 5 ounces Bell Pepper - minced
- 1 Tablespoon Parsley - minced
- 1 Tablespoon Thyme - minced
- ½ Scotch Bonnet Pepper Scotch - minced no seeds
- Oil for Frying
- & Dipping Sauces

Steps to Cook

1. Tenderize the Conch meat. Using a rolling pin or meat mallet
2. Cut into small pieces using a food processor or Dicing
3. Whisk the milk and eggs together using a whisp or eggbeater
4. In a large bowl mix the meat, parsley, celery, bell pepper, garlic, scotch Bonnet pepper, and thyme
5. Together.
6. Add egg and milk
7. In a cohesive batter add old bay seasoning, flour, and baking powder and place in the fridge.
8. Prepare your drying station using a baking dish /tray with paper towels or use a drying rack with a tray below to collect the oil drips.
9. Prepare your frying station using a heavy bottom pot or a deep fryer, add oil and bring to 350 °F/ 176 °C.
10. Once the oil is ready, add a few tablespoon-sized dollops of the batter into the oil and fry for 1-2 minutes or until golden brown. Make sure not to add too many and crowd the pot.
11. When they are finished frying, remove them with a slotted spoon to the drying station and continue frying the batter until all is finished.

Note:

Serve warm with some slices of lime and your choice of dipping sauces. The best of the Bahamas drinks you don't wish to miss is the Bahamas mamas: a co-mix of several fruit infusions to make your sunny day a worthwhile experience.

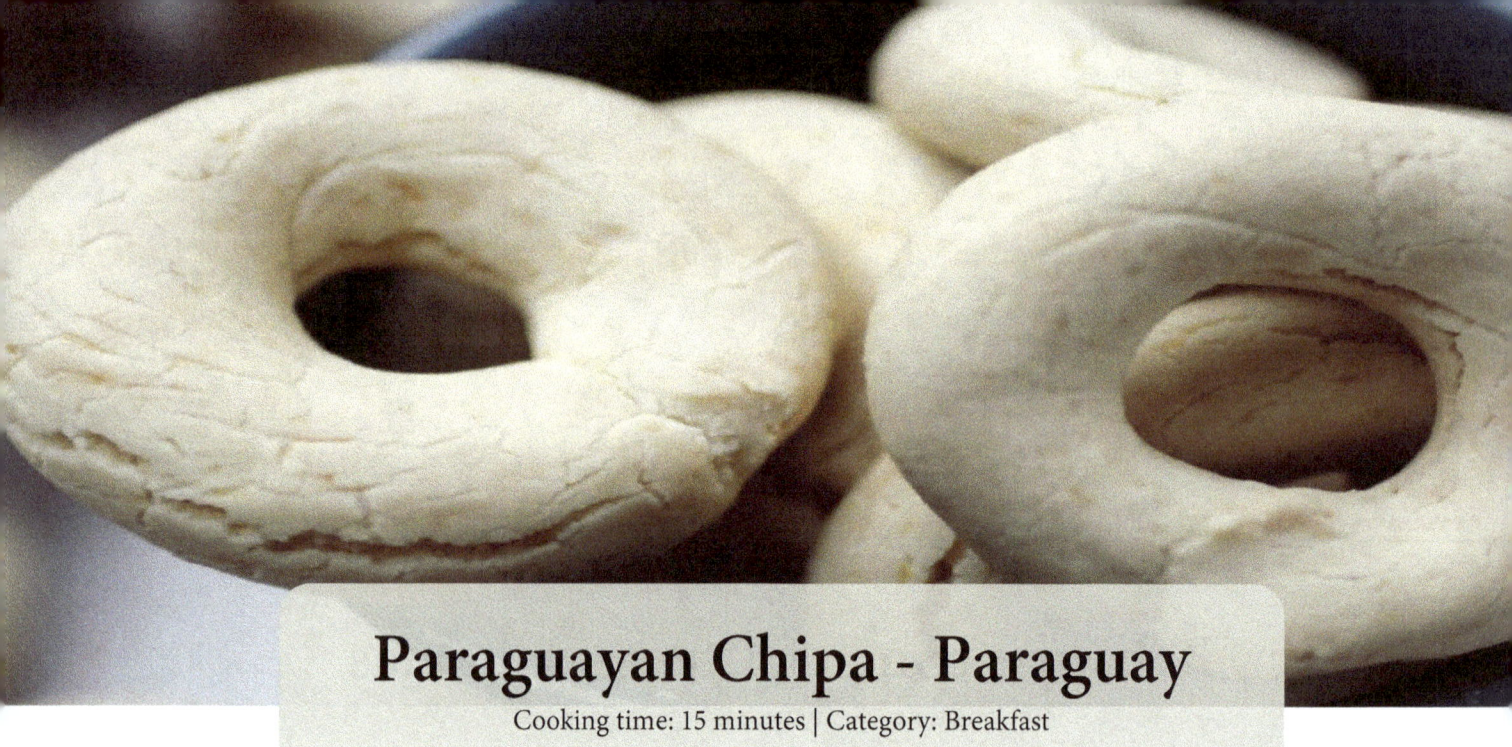

Paraguayan Chipa - Paraguay

Cooking time: 15 minutes | Category: Breakfast

Chipa is a Paraguayan-type bagel, though it can be shaped in various forms. It's traditionally made to get through a few days of fasting for Easter. Paraguayans, though, eat it year-round and it is a popular food for long trips.

Ingredients

- 3/4 cup queso fresco
- 3/4 cup shredded mozzarella cheese
- 3/4 cup shredded Pecorino Romano cheese
- 1/2 cup blue cheese
- 5 cups cassava flour
- 1 teaspoon salt
- 1 teaspoon ground anise seeds
- 1/4 cup lard or butter, at room temperature
- 1 egg
- 1 cup whole milk

Steps to Cook

1. Preheat the oven to 450F and grease 1 baking tray.
2. In a small bowl, mix all 4 kinds of cheese. Set aside 1/3 cup of this cheese mixture, to use for a topping.
3. In a big bowl, add cassava flour, salt, anise seeds, lard or butter, egg, milk, and cheese mixture.
4. The mixture might look too dry, but using your hands, bring the ingredients together until you get a uniform dough.
5. Place the dough on a flat surface and knead for about 5 minutes.
6. Divide the dough into 10 equal portions. Roll each portion into a ball between the palms of your hands. Flatten the ball slightly.
7. Place chips on the baking tray. Top each chip with some reserved cheese mixture. Bake for 25 minutes at 450F. Chips best eaten while hot.

Note:

The number of calories in chips per serving is 196. Chipa pairs well with terere, the national beverage of the Paraguayans!

Week - 10

Reflections

- How is the increased time in your practice of prayer, meditation & gratitude this week?

_____

_____

_____

_____

- What is the time of your 3 miles run for a walk?

_____

_____

_____

_____

- Did you host a luncheon or dinner?

_____

_____

_____

_____

- Describe the experience

_____

_____

_____

_____

Measuring Your Gains

Week 11

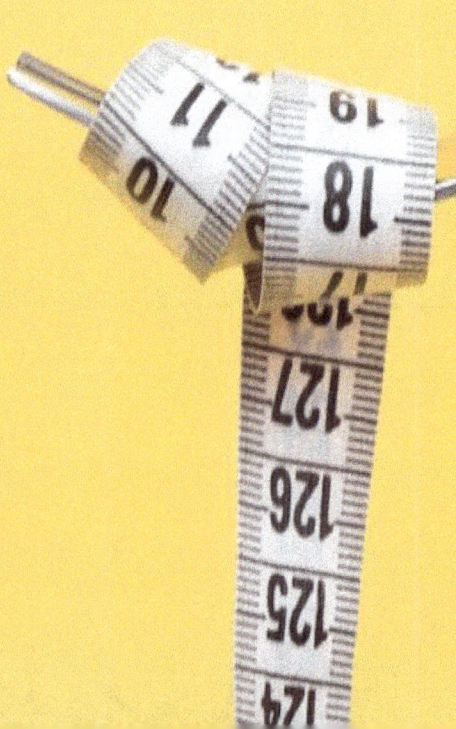

Week - 11

Take Obedient Action

- Spend 30 minutes practicing prayer, meditation & writing in your gratitude journal

- Select 3 Breakfast & 1 lunch recipes from week 11 & prepare them.

- Prepare Breakfast or Brunch for family and friends

- Increase your cardio to 3.5 miles walking or running adding 10 minutes of stretching & 5 strength training exercises

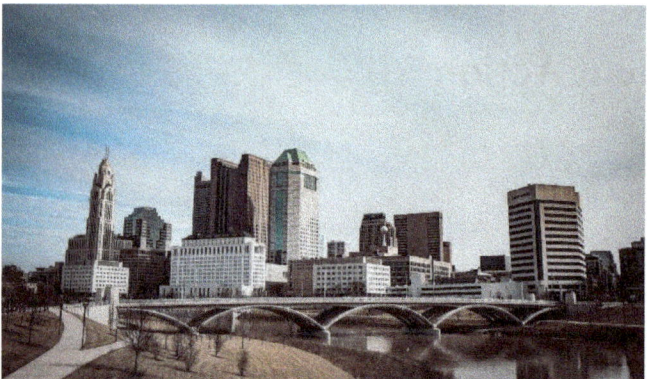

Ohio, US-Lunch

Ohio derives its name from the word O-Y-O meaning 'big river.

The Midwestern state of the United States boasts a population of nearly 11.8 million, and its capital town is Columbus.

Ohio plays home to the Rock and Roll Hall of Fame (a popular museum) a favorite hangout for tourists.

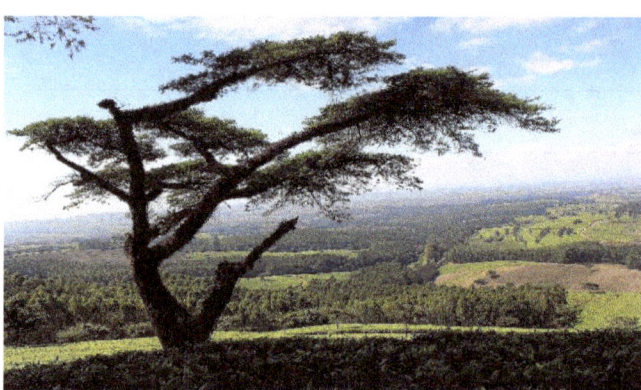

Ethiopia-Dinner

Ethiopia is Africa's oldest country, and the top honey and coffee producer in Africa. It has the largest livestock population in Africa. Ethiopia's location on the equatorial plane is another icing on the cake

It tells a story of distinct dominance and territorial influence. It is confirmed that coffee was first discovered in Ethiopia. Addis Ababa, (Ethiopia's capital city), Visit the highest capital city in Africa.

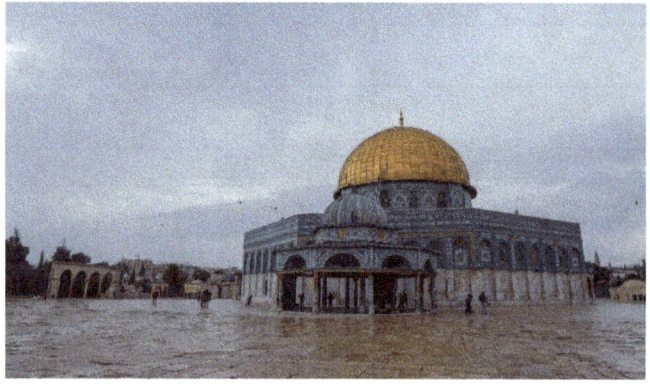

Israel- Breakfast

This country is home to the holiest city in the world (Jerusalem), also it's the capital city. The country has two official languages: Hebrew and Arabic. Israel houses about 8,871,336 people.

The small- sized country is the only Jewish nation in the world, lying on the Mediterranean Sea.

An average Israeli is active during the day hence heavy breakfasts are designed to compensate for the long stretch of work following.

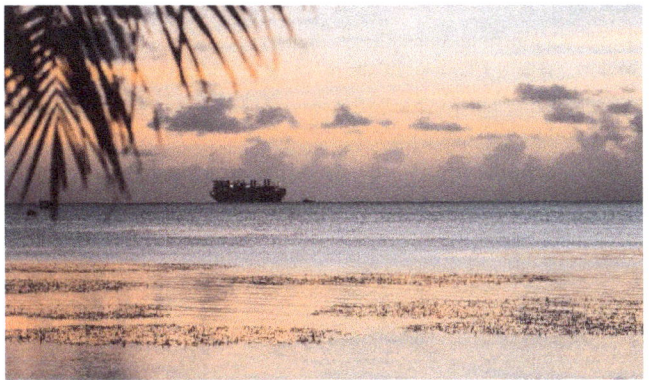

The Northern Mariana Islands-Lunch

Sandy shores and scenic mountainous glorious landscapes are typical of the Northern Mariana Islands in the South Pacific regions. This region boasts 15 volcanic Islands of which Saipan is the largest of the Marianas, as well as its capital region. The current population of this Commonwealth nation is 58,108.

An average inhabitant of this region binges on meaty foods including pork, poultry, horse meat, etc.

Most of their foods have coconut oil as a base ingredient.

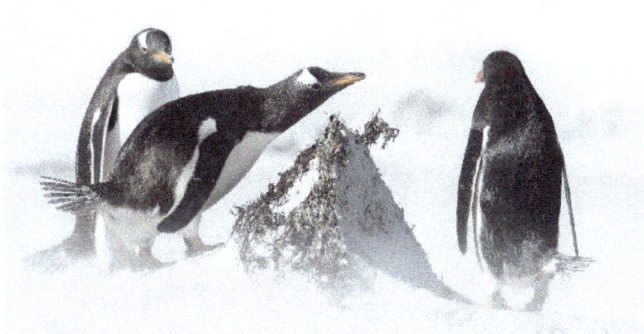

Falkland Islands (Islas Malvinas)-Breakfast

The South American country has its capital as Stanley.

There is an awesome aviary life at Carcass Islands. A visit to the Stanley will keep you spellbound on seeing the monumental Whalebone Arch. Penguins and animal husbandry in all fullness at Saunders Islands. Exotic bays and sandy beaches make your stay an unforgettable experience.

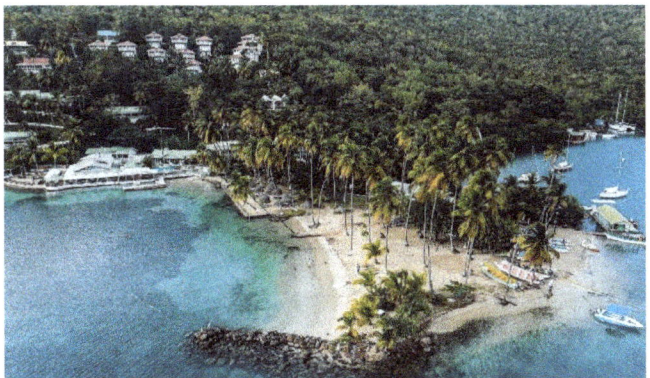

St. Lucia-Lunch

With a moderate population of 0ver 184,000 inhabitants, St. Lucia is a go-to country for lovers of the easy life. It might interest you to know that Saint Lucia is renowned for banana production, and less so for sugar cane. The Island country situated in the far reaches of the Caribbean capital city of Saint Lucia is Castries. With luxuriant agriculture, cassava, potatoes and other root crops are commonplace herein.

St. Lucian cuisine has many influences from French, British, East Indian, and West African dishes. Typical ingredients include potatoes, onions, celery, scotch bonnet peppers, coconut milk, thyme, flour and cornmeal in an ideal. To have a taste of St. Lucia, be sure to munch on Johnny Cake, a staple dough enriched with fish, pepper and onions.

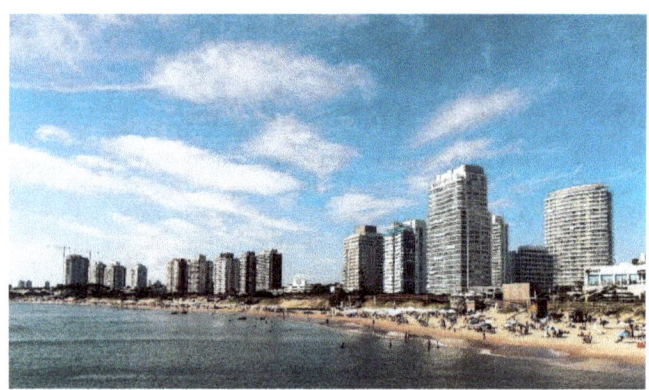

Uruguay-Dinner

This South American country has its capital in Montevideo. The name of this country has been said to mean 'rivers of painted birds'

It prides itself as home to beef lovers (being one of the largest beef producers in the world).

Animal rearing is a very common sight in this country with a population of over 3,492,968 .

A vibrant carnivore community, fine blends of seafood, and robust beef supplies are just a tip of Uruguay.

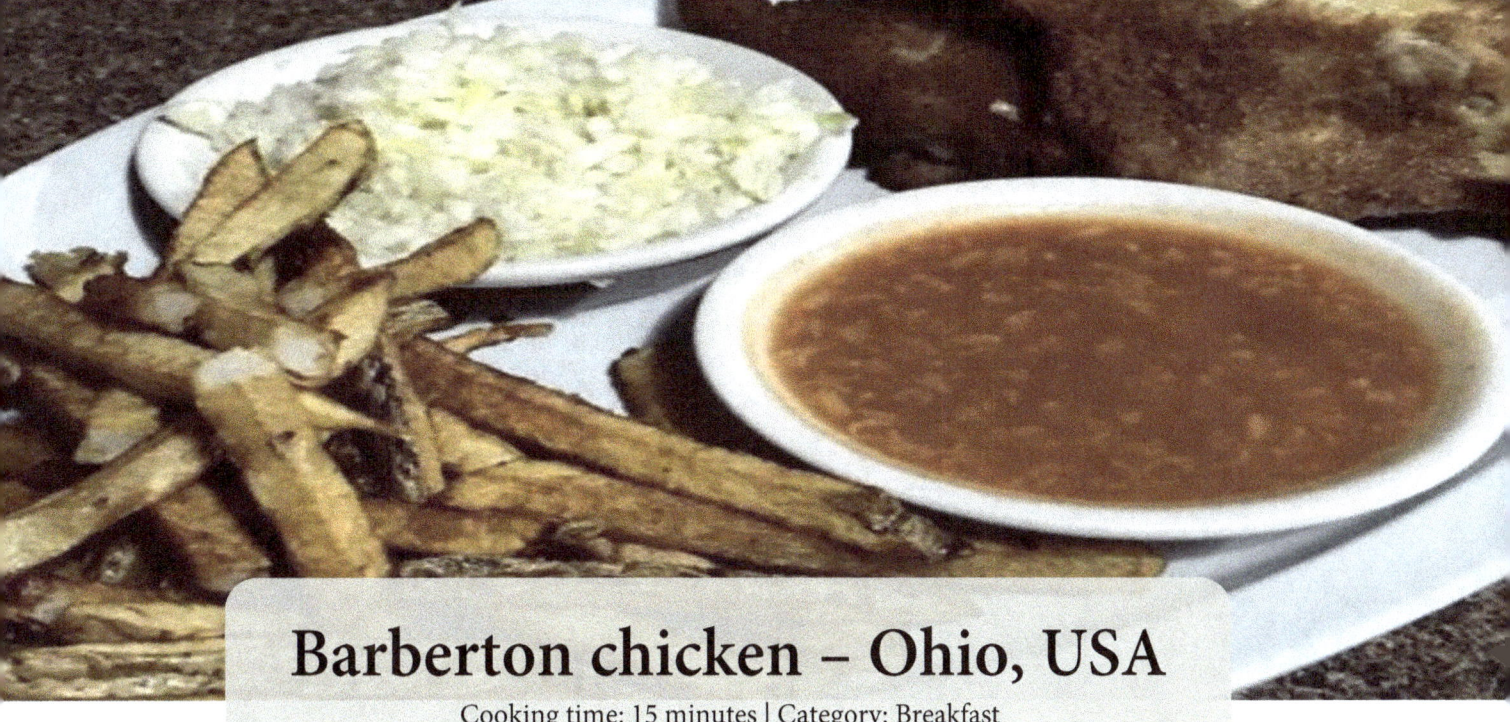

Barberton chicken – Ohio, USA

Cooking time: 15 minutes | Category: Breakfast

Barberton chicken is a household name in the city of Barberton in Summit County, Ohio. This fried chicken lunch recipe includes white bread, coleslaw, fries, and tomato sauce.

Ingredients

- 2 lb. 4 pieces boneless, skinless chicken breasts
- 3 cups buttermilk
- 1 tsp. salt

Crust Coating:

- ½ tbsp. salt
- ½ tbsp. pepper
- 1 cup all-purpose flour
- 2 ½ cups panko crumbs
- 3 large eggs beaten
- 1-quart vegetable oil

Steps to Cook

1. In a large bowl mix buttermilk and salt. Submerge chicken pieces in buttermilk, cover, and refrigerate for 2 hours.
2. Combine flour, salt, and pepper and place in a shallow bowl. Add beaten eggs into another shallow bowl and panko in another separate bowl. Remove chicken from buttermilk and dredge into the flour mixture and shake off excess. Place chicken in egg and then roll in panko until well coated.
3. Heat oil to 350°F in a heavy-bottomed Dutch oven or pot. Add chicken pieces and cook for about 5 to 6 minutes or until golden brown and cooked through. Remove and drain on paper towels. Serve with French fries and coleslaw. 5lbs of chicken quarters contain 909 calories. Ohioans are both soccer freaks and corn produce if banana leaves are not available.
4. The leaves must be heated and wilted over an open high flame to make them flexible.
5. Place the mixture of kwacoco on the leaf about ½-1 cup.
6. Then quickly fold banana leaves over it, and press sides into a rectangle shape making sure to press inwards so none of the kwacoco runs out.
7. Then fold the sides in to seal twice. Repeat the process and set them.
8. IF possible, form a steamer by placing a small cookie rack in a large pot.
9. Line with banana leaves, bring to a boil, then start placing bundles in the pot and steam for about an hour, adding water as necessary.

Note:

The number of calories per serving is 348kcal.

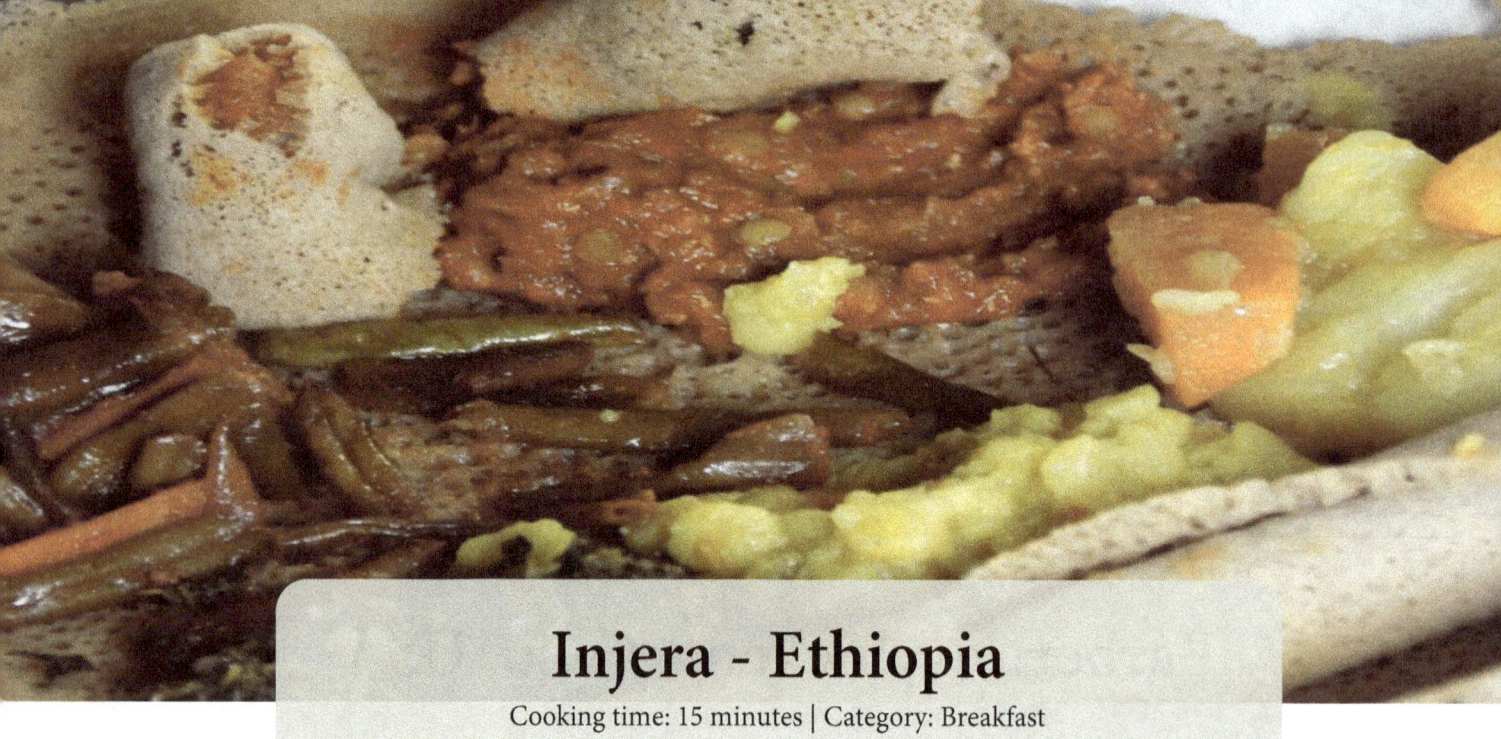

Injera - Ethiopia

Cooking time: 15 minutes | Category: Breakfast

Injera is the base behind most Ethiopian meals. Not only is Injera used to pick up your food, but it's also used to accompany stews and other dishes. Much like a sourdough flatbread, Injera is made with teff flour, an Ethiopian grain, and is fermented for three days before being fried on a griddle. Injera has a slightly tangy taste, with a texture much like a pancake.

In Ethiopian homes and restaurants, you'll find this delicious breakfast laid out on a plate, topped with a variety of stews, salads, and cooked vegetables.

Ingredients

Starter

- 1 cup Teff flour
- 2 cups of water
- Injera – The batter
- 5 cups teff flour
- 2 cups dough starter
- 1½-2 cups warm water
- 4 to 6 cups water or as needed

Absit

- 3 cups of Water
- cup Teff flour batter
- 1 cup cold water

Steps to Cook

Starter

1. Combine one cup of teff flour with one and a half cups of water. Mix well and store in a glass container or a non-reactive container with a tight-fitting lid. Leave to ferment for 3 to 4 days in a warm place.
2. Discard the muddy water above the starter and stir well. It's ready to be used!

Dough

1. Combine 2 cups of dough starter with 5 cups of teff flour and add the 2 cups of warm water gradually. You may end up using about 1½ (the consistency should be thick but smooth) Mix with a stand mixer on medium speed for 5 minutes or mix with your hands.
2. Pour 5 to 6 cups of water over the dough or pour enough to cover it about half an inch deep Don't mix. Cover it up and leave it to ferment for three days.
3. Discard the old water and replace it with a new one. Leave to ferment again for another 3 days.
4. Discard the water again. Add 2 cups of water, then mix the batter very well.

Absit

5. Prepare the absit by boiling 3 cups of water. Turn off the heat.
6. Add 1-1/2 cup of the batter to the boiled water. Mix well to dissolve.
1. Turn on the heat and cook till the absit bubbles—about 5 minutes.
2. Remove from heat and add 1 cup of cool water to bring down the temperature of the absit.

Note:

Ethiopia tours are a wonderful way to explore this African country.

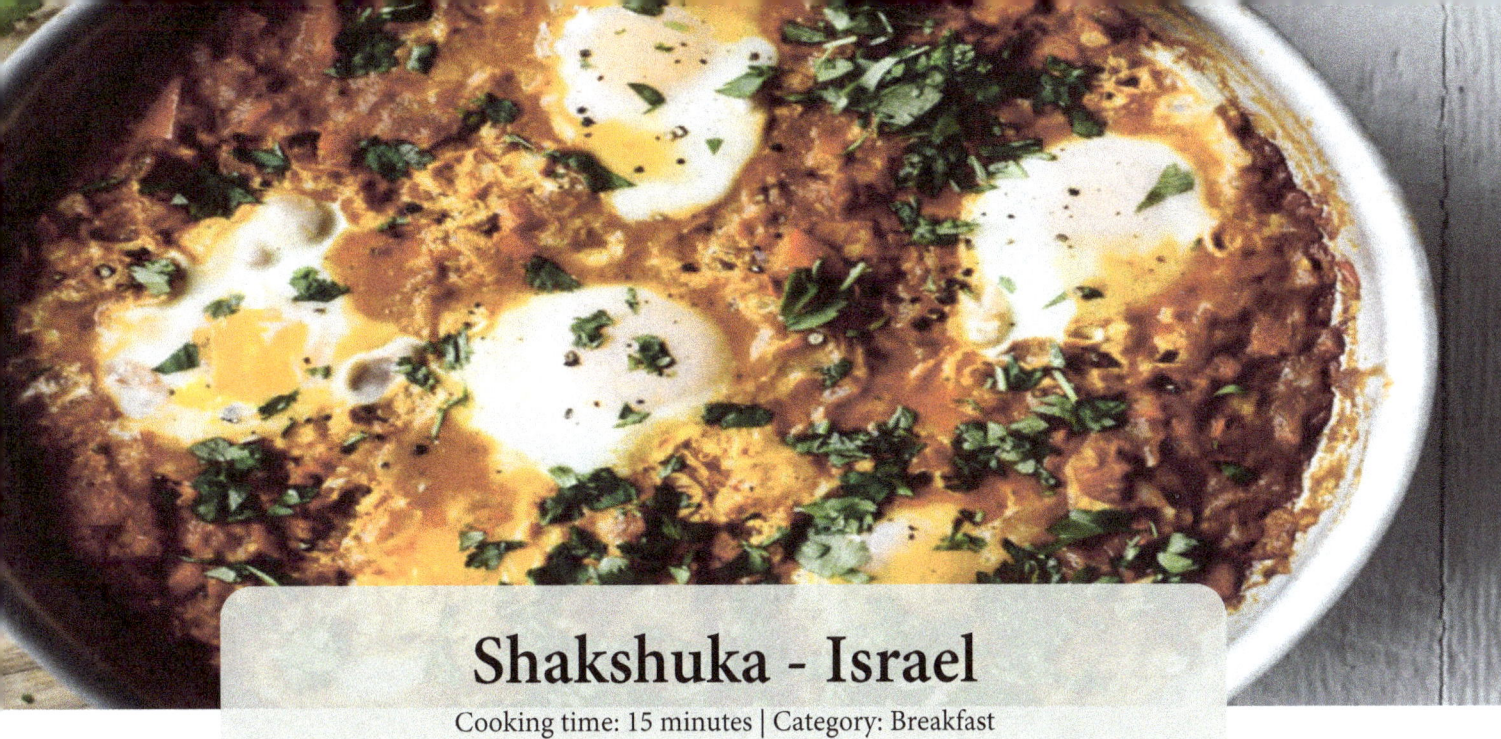

Shakshuka - Israel

Cooking time: 15 minutes | Category: Breakfast

The Mediterranean dish has got many sides to preparation. You have a choice of tomato or veggies as a carrier sauce. Truthfully, this breakfast dish is a mixture of poached eggs.

Ingredients

- 1 teaspoon ground cumin
- A little dried paprika
- Pinch red pepper flakes
- Kosher salt
- 1 can of tomatoes
- 5 large eggs
- warm pita bread, for serving
- 2 spoonsful of extra-virgin olive oil
- 1 sliced onion, chopped
- ¼ thinly sliced red bell pepper
- 1 chopped cilantro stems
- 1/2 minced garlic

Steps to Cook

1. Into a casserole, heat the olive oil on low heat.
2. Add sliced onion & bell pepper and gently stir for about 5mins
3. Pour in the cilantro stems, garlic, cumin, paprika, and red pepper flakes.
4. Season veggies with a pinch of salt and a few grinds of pepper.
5. Continue until all the veggies are soaked in the spices and the garlic is translucent.
6. Preheat the oven to 400 degrees F. Stir the tomatoes into the cooking pan and stir occasionally until the sauce has a slightly thick consistency. This should take about 15 minutes.
7. Use the back of a spoon to make 4 wells in the sauce, 2 inches apart in distance.
8. Crack eggs, filling each egg into each well. Run the edge of a rubber spatula through the egg whites to break them slightly, try to avoid dispersing the yolks (this allows rapid cooking of the egg whites).
9. Transfer the skillet to the oven and bake until the egg whites are just set, 20 minutes.
10. Season with salt and pepper and garnish with the cilantro leaves. Serve with pita bread.

Note:

Be submerged in Israel's summer experience binging on the limonana drink.

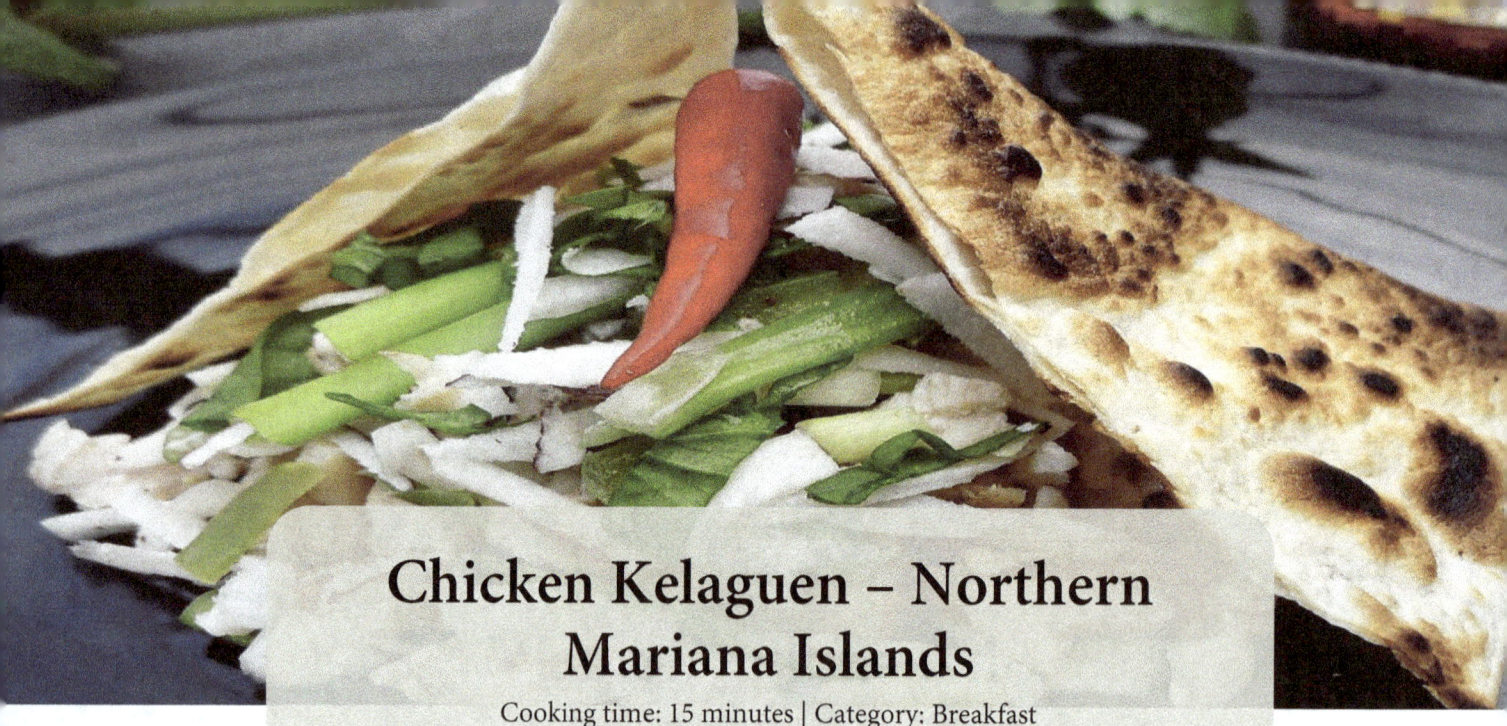

Chicken Kelaguen – Northern Mariana Islands

Cooking time: 15 minutes | Category: Breakfast

Kelaguen is a signature dish in the Northern Mariana Islands. Populare chicken kelaguen can also be made with fish or shrimp. The desired protein is mixed with coconut, onions, and peppers, then pickled in lemon juice, much like ceviche.

Ingredients

- 3 chicken leg quarter
- 2 tsp. Salt
- 1 coconut, grated
- 5 sliced peppers
- 3 chopped springs onions & 1 yellow onion
- 1 pressed lemon juice

Steps to Cook

1. Preheat the stove at 400 F for 40 minutes. Bake Chicken therein and allow it cool.
2. Using a bone or knife, debone chicken and tear it into shreds.
3. Combine green onions and peppers in the bowl. Squeeze lemon and mix everything.
4. Taste and adjust seasoning and serve.

Note:

A visit to Buffet World Restaurant is a quest to sample the delights of Mariana's cuisine in one place.

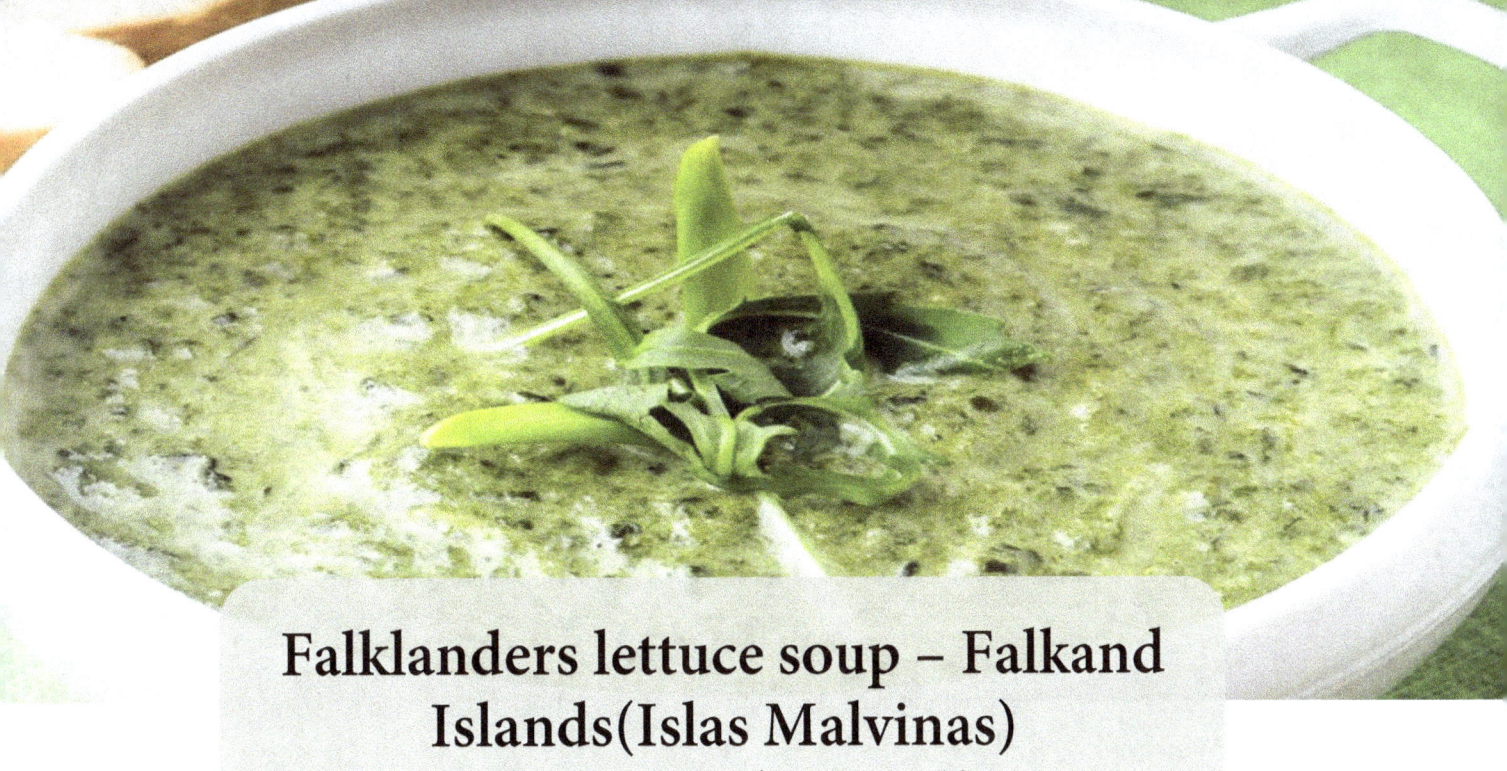

Falklanders lettuce soup – Falkand Islands(Islas Malvinas)

Cooking time: 15 minutes | Category: Breakfast

Lettuce soup is a super creamy vegan recipe. You have choices of eating this soup hot or cold. Parsley is responsible for the rich green color of lettuce soup.

Ingredients

- 10 pieces of lettuce leaves
- 4 cups chicken stock
- 1 cup of milk
- salt and pepper to taste
- 1 tsp butter
- 1 small onion
- 1 spoonful of flour

Steps to Cook

1. Fry onions in a pan on which a little butter has been melted.
2. When the onions turn pale yellow, add the lettuce leaves to the pan
3. Stir gently continuously, until the lettuce leaves have a weak look.
4. Into the pot of chicken stock, pour the flour. Let it simmer gently for 30 minutes, blend and then return to the stockpot.
5. Add the milk and seasonings and bring back to gentle cooking. Serve hot.

Note:

The number of calories per serving is 114.

Binging on your favorite brand of Falkland's local ale is a must-try. More still, you might wish to worship at the Christ Church Cathedral too.

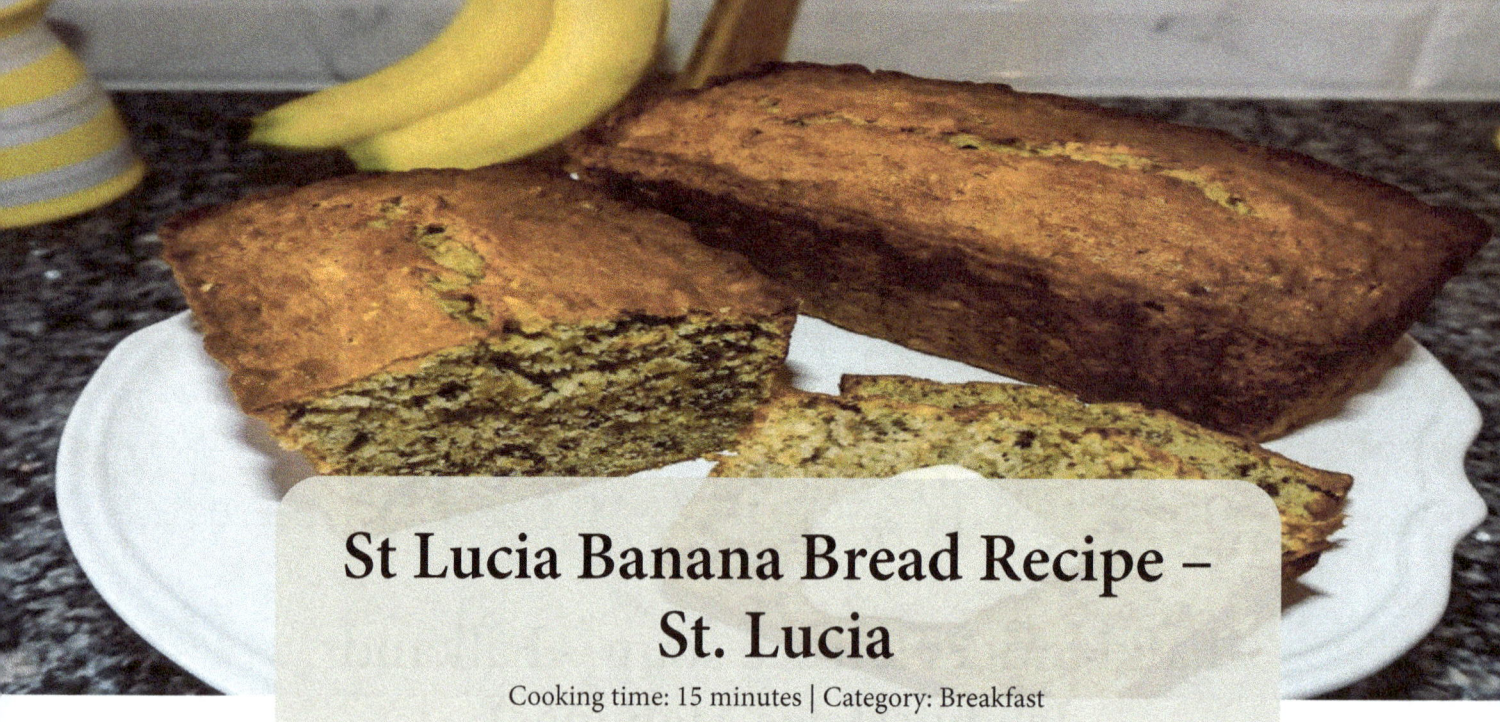

St Lucia Banana Bread Recipe – St. Lucia

Cooking time: 15 minutes | Category: Breakfast

St Lucia boasts of a plethora of banana plantations. Hence, banana bread paired with rum punch is not missing in many kitchens as a healthy lunch snack for tourists. Healthily satisfy your sugar cravings with this richly alkaline delicacy. Added flavorings of nuts and spices are a game-changer sumptuous treat.

Ingredients

- 1 1/2 cups all-purpose flour
- 1 teaspoon Baking Soda
- 1 teaspoon salt
- 1/2 teaspoon Nutmeg
- 1/2 teaspoon cinnamon
- 1/4 teaspoon allspice
- 1/2 cup unsalted butter; softened
- 1/2 cup sugar
- 1/2 cup Light brown sugar
- 2 large eggs
- 1 1/4 cups mashed ripe banana
- 1/2 cup Light sour cream
- 1 Teaspoon Vanilla extract
- 1/2 cup chopped walnuts or pecans
- 1/4 cup chopped dates or dried apricots: optional

Steps to Cook

1. Grease a sizable pan with butter.
2. Preheat oven to about 3oo degrees.
3. Measure out your flour, baking soda, salt, nutmeg, cinnamon, and allspice, into a large bowl, stir together and set aside.
4. Get a second bowl and mix the butter and sugars until the consistency and color is lighter. Add in the eggs, stirring one at a time. Join together the mixture, alternating with the mashed banana, sour, cream and vanilla.
5. Into the resultant mixture, add in and stir the nuts, dates, and apricots.
6. Pour the batter into a loaf pan and bake for about 70mins.
7. Transfer the bread to a wire rack and leave to cool.

Note:

Spice-infused rum punch is a household name amongst the locals in the Caribbean. Unwinding is easy with rum punch, whilst relaxing on the marina around Rodney Bay. An island nation in the Caribbean popular for its beachside escapades and street festivities. Saint Lucia is a melting pot of African, English, and Dutch influence. This island's rich history can only be rivaled by its natural wonders.

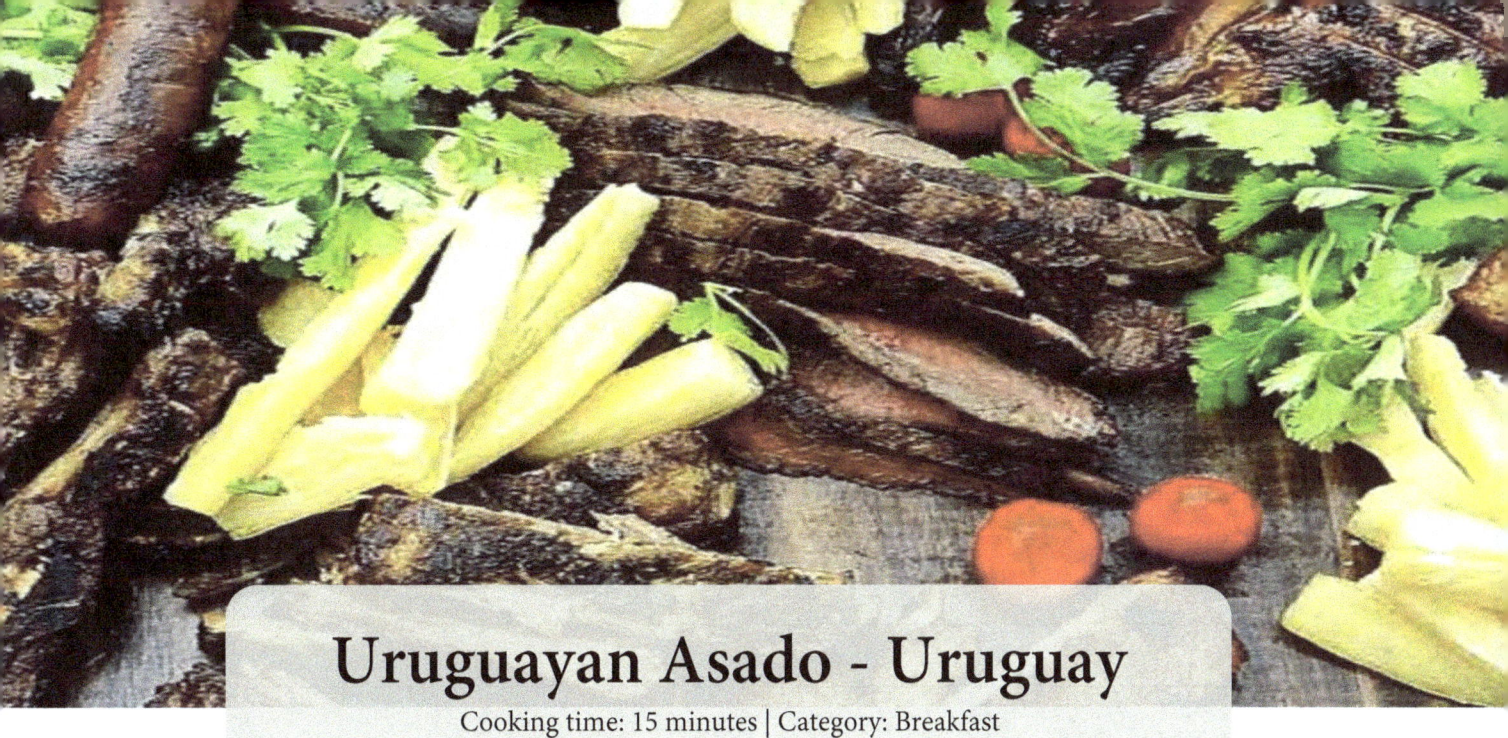

Uruguayan Asado - Uruguay

Cooking time: 15 minutes | Category: Breakfast

Asado is an important and patriotic Uruguayan food. Although its preparation is time-consuming, nothing compares to that traditional feel over a platter of delicious Asado.

It is an assembly of beef, sausages, and other meats that are gently steamed over a parrilla.

Ingredients

- Top sirloin (tapa cuadril)
- Flank steak (vacio)
- Tri-tip, rump tail, sirloin bottom, or tip roast (colitacuadril)
- Beef ribs (costillaancha)
- Parrillero (beef and pork chorizo sausage)
- Morcilla (blood sausage)

Steps to Cook

1. Season the meat with rock salt.
2. Slow cook the meat on a barbecue for a few hours. The meat must first be placed with the fat side down and must be flipped only once.
3. Grill the sausages toward the end. You can also grill the sausages at the beginning and snack on them while waiting for the meat to finish cooking.
4. Serve with mandioca, salad, sopaparaguaya and/orchipaguasu.

Note:

Your trip to Uruguay is incomplete without a taste of chilled Caña, (a refreshing distillate from fresh sugarcane).

Week - 11

Reflections

- How was your practice of prayer, meditation & gratitude this week?

_____
_____
_____
_____

- What new recipes did you try?

_____
_____
_____
_____
_____

- How have experiencing and embracing new cuisines and cultures changed and shaped your lifestyle

_____
_____
_____
_____
_____

- Have you noticed and felt improvement in your health?

_____
_____
_____
_____
_____

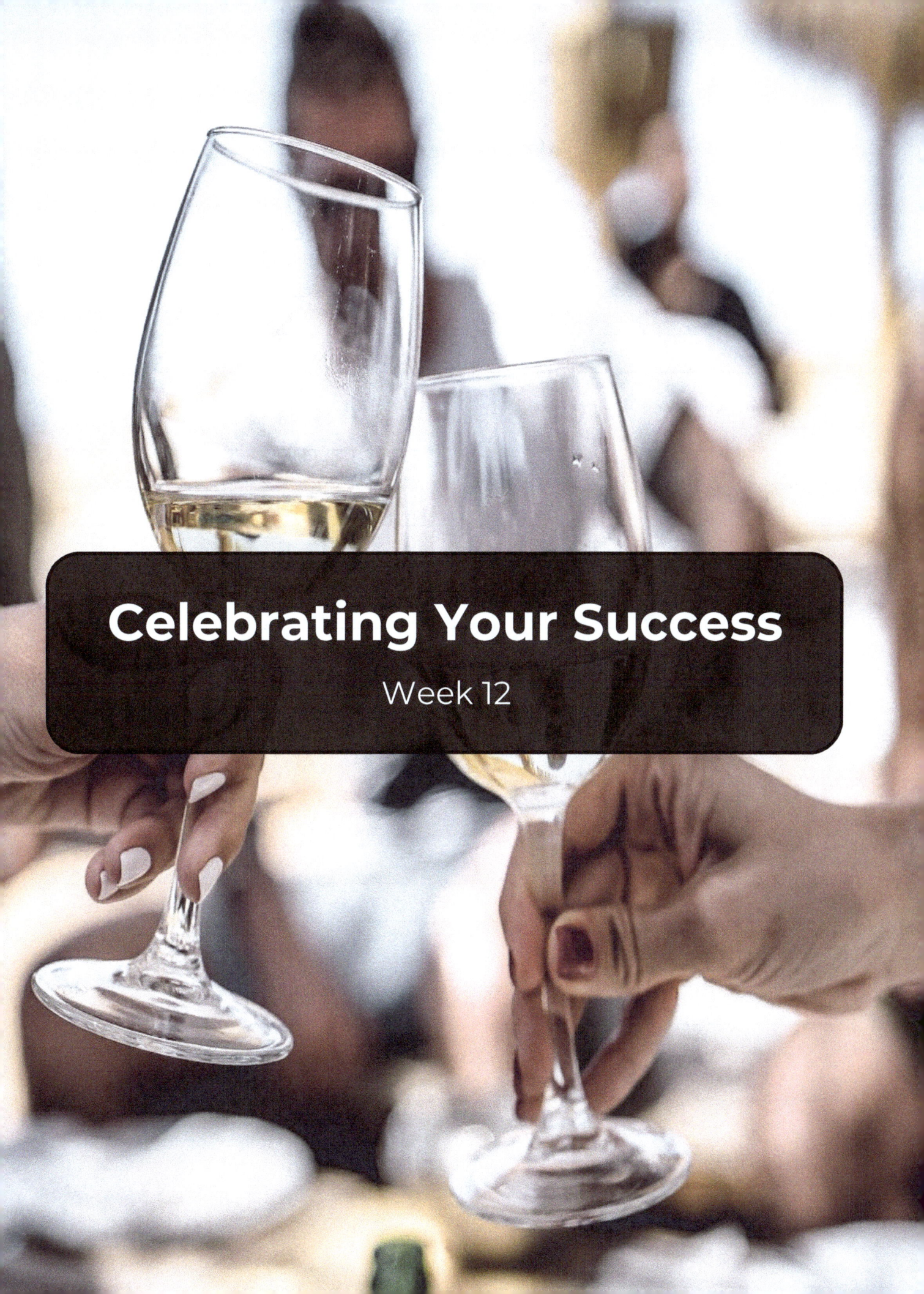

Week - 12

Take Obedient Action

- Spend 30 minutes practicing prayer, meditation & writing in your gratitude journal

_____
_____
_____
_____

- Select 3 Dinner recipes from week 12 & prepare them this week.

_____
_____
_____
_____

- Connect with people from different countries digitally or in person

_____
_____
_____
_____

- Share a meal with someone from one of countries

_____
_____
_____
_____

- Visit a new supermarket this week

_____
_____
_____
_____

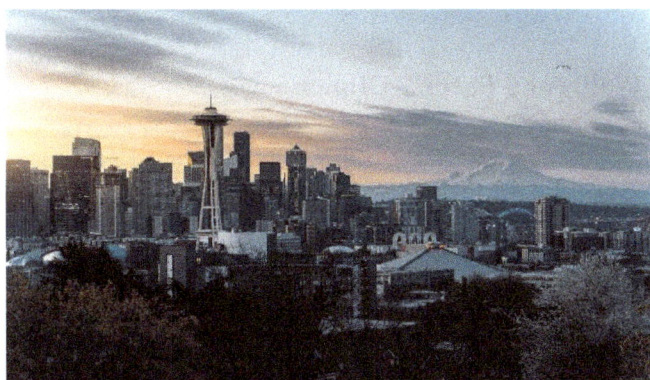

Seattle-Diner

Seattle (also known as Emerald City) is a city in the Pacific Northwest, that is graced with lush water bodies, graceful hills, cascading mountains, and buoyant forests.

It plays host to digital platforms like Microsoft, Amazon and Others like the coffee chain Starbucks.

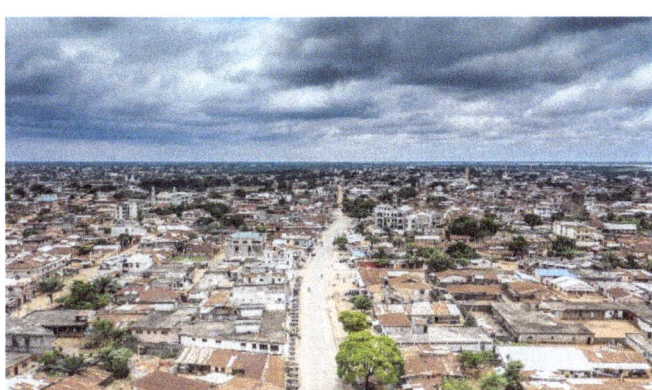

Benin-Breakfast

Formerly called Dahomey. This West African country has its official capital in Porto-Novo. However, Benin's largest city is Cotonou. With a dense population of over 12,629,899 inhabitants, multi-diverse landscapes, and an ecosystem.

A taste of Beninese snack is a taste of Kuli-kuli (Benin's national dish). This portentous goodness satisfies the hunger cravings of most of the locals. The same goes for Masa (popular also in Nigeria).

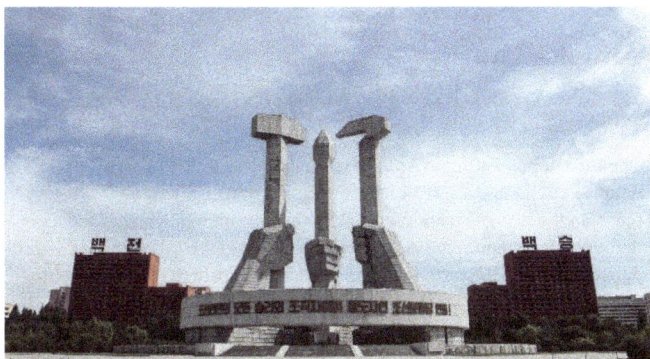

North Korea-Lunch

The East Asian country has its capital in Pyoungvang. It is famous for its production of nuclear weapons. The current population of this most secluded country in the world is 25,959,349. Little wonder, it is also called the hermit kingdom.

Important food staples are grains—notably rice, corn (maize), wheat, and barley.

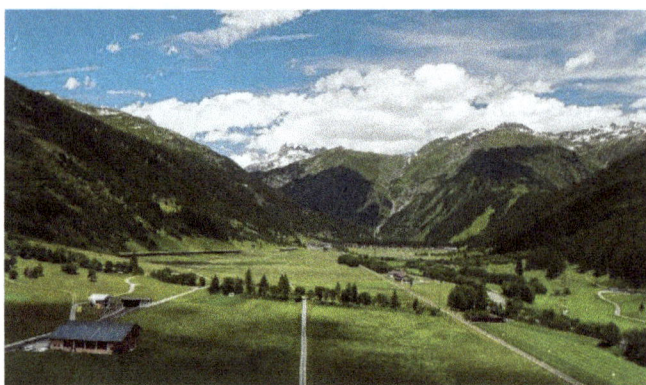

Wallis and Futuna-Dinner

Wallis and Futuna is a South Pacific French Islands, the capital and largest city is Mata Utu. The people are known for their traditional sword dance.

A population of Wallis and Futuna are proud cultivators of yams, taros, bananas, and other food crops. Livestock reared is mainly pigs.

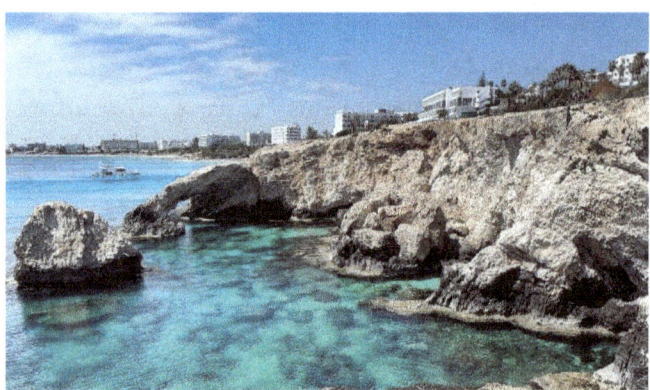

Cyprus-Breakfast

Cyprus is number 3 in terms of the sizes of islands in the Mediterranean Sea. Its capital city is Nicosia. Cyprus is renowned for its rich mineral reserves and fine flavors of brewery. The graceful archaeological site in Paphos is sure to keep you spellbound for a long time.

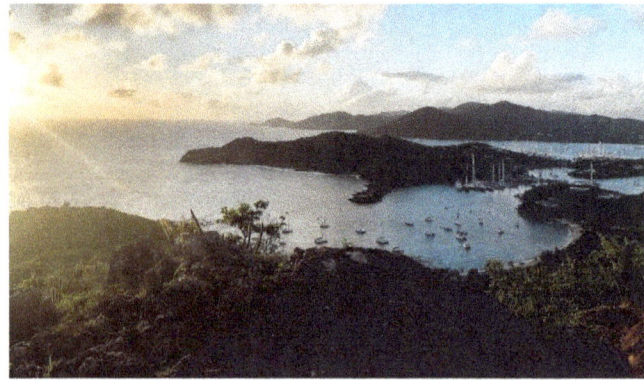

Antigua-Lunch

This Caribean nation is also called Waladli or Wadadli by the locals. Its state capital is Saint John's.

The current population of Antigua and Barbuda is 99,211. Vast aviary, unique cuisines and sandy beaches are typical of Antigua. Fruit lovers wily binge on the Antigua black pineapple. When it comes to Antigua and Barbuda's food, Ducana is almost as traditional as it gets. Ducana is a sweet potato dumpling or pudding that is loved by most who try it. Chances are, you'll love it too!

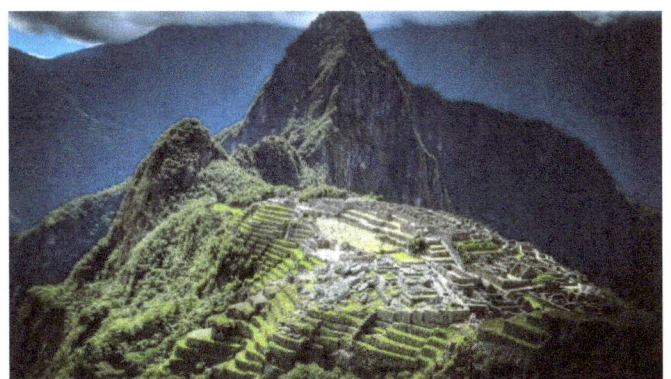

French Guiana-Dinner

This South American country has its capital city in Cayenne. Roadside markets, creoles and clustered settlements are common. Devils Islands, Guiana Amazonian Park, hattes beach, and recreational zoos are favorite hangout spots for visitors. Seafood and a vibrant game life are seen in French Guiana. Common staples from starchy carbs form most of the dieting habits of people.

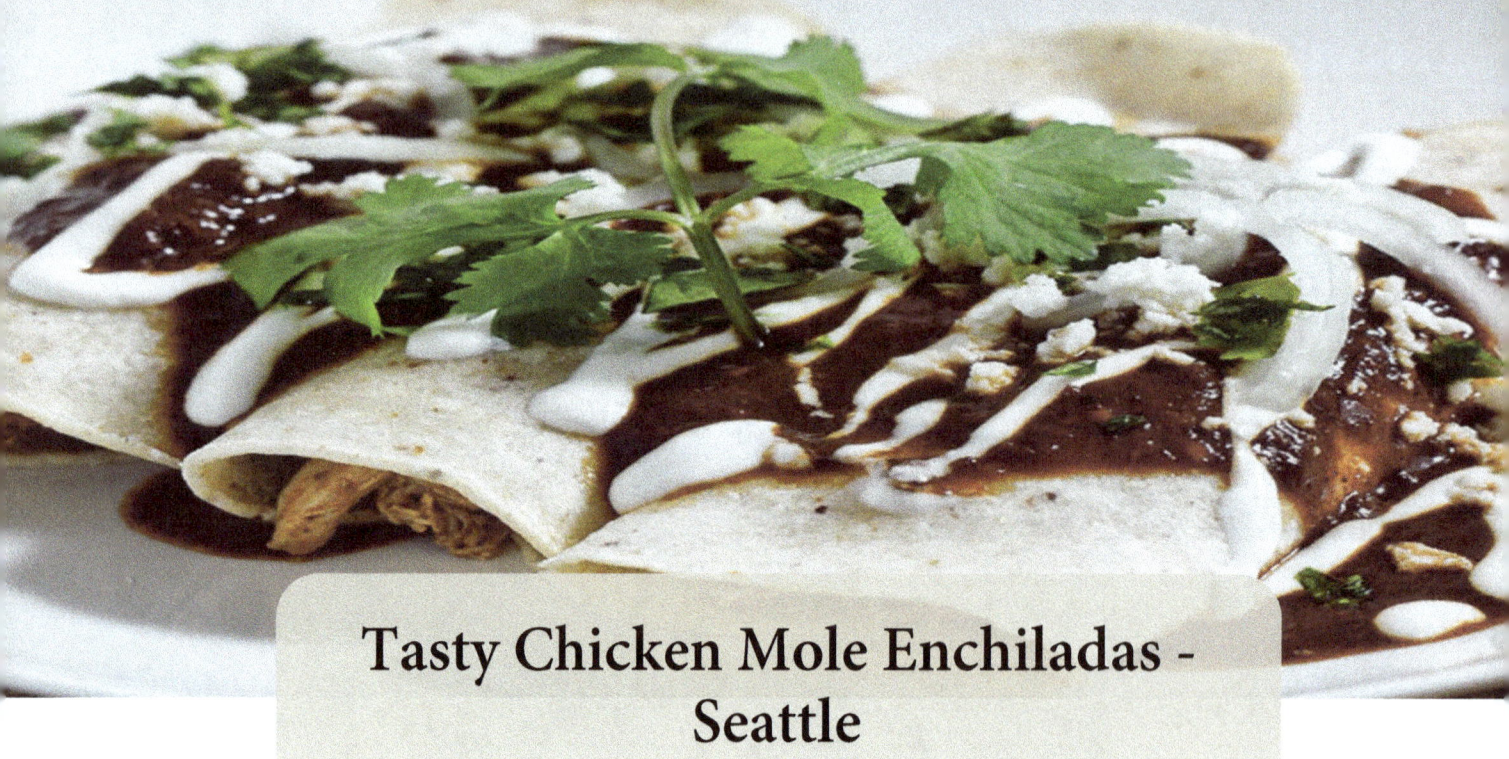

Tasty Chicken Mole Enchiladas - Seattle

Cooking time: 15 minutes | Category: Breakfast

This heatless delicious mole sauce is a popular favorite for a fast Mexican dinner party.

Ingredients

For the Mole Sauce:

- 2 cups of hot water
- 15mls honey
- 2.5mls kosher salt
- Half cup melted chocolate chips,
- 3 spoons of groundnut butter
- 1 spoon of ground cinnamon
- 3 chiles
- 3 sliced onions
- 3oml can tomatoes
- 3 cloves minced garlic

To Assemble the Enchiladas:

- 7 flour tortillas
- 3 cups shredded chicken
- 1 sliced onion
- 3 cups shredded cheese
- 2 cups mole sauce

Steps to Cook

For the Mole Sauce:

1. Blend the onion, tomatoes, garlic, honey, and kosher salt and
2. Submerge the chiles in the water, in a high-powered blender, add the hot water.
3. Allow immersing for 10mins
4. Into the mixture, add the chocolate chips, peanut butter, and cinnamon and blend for 30 mins

To Make the Enchiladas:

5. Allow the oven to heat.
6. Add 1 cup of the mole sauce, into a baking dish, swerving the dish to allow for even distribution.
7. Line the tortilla bread with shredded cheese and chicken.
8. Sprinkle with more mole sauce and spread some sliced onion. Place the enchilada seam side down in the pan, laying them one on top of another.
9. pour a generous amount of sauce over the middle of the enchiladas and cover with some shredded cheese.
10. Bake until heat melts the cheese, ensuring the wrap is covered with aluminum foil.
11. Remove the aluminum foil and bake for an extra 15 minutes.
12. Garnish with the chopped avocado, onion, cilantro, and cotija cheese if desired.
13. The meal can be garnished with avocado, green onions, cilantro, etc.

Note:

The number of calories per serving is 1412kcal A sneak peek at Snoqualmie Falls leaves one wanting more of Seattle city. Pearls Tea & Coffee is a must-try for a complete feel of Seattle culture.

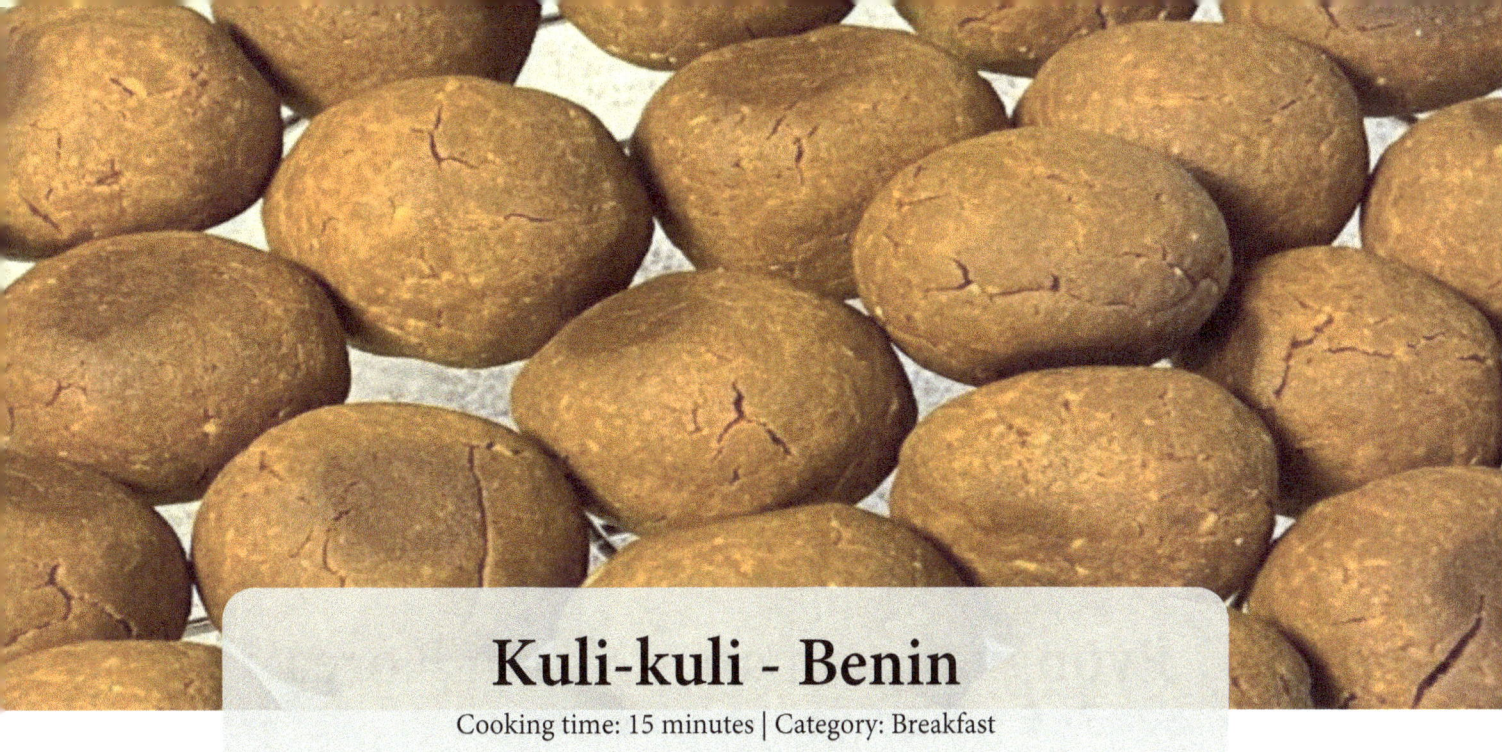

Kuli-kuli - Benin

Cooking time: 15 minutes | Category: Breakfast

Massa is fermented rice crepe mixed with cereals flour. Other countries have their locally made crepes however, Massa is unique to Benin citizens.

Ingredients

- 1 lb millet flour
- 1 ripe banana, mashed
- ¼ cup rice
- 1½ cup sugar
- Vegetable Oil

Steps to Cook

1. Combine millet flour and water. The dough must not be liquid but firm enough to form a ball.
2. Cover this ball and let it sit for 8 hours or overnight.
3. The next day, add ¾ to 1 cup (180-240ml) of cold water to the dough. The consistency of the dough must be a little thicker than a pancake batter. Mix well with a stand mixer or food processor so that the dough increases in volume. Let stand for 15 minutes.
4. Cook rice with ½ cup (130ml) of water over medium heat for 15 minutes. Make porridge by mixing the cooked rice.
5. Add the mixed rice to the dough and mix well in a food processor.
6. Add banana and sugar and continue mixing.
7. Add about ¾ cup (180ml) of water and mix to obtain a liquid mixture.
8. Oil a non-stick pan and cook ladles of dough for 2 minutes on each side (in the same way as pancakes).

Note:

Each serving of Massa contains about 79 calories.

You don't want to miss sampling the delights of legendary elephants at Pendjari National Park.

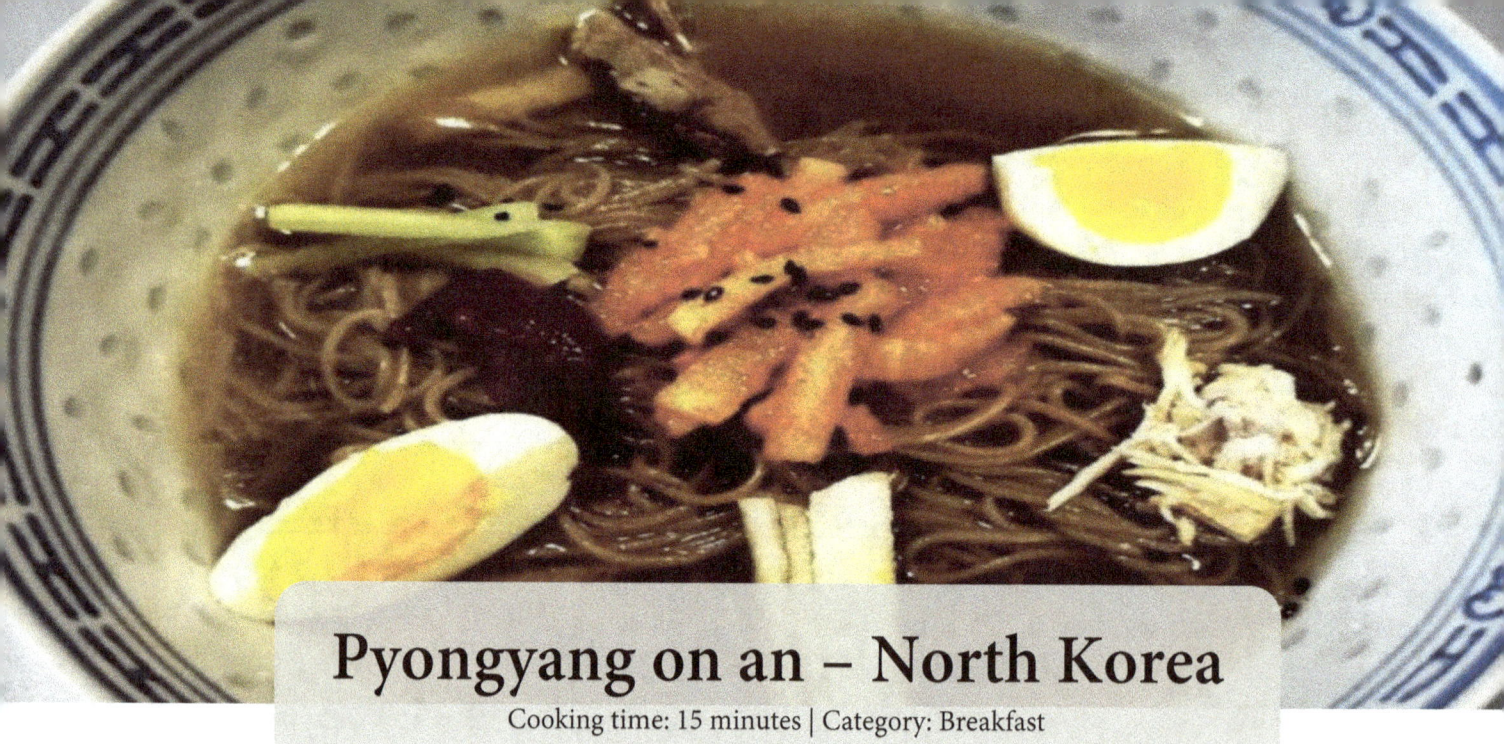

Pyongyang on an – North Korea

Cooking time: 15 minutes | Category: Breakfast

This food is a local lunch delight of the Pyongyangans. It consists of steamed rice that is garnished with eye-popping dressings like shredded chicken, mushrooms, sliced leeks, garlic, sliced eggs and green beans dough.

Ingredients

- 2 2/3 cup sushi rice
- 7 oz chicken breast
- 2/3 cup dried mushrooms
- 8 oz chicken bones
- 1/4 cup leeks
- 2 tbsp sesame oil
- 1 tsp sesame seeds
- 1 tbsp lard
- 2 tsp shredded egg
- 2 tsp ground Cayenne pepper

Steps to Cook

1. Cook rice.
2. Prepare chicken broth with cut chicken breast& bones. Add Season to the broth with soy sauce and salt to taste. Get rid of bones.
3. Soak the dried mushrooms &pan-fry them with leeks, garlic, and soy sauce. Add green beans remove seeds, and then mill to make bean flour.
4. Prepare a batter of green bean flour, salt, & leeks. Grease skillet with lard and mold batter into a circle shape, to make a pancake. Cook the pancake until lightly brown
5. Place rice in a bowl and with chicken, mushrooms, and the pancake on top. Garnish with eggs and cayenne pepper. Pour broth on top with sprinkle sesame seeds and serve hot.

Note:

Visiting North Korea on a cold day? The Pyongyang on an is a perfect lunch recipe for you!

- 2/3 cup green beans dried
- 2 tbsp minced garlic
- Salt to taste
- 2 tbsp soy sauce

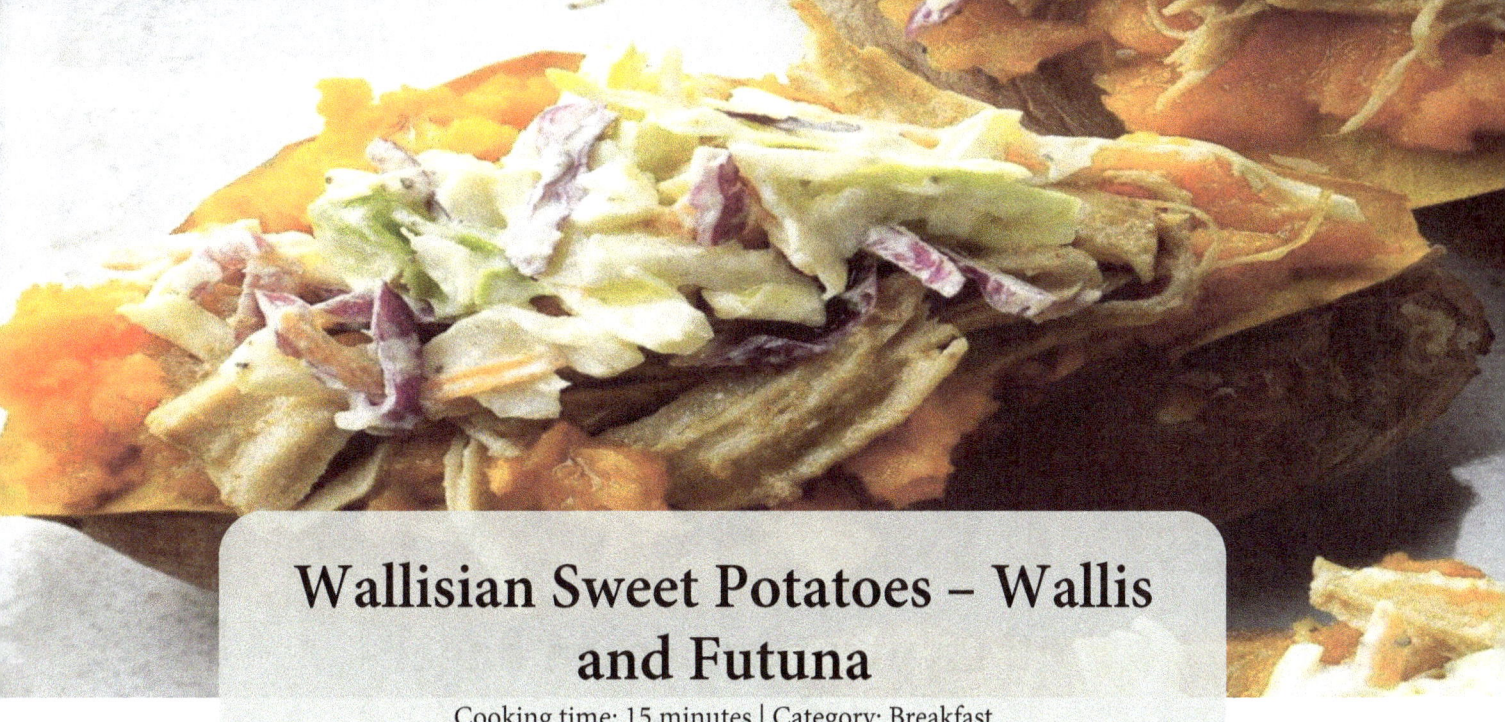

Wallisian Sweet Potatoes – Wallis and Futuna

Cooking time: 15 minutes | Category: Breakfast

Sweet Potatoes is a well-enjoyed dinner recipe for the Wallisans. It can be paired with milk and/or eggs for protein gain.

Ingredients

- 1/2 clove garlic
- 1 spoonful of ginger
- 3 eggs
- 1 cup coconut milk
- 5 sweet potatoes
- 2 medium onions

Steps to Cook

1. Peel and cut the sweet potatoes into chunks. Boil for 15 or 20 minutes or until moderately soft.
2. Pick out potatoes and set aside.
3. Into a frying pan of little oil, sauté the onions and garlic.
4. Add the coconut milk, sweet potatoes and boiled eggs.
5. Stir and serve.

Note:

Kava is the indigenous Polynesian beverage in Wallis and Futuna mostly enjoyed by most of the people.

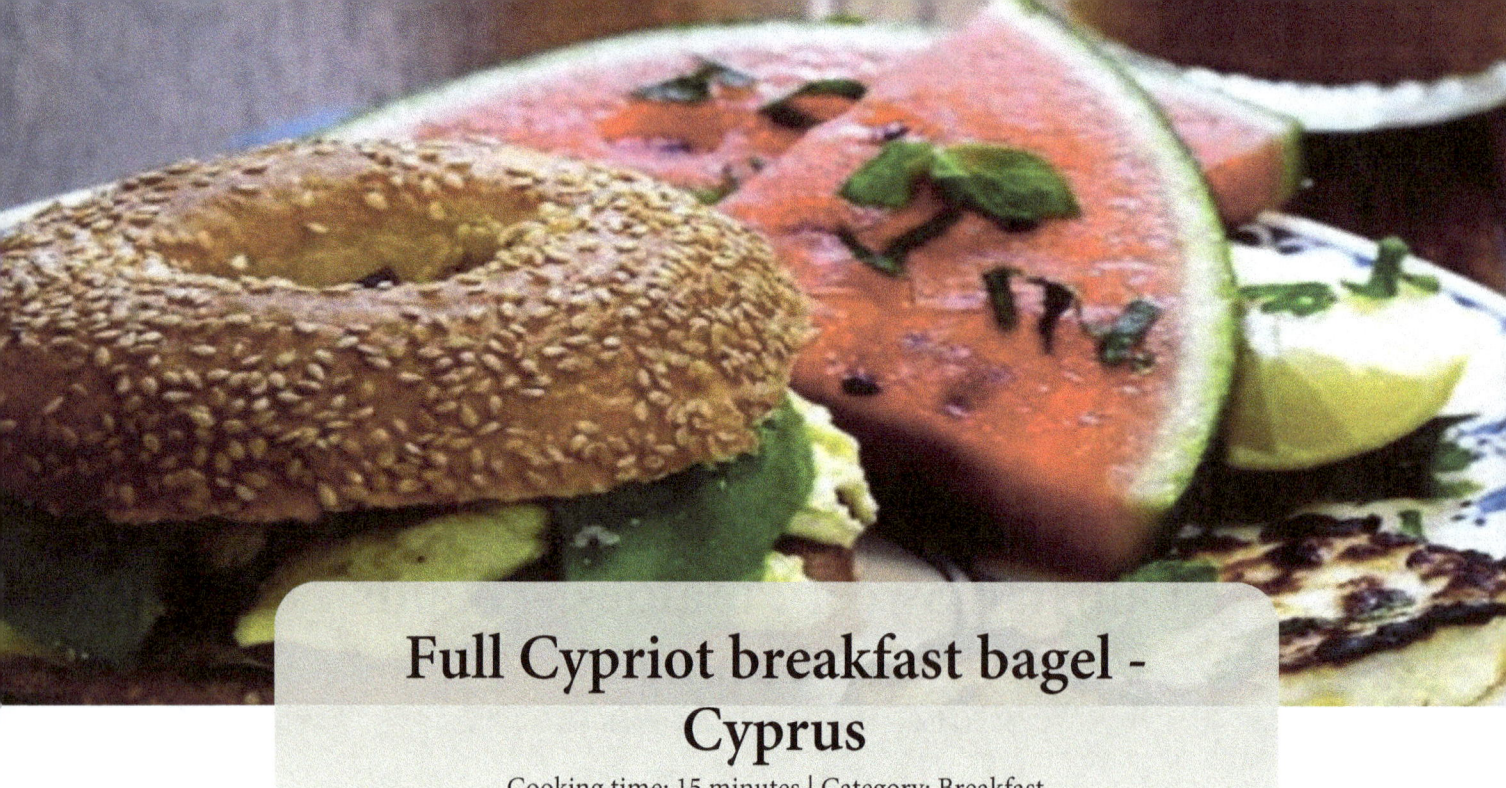

Full Cypriot breakfast bagel - Cyprus

Cooking time: 15 minutes | Category: Breakfast

The full Cypriot breakfast bagel is a beautiful combo of tomato, lettuce, avocado, olives, smoky bacon, and scrambled eggs. Gluten can be removed using no-gluten bagels.

Ingredients

- 7 smoked bacon
- 1 avocado
- 1 tomato, sliced
- 6 dried tomatoes
- 4 roasted seed bagels
- Mayonnaise
- 4 eggs
- salt and pepper
- olive oil
- unsalted butter

Steps to Cook

1. Into a deep bowl, add eggs, plenty of cream, a pinch of salt and black pepper. Whisk well.
2. Add a spoon of olive oil in a non-stick pan on medium heat. Add little butter till it melts and spreads.
3. Then add in the eggs and cook well. Scrape the cooked eggs onto a plate and set them aside. Add the bacon to the pan - you don't need to add any oil. Keep frying and turning over till you achieve your desired color of brown.
4. Remove the pan from the heat.
5. To assemble a breakfast bagel:
6. Spread some mayonnaise on the lower half of the bagel, Smear with dressings of tomato, lettuce, bacon, some scrambled egg, avocado, some sliced olives, tomatoes, and finally the top half of the bagel.
7. And that's it. Enjoy!

Note:

A feel of Cyrus is a feel of the Nissi beach and coral bay whilst sipping your retsina wine.

Every gulp of the ouzo drink will leave sweet memories of Cyprus in your head!

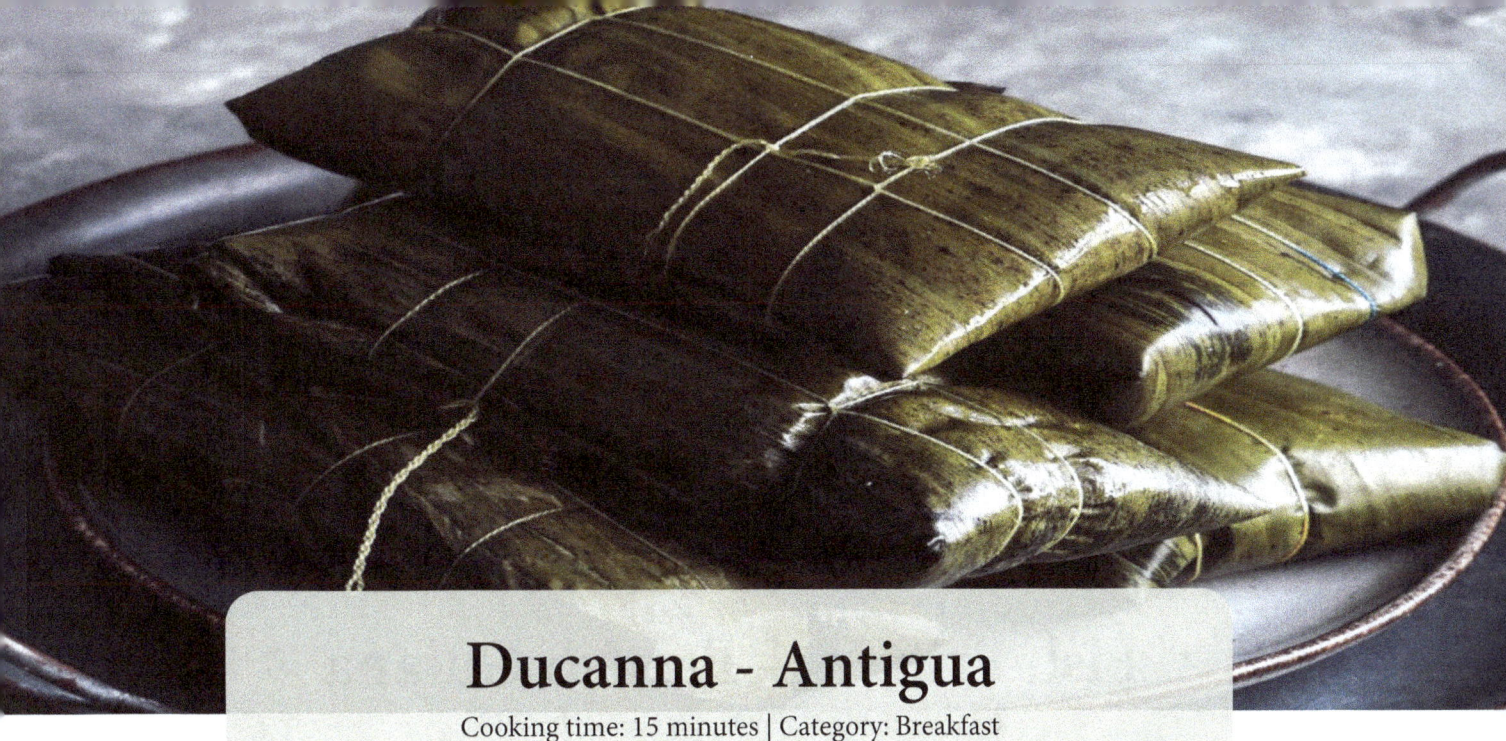

Ducanna - Antigua

Cooking time: 15 minutes | Category: Breakfast

Ducana is made with grated sweet potatoes, grated coconut, sugar, flour, coconut milk, raisins, ginger, nutmeg, and a variety of other seasonings and ingredients.

Ingredients

- 1 3/4 cups all-purpose flour
- 1 teaspoon ground cinnamon
- 1 teaspoon vanilla extract
- 1/2 teaspoon ground nutmeg
- 1/4 cup raisins
- 1/4 cup water
- Banana leaves wraps
- 3/4 cup finely grated potato
- 2 spoonsful of unsalted butter
- 3/4 cup grated coconut
- 1 cup finely ground sugar

Steps to Cook

1. Boil some water in a large pot
2. Mix in the sugar, butter, cinnamon, vanilla, nutmeg, and raisins.
3. Pour in the grated sweet potato and coconut.
4. Add in enough flour for a thick consistency. Add some water if it's too dry.
5. Cut the banana leaves into desired shapes. Run the banana leaves under warm water till soft.
6. Transfer some of the mix into the center of a banana shaped structure. Fold the banana over the dough to cover on all sides, then wrap with the twine to secure or wrap with foil. Repeat with remaining dough.
7. Reduce the boiling water to medium-high for a gentle boil. Add the packets of dough and cook for 40 minutes
8. Remove from heat and leave to cool before removing the wraps

Note:

Wadadli and local rum punch are two compulsory beverages to sample on your visit to Antigua. It's always a blast.

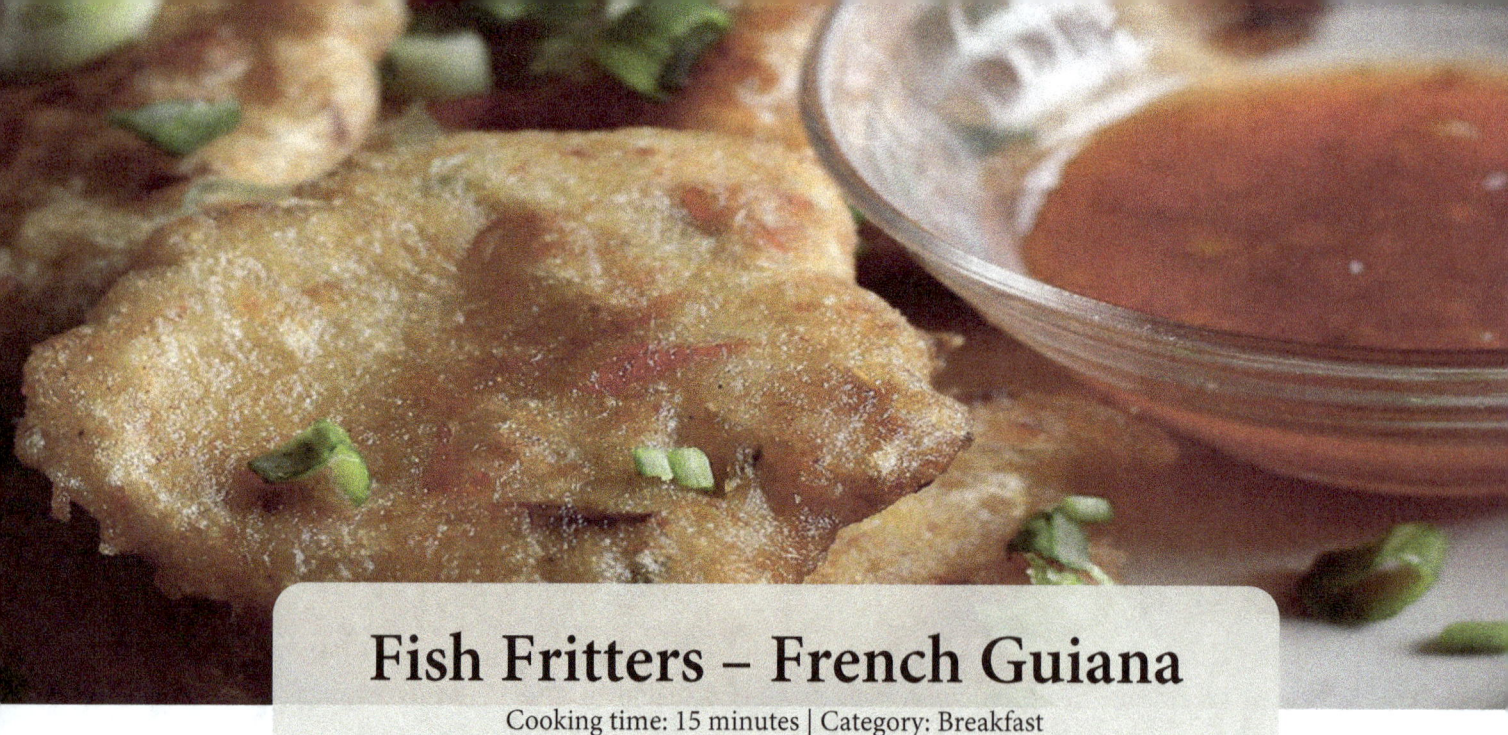

Fish Fritters – French Guiana
Cooking time: 15 minutes | Category: Breakfast

This French Guianan recipe is traditionally made with salt cod or fresh cod. You might want to add a little more pepper to project a spicy feel. These deep fritters are very heavy and can serve as a quick filling snack.

Ingredients

- 2 cups flour
- 1 cup water
- 2 eggs
- 1 spoonful baking soda
- Olive oil
- 2 ounces salt cod
- 2 minced onions
- 2 minced garlic
- 1 hot pepper
- Cut parsley leaves
- 1 tablespoon lime juice
- salt and pepper

Steps to Cook

1. Soak the salt cod in a bowl of cold water in the refrigerator for 1 day replacing the water at intervals to remove the salt.
2. Place the no-salt fish in a pot of water and boil until the fish is soft. Remove from heat and leave to cool.
3. Debone the fish, and separate the skin, using a fork.
4. Use onions, garlic, hot pepper, parsley, lime juice, salt and pepper to mix the fish
5. Mix in water and egg yolks& add flour, then the baking soda.
6. Add the separated egg whites until stiff, then fold them into the batter.
7. In a Dutch oven or similar sturdy cooking vessel, smear with melted butter or oil until it is hot. Drop the batter in batches into the hot oil, slight distances apart. You need to do several batches. Cook until golden brown, turning once for about 3 minutes. Remove and strain on paper towel.
8. Serve hot with a tasty dipping sauce.

Note:

Each serving has a calories content of 281.

French Guiana's soda punch is a drink to binge on whilst sampling the sandy white beaches of French Guiana.

Week - 12

Reflections

- How was your practice of meditation & gratitude this week?

_____
_____
_____
_____

- What new recipes did you try?

_____
_____
_____
_____

- Describe the lessons learned from exploring new countries

_____
_____
_____
_____

- Reflect on your fitness journey

_____
_____
_____
_____

Bonus: Go the Extra Mile

Week 13

Week - 13

Take Obedient Action

- Spend 30 minutes practicing prayer, meditation & writing in your gratitude journal

_____

- Invite friends or family members to your Taste of Global Cuisines
- Sign up to run or walk a 5k race
- Invite a friend or family member to retake this journey through the book with you.

_____

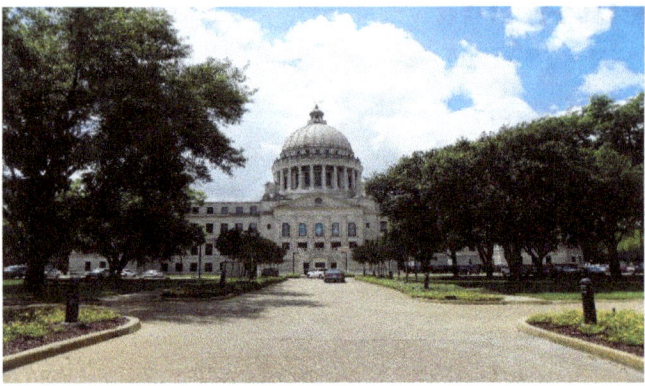

Mississippi-Breakfast

This state was called the Magnolia state due to its abundance of magnolia trees. Its vibrant aquatic community made catfish very abundant.

This southern United States state is known for the birth experiences of blues music. Jackson is the state capital, with a population of over 3 million inhabitants.

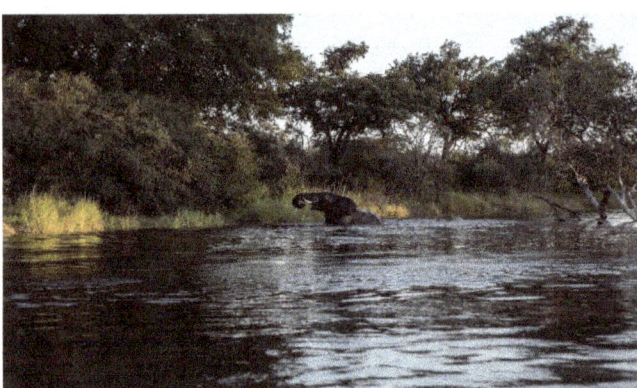

Zambia-Lunch

The famous Victoria Falls Bridge is home to this East African country. The capital city is called Lusaka. With a current teeming population of over 19million inhabitants,

Zambia is known for being secluded and somewhat unexplored by tourists. Wildlife husbandry is continually enjoyed in Zambia as almost half of the country is made of national parks

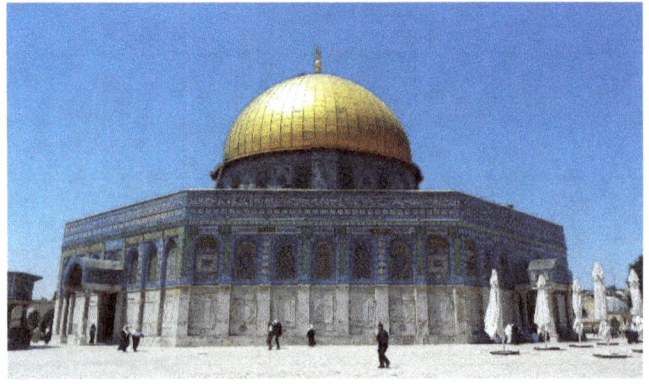

Palestine Dinner

This East Asian country has two capitals: Jerusalem and Ramallah with a current population of over 5 million residents.

Judaism and Christianity found roots firstly in Palestine. Olive trees are common, signifying peace and progress.

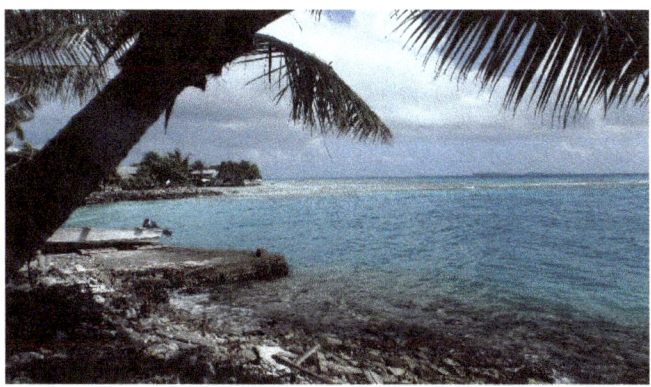

Tokelau-Breakfast

This Island territory of New Zealand has three atolls in the South Pacific Ocean, namely Atafu (largest city), Nukunonu, and Fakaofo. Tokelau is a world leading nation in renewable solar power.

Its capital is Nukunonu Lovers of pork and aquatic delicacies will love it at Fakaofo.

Tokelauns are selfless and ardent nutritionist ensuring equality in food supply distribution to all inhabitants.

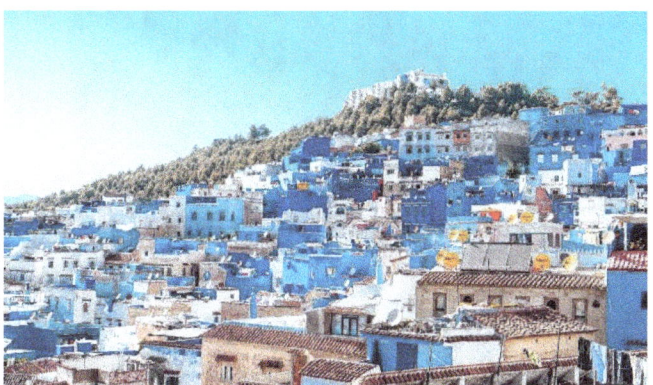

Morocco-Lunch

This North African nation has its capital as Rabat. The proud producers of jewelry and unique pottery boast of an average of 37755260 inhabitants. Scintillating about Morocco are the Moroccan spices and mint, argan oil, the famous Sahara Desert, and the Atlas Mountains.

Cinnamon, cumin, turmeric, and ginger are all lavish, mouth-watering, and healthy Moroccan dishes to suit any palette.

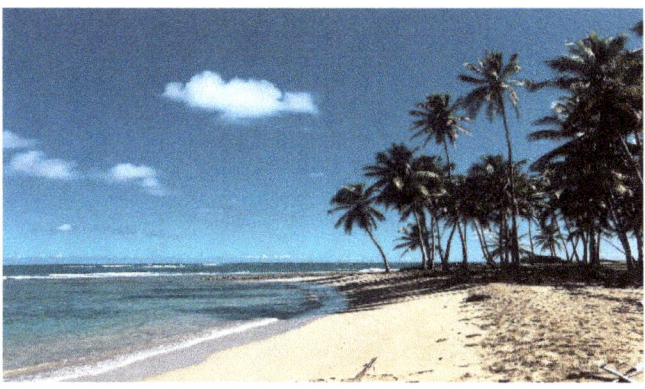

Dominica Republic-Dinner

This 2nd largest Caribbean nation welcomes all lovers of golf and opens its doors to tourists!

The name of its present capital is known as Santo Domingo.

The largely self-sustaining nation boasts of a teeming population of over 10,614,000 inhabitants.

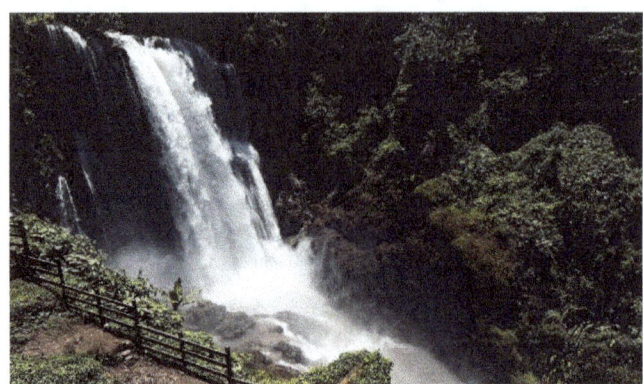

Honduras-Breakfast

Honduras is a country in Central America. The capital city is Tegucigalpa. The country was nicknamed the banana republic, maybe because exported bananas and coffee.

Honduras has four distinct regions: the central highlands, Pacific lowlands, eastern Caribbean lowlands, and northern coastal plains and mountains.

Typical Honduran dishes also include an abundant selection of tropical fruits such as papaya, pineapple, plum, sapote, passion fruit, and bananas which are prepared in many ways while they are still green

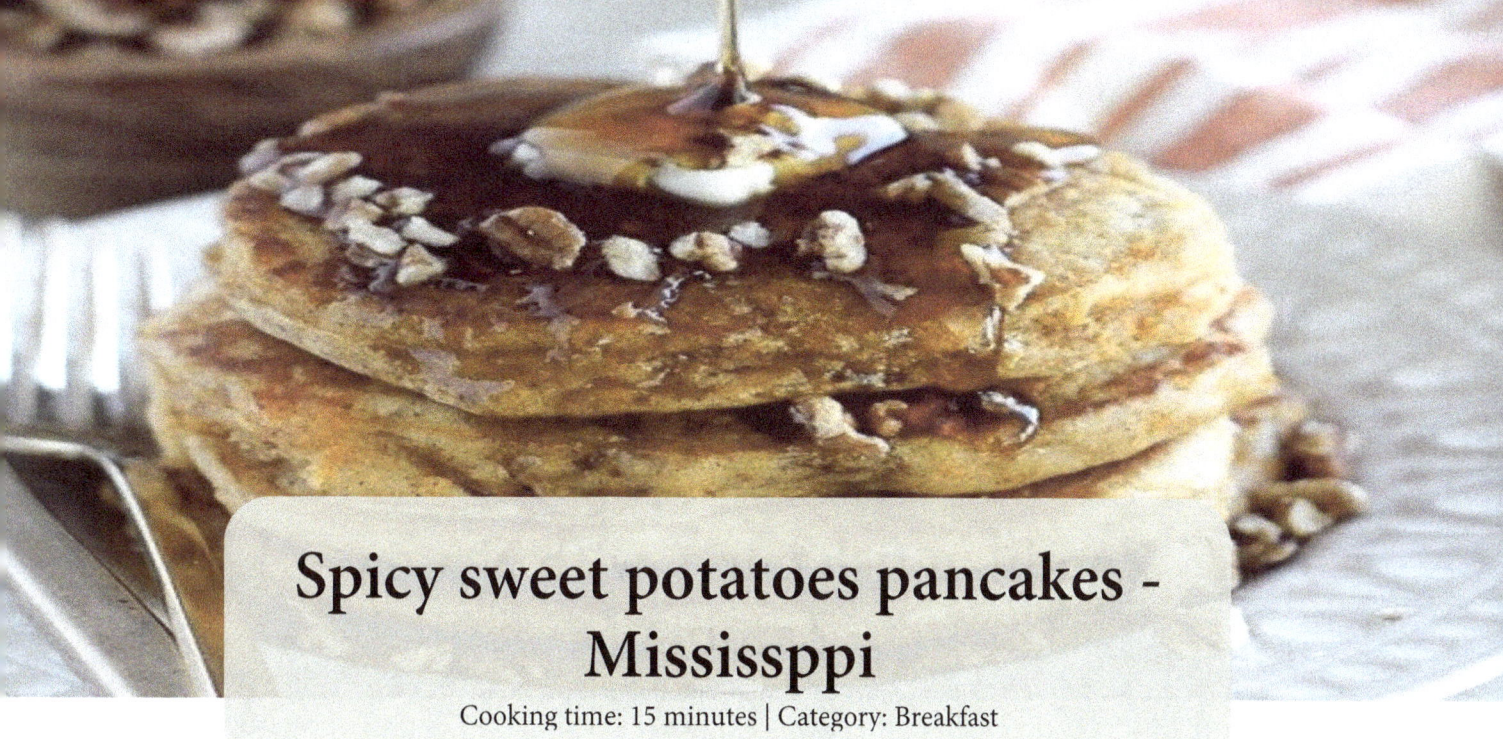

Spicy sweet potatoes pancakes - Mississppi

Cooking time: 15 minutes | Category: Breakfast

These spiced sweet potato pancakes are adapted from the version served at the historic Arcade Restaurant in Downtown Memphis. Enjoy them soaked with syrup and pecan butter, or pair them with bacon, eggs, and grits like they do in Memphis.

Ingredients

- One 14-oz. sweet potato
- 1 cup all-purpose flour
- 1 cup whole-wheat flour
- ¼ cup dark brown sugar
- 1 tbsp. plus 1 tsp. baking powder
- 1 tsp. ground cinnamon
- 1 tsp. kosher salt
- ½ tsp. ground green cardamom
- ¼ tsp. ground cloves
- ¼ tsp. freshly grated nutmeg
- 12 tbsp. unsalted butter, melted, divided, plus more for serving
- 2 large eggs beaten
- 2 cups whole milk
- Maple syrup

Steps to Cook

1. Position a rack in the center of the oven and preheat to 400°F. Use a fork to prick the sweet potato a few times on each side, then place it on a baking sheet.
2. Bake until very tender when pierced with a fork, about 1 hour. Set aside to cool, then remove and discard the skin. Transfer the flesh to a food processor and purée (or mash well with a fork).
3. In a large bowl, beat the all-purpose and whole wheat flour, baking powder, cinnamon, salt, cardamom, cloves, and nutmeg.
4. In a bowl, combine the sweet potato mixture, brown sugar, and ¼ cup of melted butter, eggs, and milk. Pour the sweet potato mixture into the flour mixture and whip until completely combined (the batter should be thick and fluffy).
5. To a large cast-iron skillet over medium-low heat, add 1–2 tablespoons of the melted butter and swirl to coat the surface.
6. When the foam calms, scoop ⅓ cup of batter into the skillet for each pancake, cook until they begin to pull away from the bottom of the pan, about 4 minutes, then use a spatula to flip. Continue cooking until golden brown on both sides and the batter is cooked through, 3–4 minutes.
7. Transfer the pancakes to a serving platter and tent with foil while you cook the rest of the pancakes, adding more butter to the skillet between batches.
8. Serve immediately, with additional butter and maple syrup, if desired.

Note:

Be sure to have a taste of Mississippi's punch to have a taste of Mississippi.

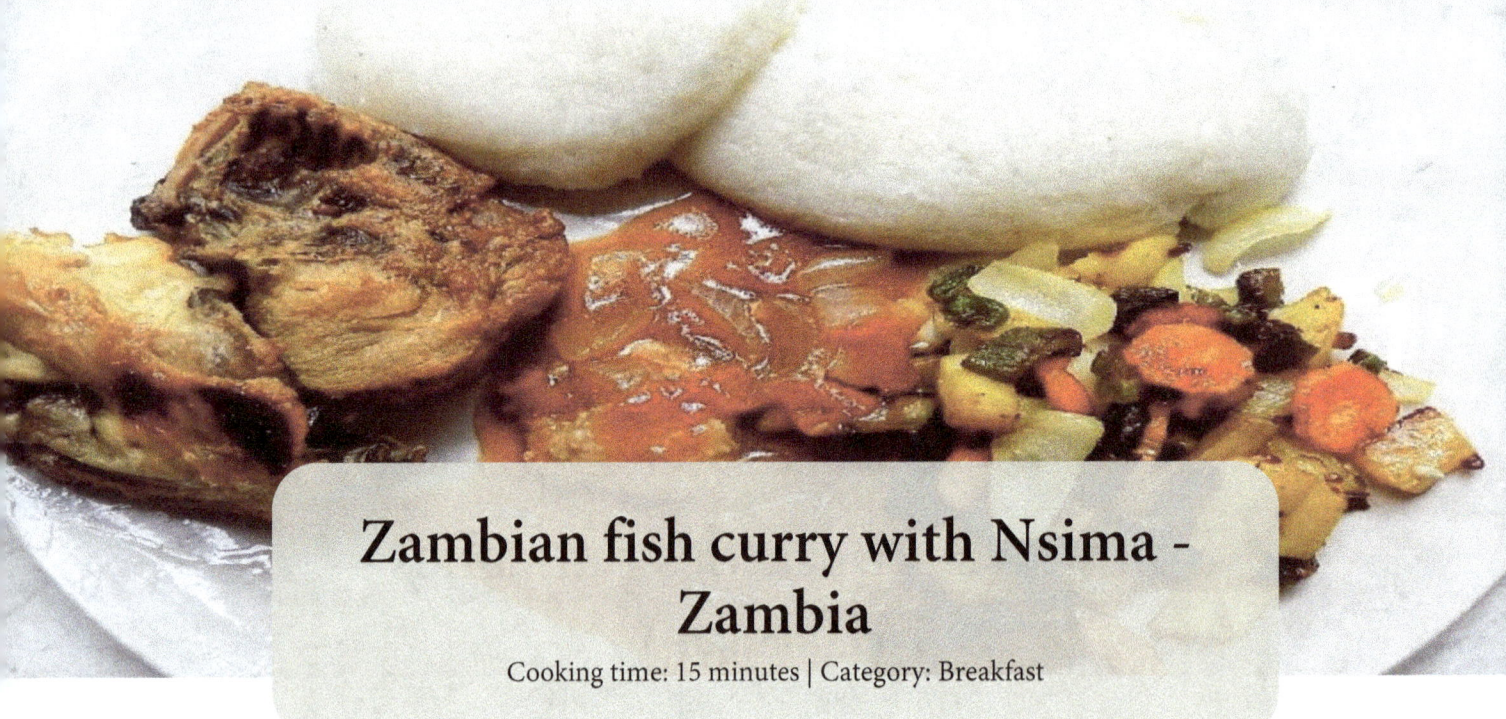

Zambian fish curry with Nsima - Zambia

Cooking time: 15 minutes | Category: Breakfast

Nshima, locally known as Ubwali, is a staple in Zambia. It can be made using maize meal, which is the most common, or with cassava, millet, and/or sorghum meal.

Ingredients

For the fish curry and cabbage

- 2 Large tilapia or bream, gutted and cleaned
- 2 tsp Curry powder
- 1 tsp Your favorite mixed herb blend
- 2 Fresh chilies
- 1 tsp Black pepper
- 2 Tomatoes, grated
- 2 tbsp Tomato paste
- 1 Onion
- Salt, to taste
- 4 Garlic cloves, crushed
- 2 Bunches of Chinese cabbage

For the nshima

- 4 cups Maize meal/mealie meal (any brand is fine)
- Cold water
- Boiling hot water

Steps to Cook

1. In a clean pot, add salt and curry. Put the fish, and meat side down, on top of the curry and salt.
2. Add more curry on top of the fish and pour enough water into the pot until it covers the fish.
3. Boil it on high for 10 minutes.
4. In a separate pan, fry onion and garlic until fragrant.
5. Add tomatoes and tomato paste and mix well. Add the herbs and fresh chilies and continue to cook the mixture together, over medium heat.
6. Once the mixture thickens pour over the boiled fish and simmer it on low heat for 10 minutes.
7. Wash and cut the Chinese cabbage into small pieces.
8. In a clean pot, fry the chopped onion in oil. Once cooked, add Chinese cabbage and salt to taste. Cook for 5 minutes and remove from heat and keep warm.
9. In a pot, add one cup of maize/mealie meal and a cup of cold water to make a paste.
10. Pour 2 1/2 cups of boiling water into the paste and mix well. Bring the mixture to a boil for at least 10 minutes.
11. Then, slowly start to add the remaining 3 cups into the pot, while stirring the mixture carefully until completely combined, about 15 extra minutes. Once a stiff consistency is achieved and you're able to form the nshima into a shape, it's ready.
12. Serve the fish with plenty of curry sauce, a side of cabbage, and a generous helping of nshima for a complete meal.

Note:

Be sure to drink a refreshing glass of Chibuku (beer distillate from maize or sorghum).

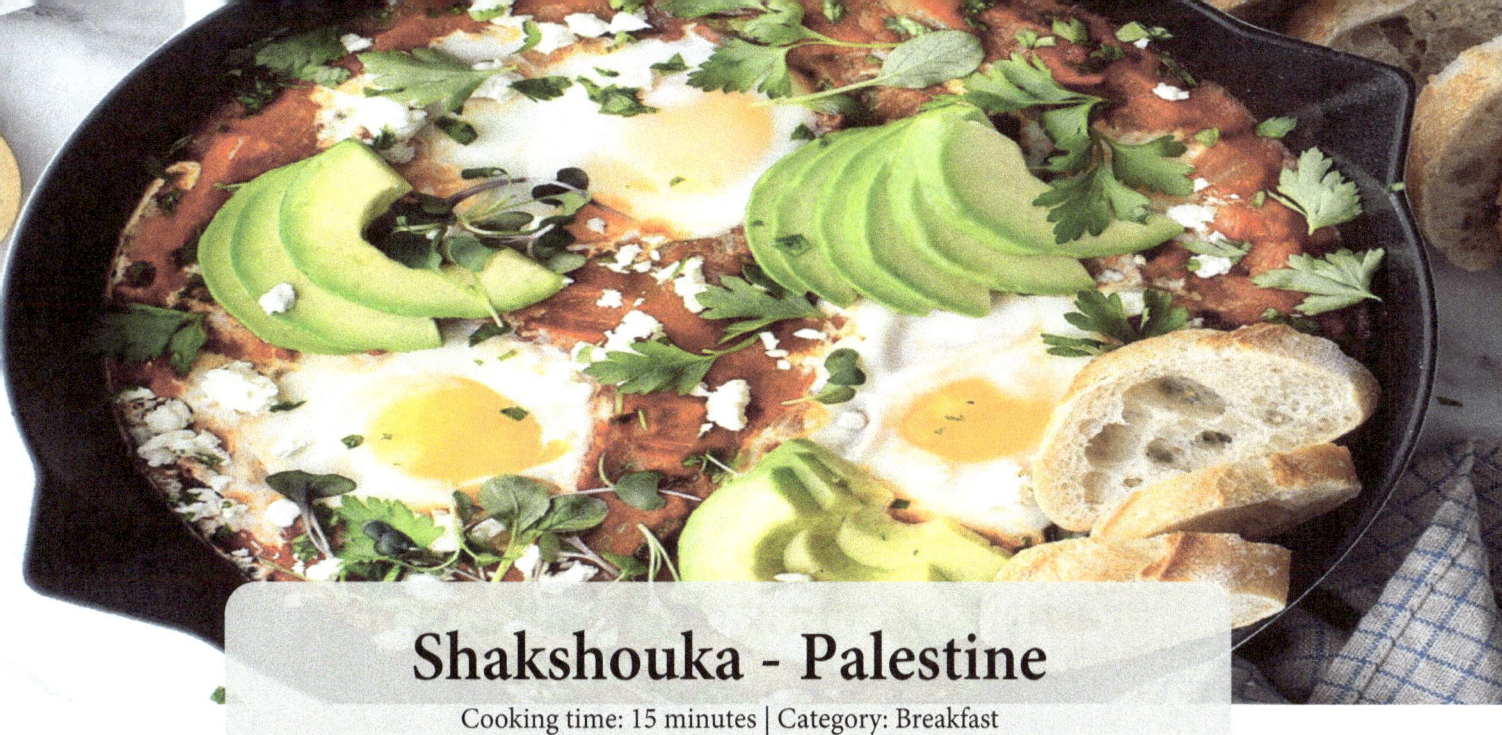

Shakshouka - Palestine

Cooking time: 15 minutes | Category: Breakfast

Shakshouka is a delicious combination of eggs poached in a spicy tomato sauce. Although it has an unusual name, the dish is easy to make. It is usually made in a skillet in which onions, tomatoes, and spices are cooked until they form a delicious tomato sauce.

Ingredients

- 2 teaspoons olive oil
- 3 cardamom pods
- 1 - 3 hot peppers (optional or to taste — spicy food is popular in Gaza)
- 1 cinnamon stick
- 1 1/2 to 2 pounds chicken thighs
- 2 Teaspoons tomato paste
- 1 cup rice
- 1/2 teaspoons salt
- Water
- 1/2 cup raisins
- 1/2 cup almonds
- 2 bay leaves
- 2 onions — 1 sliced, 1 diced
- 1 medium carrot

Spice mix

- 1/2 t dry ground coriander
- 1/2 t of turmeric
- 1/2 t of ginger
- 1/2 t of cumin
- 1/2 t of paprika
- 1/2 t of ground black pepper
- 1/2 t of ground cloves
- 1/2 t of cinnamon
- 1/4 t of dried lime

Steps to Cook

1. Add 2 Teaspoons of oil to a pot. Heat it and add the onions, chicken, salt, cinnamon stick, cardamom pods, bay leaves, and a few hot peppers.
2. Brown the chicken a bit and soften the onions. Add water to cover the chicken & tomato paste. Let Simmer. Cook for a half hour (or until the chicken is cooked).
3. In a separate pot, add the rice, dried spice mix, carrots, and 2 cups of chicken broth strained from the other pot. Cook, cover, lower heat, and cook until rice is done.
4. In a frying pan heat diced onion until caramelized. Add raisins and heat through
5. Add a little more oil to the pan and sauté the almonds until slightly browned.
6. brown the chicken.
7. Put the rice on a platter with chicken. Add raisin and onion mix and then the almonds on top. Serve with a side of plain yogurt.

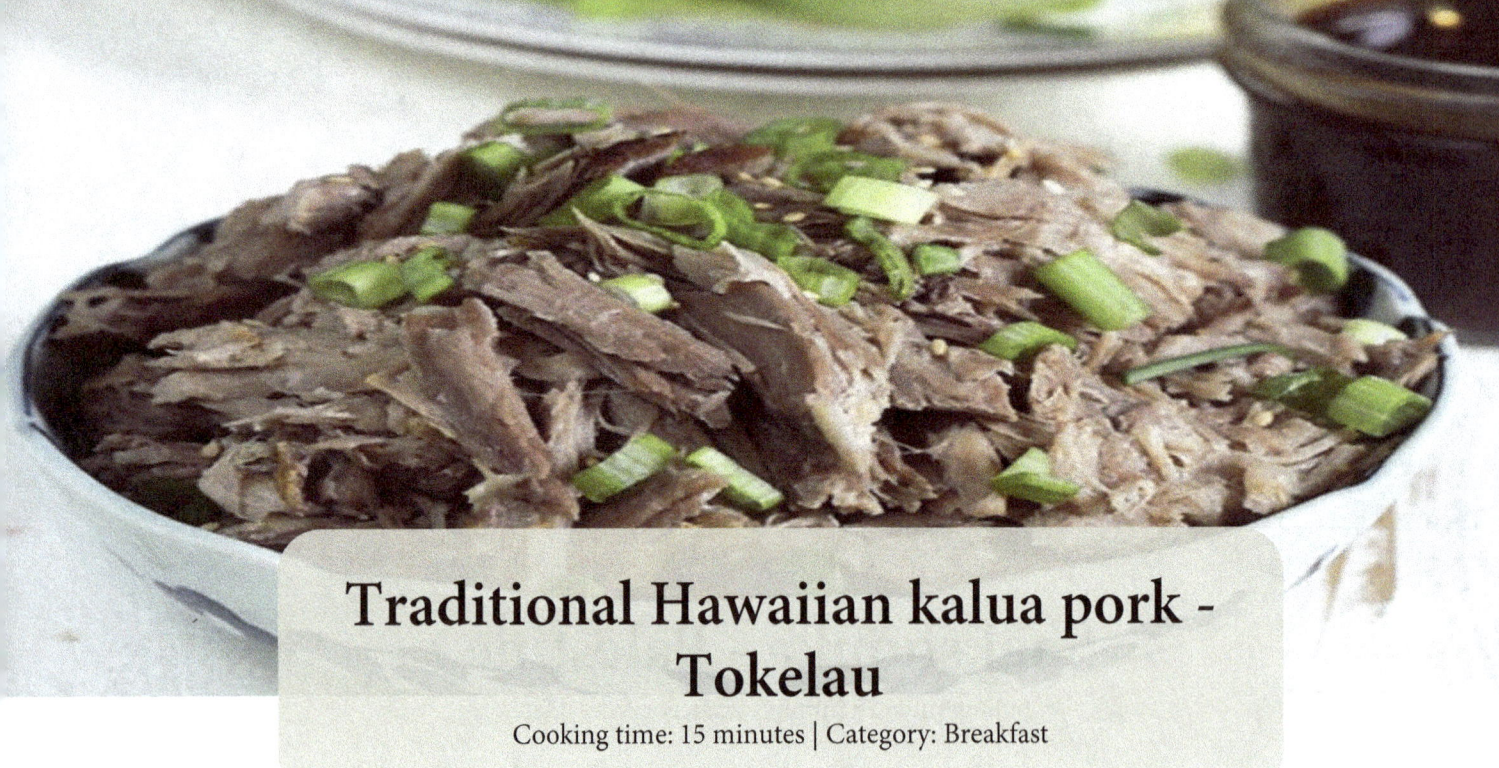

Traditional Hawaiian kalua pork - Tokelau

Cooking time: 15 minutes | Category: Breakfast

Traditional Hawaiian Kalua pig is cooked in an underground oven called an Imu. An Imu is a 2- 4-foot-deep pit dug and filled with kindling and rock, most often lava rock or basalt, and lit on fire. It takes a few hours for the kindling to turn to coal and the stones to get to an even heat and once they are ready to cook the pig, tropical leaves are placed on top to steam cook the pork.

Ingredients

- 1 4–6-pound pork shoulder or Boston butt roast
- 1 Tablespoon liquid smoke, Hickory, or Mesquite flavor
- 2-3 teaspoons red Hawaiian
- Banana leaves - optional

Steps to Cook

1. Rinse and pat the pork shoulder dry with paper towel, do not trim off excess fat and place in the slow cooker.
2. Pierce all over with a fork, pour the liquid smoke evenly over the roast and sprinkle liberally with the sea salt.
3. Place the lid of the slow cooker on and set the time for eight to twelve hours on LOW.
4. Check at about eight hours for doneness. If not done let go the full 12 hours, checking every hour.
5. If you have used banana leaves you can remove them before shredding the pork.
6. Remove around 2 cups of liquid (500ml) and set aside. This should be most of the cooking liquid removed. Shred the pork with forks and then add some of the liquid back in to keep the pork from drying out. You might not add all the liquid back in, save it for storing the pork if there are leftovers.
7. The pork should be kept warm in the liquid before serving. You can place the banana leaves on a platter then serve the pork on top of them or use fresh banana leaves for serving. Do not eat the banana leaves.
8. The pork saves well-kept in an airtight container in the refrigerator or freezer, keep some of the cooking liquid with it. Thaw in the refrigerator if frozen. It can be reheated on low in the slow cooker.

Note:

At Fakaofo, the delight of seeing swimming pigs is an attraction visitors can attest to. Tokelau has been reported to be the wealthiest Polynesian nation.

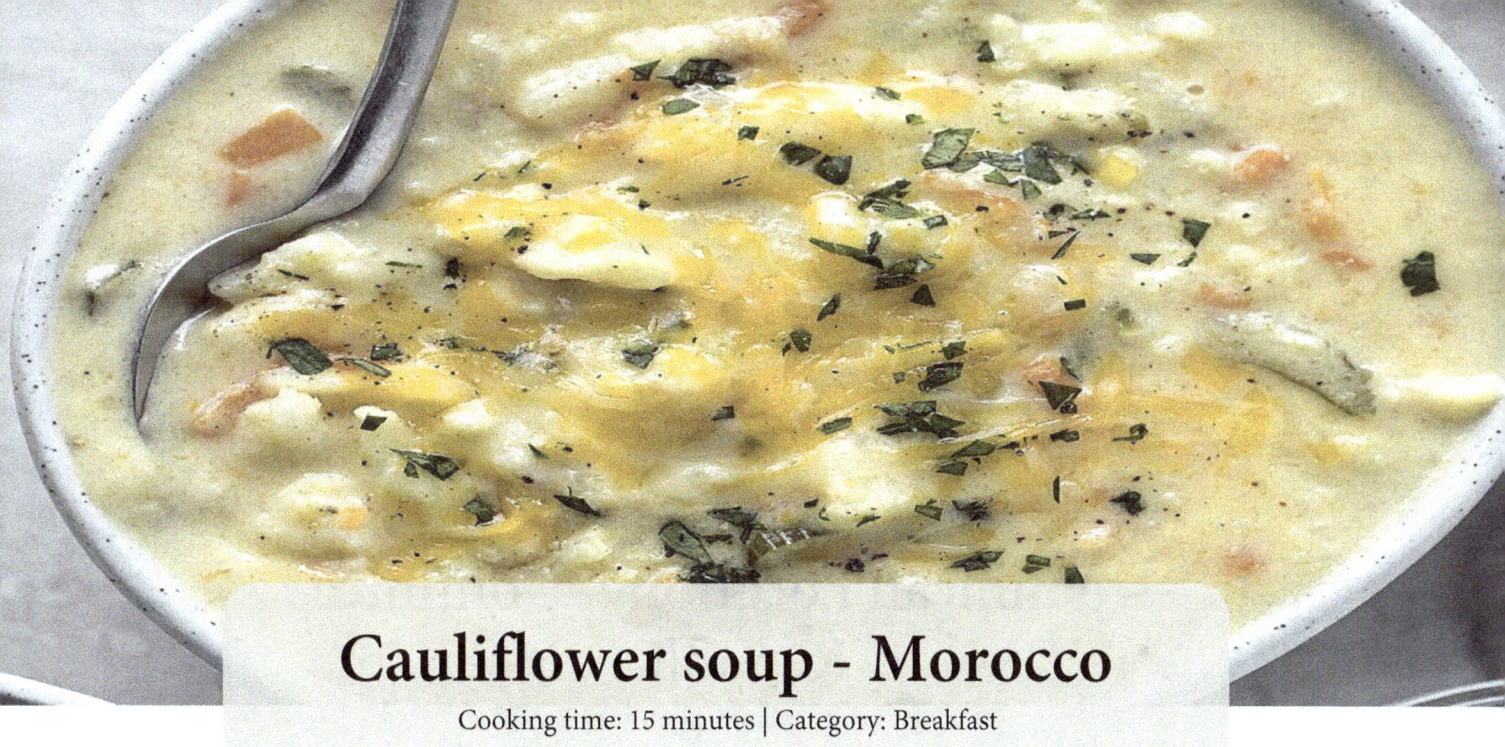

Cauliflower soup - Morocco

Cooking time: 15 minutes | Category: Breakfast

This cauliflower soup recipe is healthy condiments like ginger and turmeric. It's a healthy soup that's easily prepared

Ingredients

- 7 cups vegetable broth
- 1 carrot
- 6 garlic cloves
- 3 lbs. of Cauliflower
- 2 teaspoon salts
- 1 teaspoon ginger
- green onion
- 1 large yellow onion
- 8 tablespoons olive oil
- 1 teaspoons cumin
- 1 teaspoons coriander
- 1 teaspoon turmeric
- Half teaspoon black pepper
- 1 teaspoon cinnamon
- Paprika

Steps to Cook

1. Set the oven to 450F.
2. Put the cauliflower and garlic in a bowl and together with 3 tablespoons olive oil and 1 teaspoon. Peel the garlic
3. Cutup cauliflower
4. Roast the cauliflower in pan for half an hour.
5. Slice carrots and onions
6. Sauté the onion, oil& carrot for 3 mins. Add 7 cups vegetable broth and the cumin, coriander, ginger, turmeric, cinnamon, and black pepper, Simmer for 15 minutes while the cauliflower
7. roast the cauliflower is done, use a spoon to reserve some parts for toppings. Then pour the remaining roasted cauliflower and garlic into the broth mixture. Add broth, olive oil, and teaspoons.
8. Blend mixture
9. Serve hot

Note:

The number of calories per serving of cauliflower soup is 322.

Fully immerse yourself into the Moroccan culture with a glass of Moroccan mint tea. This national drink always leaves a refreshing experience.

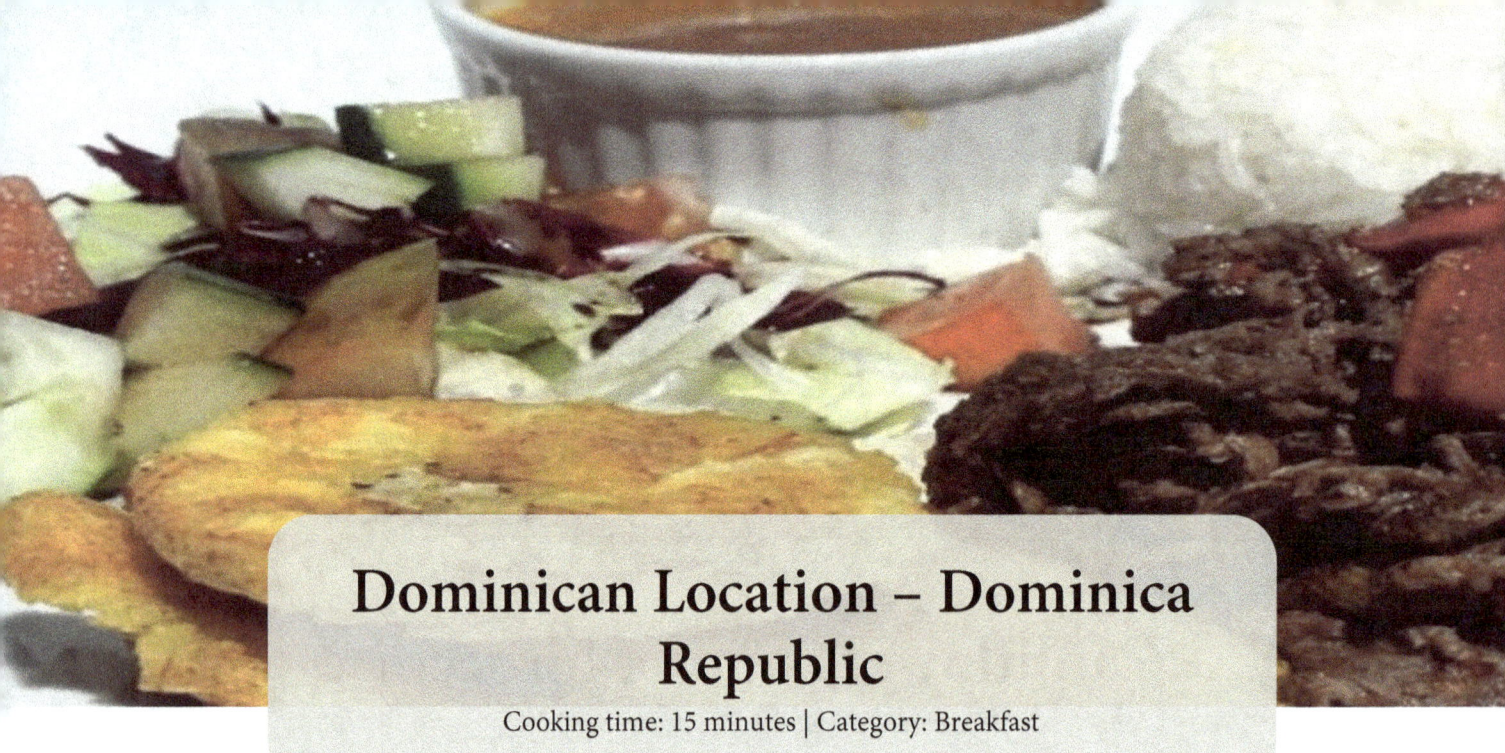

Dominican Location – Dominica Republic

Cooking time: 15 minutes | Category: Breakfast

Locrio gets its color from tomato sauce. There are many types of locrio depending on the meat it's served with. Some of the most common include locrio de pica-pica (spicy sardines), locrio de camarones (shrimp), locrio de arenque (smoked herring), and locrio de salami (Dominican salami). In general, Dominican rice dishes made with meat or seafood are called locrio.

Ingredients

- 2 cups long-grain white rice
- 1 3 1/2 lb. skinless chicken, cut into 12 pieces.
- 2 celery
- 1 cubanelle pepper
- 1 small yellow onion
- 2 small cloves of garlic
- 1/2 cup green olives
- 2 tablespoons lime juice
- 1 can (8 oz each) Hunt's tomato sauce
- 1 packet (0.17 oz each) sazon with coriander and annatto seasoning blend
- 2 teaspoons adobo seasoning
- 2 teaspoons salt
- 1 teaspoon Mexican oregano
- 1/2 teaspoon black pepper
- 2 teaspoons granulated sugar
- 2 tablespoons canola oil
- 3-1/2 cups of water

Steps to Cook

1. In a large bowl, stir together cubanelle, onion, garlic, celery, olives, lime juice, sazon packet, adobo seasoning, salt, oregano, and pepper. Add chicken pieces and marinade for 20 minutes.
2. In a heavy-bottomed lidded pot, heat oil over medium-high heat. Add sugar and cook until it caramelizes, about 30 seconds to 1 minute. Remove just the chicken from the marinade and add to the pot. Cover and Simmer. Browned Chicken on all sides, about 5 to 7 minutes.
3. Add vegetables and marinade, until vegetables are tender, about 3 to 5 minutes.
4. Add water and tomato sauce to the pot and stir. Increase heat to high and bring to a boil. Add rice and return to a boil. Reduce heat to medium and continue to cook for about 7 minutes.
5. Simmer 15 minutes. Recover and continue to simmer until rice is tender and chicken is cooked through about 5 to 10 additional minutes.

Note:

The number of calories per serving is 767

Mamajuana, a herbal infusion believed to promote sexual libido is worth trying to have a traditional feel of Dominica Republic.

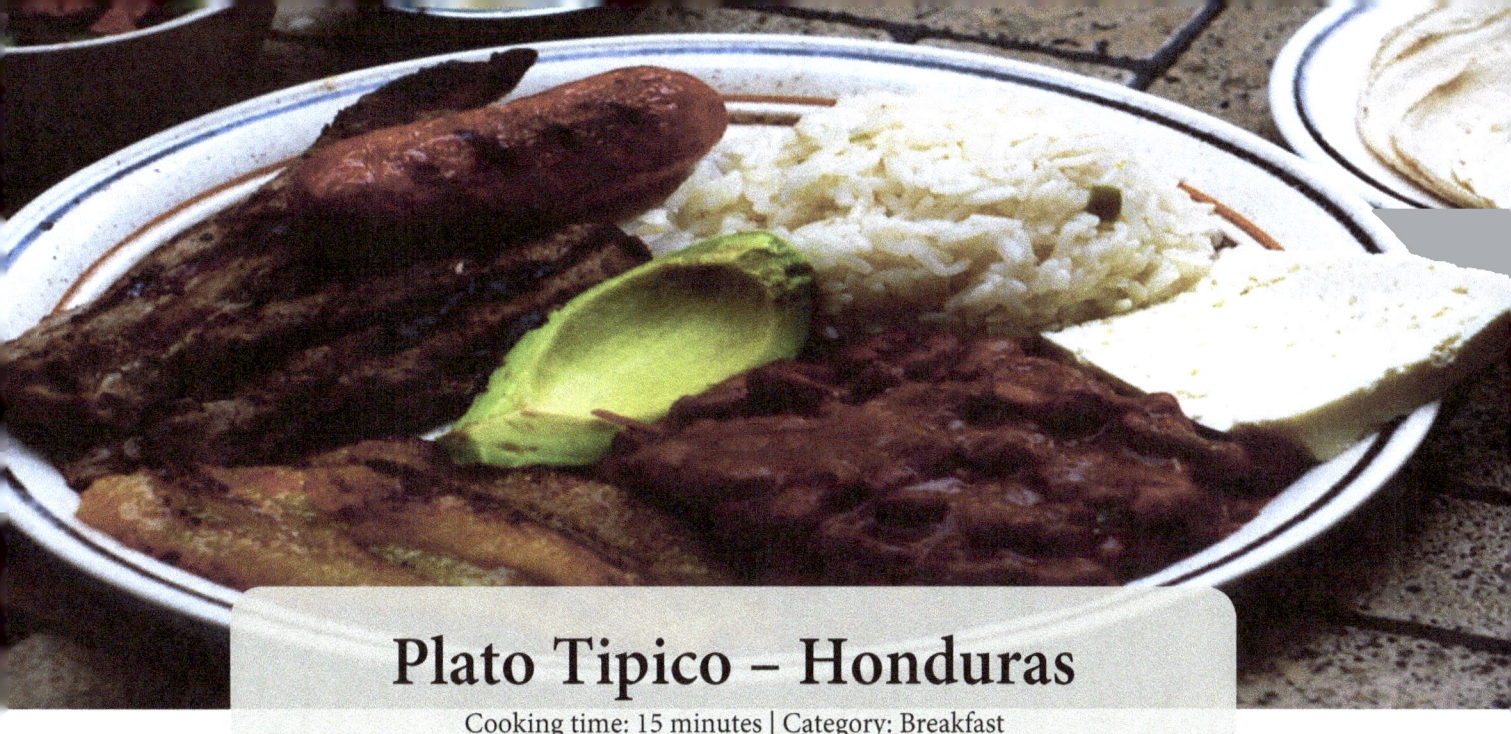

Plato Tipico – Honduras

Cooking time: 15 minutes | Category: Breakfast

Plato Tipico (typical dish) is the national dish of Honduras. And is one of the most popular because it combines the most liked and used ingredients in a dish that will satisfy most tastes! It includes a variety of foods, which are prepared separately, but form a complete meal: Grilled meat and pork sausages, stewed beans, chimol, fried plantain, and rice.

Ingredients

For the meat:

- 450g beef sirloin, cut into long strips
- 450g pork (recipe said sirloin, we used belly), cut into long strips
- 4 chorizo sausages
- 1/2 tsp salt
- 1/2 tsp pepper
- 2 cloves garlic, minced
- 2 tbsp olive oil
- 3 tbsp white vinegar

For the stewed beans:

- 2 cans of kidney beans, drained
- 1 red onion, thinly sliced
- 3 peppers (1 green, 1 yellow, 1 red), thinly sliced
- 2 cloves garlic, minced
- 2 tbsp olive oil
- 1 tsp oregano
- 1/4 tsp salt
- 1/4 tsp white pepper
- Pinch cayenne pepper
- 1/4 tsp dried thyme
- 1/4 tsp paprika
- 250ml ketchup

Steps to Cook

For the meat:

1. Put the beef and pork into a bowl and mix in the salt, pepper, garlic, olive oil and vinegar. Marinate for at least one hour.
2. When ready, barbecue with the sausages.
3. For the stewed beans:
4. Heat the olive oil in a pot over medium-high heat and add the onion, peppers and garlic. Sauté for about 3 minutes or until tender.
5. Add the beans. Stir and lower the heat to medium.
6. Add the spices and ketchup, mix thoroughly, and add the water.
7. Lower the heat to medium-low and simmer for 15 minutes.
8. For the chismol:
9. 1. Mix everything.

For the plantains:

1. Peel the plantains and cut them in half. Then cut each half lengthwise into 1/2 cm slices (about 4 slices from each half).
2. In a frying pan, heat the vegetable oil over medium heat. Fry the plantains until each side is slightly browned (about 3 minutes on each side). Remove from the pan and keep warm.
3. For the rice:

- 250ml water

For the chismol:

- 2 large tomatoes, diced
- 1 large green pepper, diced
- 1 red onion, diced
- 3 sprigs of coriander, chopped
- 1/2 tsp salt
- 1/2 tsp black pepper
- 1/4 tsp cumin
- 2 tbsp lemon juice

For the plantain:

- 2 plantains
- 4 tbsp vegetable oil

For the rice:

- 200g white rice
- 1 tbsp chopped green pepper
- 1 tbsp chopped red onion
- 1 clove of garlic, minced
- 1/2 tsp salt
- 1 tbsp vegetable oil
- 500ml hot water

To serve:

- Sliced avocado
- Sour cream
- Fresh farmer's cheese (we used cottage cheese)
- Soft corn tortillas (we used wheat ones)

4. In a pan, heat the vegetable oil over medium heat and add the green pepper, onion and garlic. Sauté for 2 minutes.
5. Add the rice and salt and continue stirring for 2 more minutes.
6. Add the water. When it starts to boil, lower the heat to medium-low and cover. Simmer until all water has been absorbed and rice is cooked (about 20 minutes).

Note:

There are 387 calories per serving. A nice idea will be to have fun at Utila, Bay Islands. Central America's second-largest country continues to dazzle even seasoned travelers with its beautiful beaches, bird-rich jungles, underwater wonders and wild encounters.

Honduras is also home to the Copan Ruins, the most studied Maya city in the world which dates back 2,000 years.

Week - 13

Reflections

- Record a video of your practice of prayer, meditation & gratitude session of yourself.

_____
_____
_____
_____
_____
_____
_____
_____

- Write a note encouragement to your old self about the importance of taking daily & weekly small steps

_____
_____
_____
_____
_____
_____
_____
_____

- What cause will run your 5k for?

_____
_____
_____
_____
_____
_____
_____
_____

Next Step

Thanks for purchasing this book, reading it, and taking obedient action as you reflect on your food experiences & relationships. I hope it was enlightening and encouraging and that your life flourishes, one small step and one week at a time.

As you connect with more people & your lifestyle becomes healthier, you will influence many others around you, just like my friends in college influenced me with unique food experiences that led me to create this book.

I would love to hear from you about how this book has impacted you. Your feedback will help me in improving this book and other books in the future.

Receiving your review is important to me, it will help this book reach more people and change lives around the world.

www.ingramcontent.com/pod-product-compliance
Lightning Source LLC
Chambersburg PA
CBHW051803100526
44592CB00016B/2546